Clinical Decision Making in Mental Health Practice

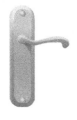

Clinical Decision Making in Mental Health Practice

Edited by Jeffrey J. Magnavita

American Psychological Association
Washington, DC

Copyright © 2016 by the American Psychological Association. All rights reserved. Except as permitted under the United States Copyright Act of 1976, no part of this publication may be reproduced or distributed in any form or by any means, including, but not limited to, the process of scanning and digitization, or stored in a database or retrieval system, without the prior written permission of the publisher.

Published by
American Psychological Association
750 First Street, NE
Washington, DC 20002
www.apa.org

To order
APA Order Department
P.O. Box 92984
Washington, DC 20090-2984
Tel: (800) 374-2721; Direct: (202) 336-5510
Fax: (202) 336-5502; TDD/TTY: (202) 336-6123
Online: www.apa.org/pubs/books
E-mail: order@apa.org

In the U.K., Europe, Africa, and the Middle East, copies may be ordered from
American Psychological Association
3 Henrietta Street
Covent Garden, London
WC2E 8LU England

Typeset in Goudy by Circle Graphics, Inc., Columbia, MD

Printer: Bang Printing, Brainerd, MN
Cover Designer: Beth Schlenoff Design, Bethesda, MD

The opinions and statements published are the responsibility of the authors, and such opinions and statements do not necessarily represent the policies of the American Psychological Association.

Library of Congress Cataloging-in-Publication Data

Clinical decision making in mental health practice / edited by Jeffrey J. Magnavita. — First edition.
    p. ; cm.
Includes bibliographical references and index.
ISBN 978-1-4338-2029-8 — ISBN 1-4338-2029-3
I. Magnavita, Jeffrey J., editor. II. American Psychological Association, issuing body.
[DNLM; 1. Mental Disorders—diagnosis. 2. Mental Disorders—therapy. 3. Decision Making. 4. Evidence-Based Practice. 5. Psychotherapy—methods. WM 141]
RC454.4
616.89—dc23
                         2015004772

British Library Cataloguing-in-Publication Data

A CIP record is available from the British Library.

Printed in the United States of America
First Edition

http://dx.doi.org/10.1037/14711-000

This book is dedicated to the memory of Vincent Stephens, MD,
a loyal friend, consummate psychiatrist, and passionate psychotherapist.

CONTENTS

Contributors ix

Foreword xi
Gerald P. Koocher

Preface xiii

Chapter 1. Overview and Challenges of Clinical Decision
Making in Mental Health Practice 3
Jeffrey J. Magnavita

Chapter 2. Clinical Expertise and Decision Making:
An Overview of Bias in Clinical Practice 23
Jeffrey J. Magnavita and Scott O. Lilienfeld

Chapter 3. A Dual Process Perspective on the Value of Theory
in Psychotherapeutic Decision Making 61
Jack C. Anchin and Jefferson A. Singer

Chapter 4. Clinical Practice Guideline Development and Decision Making 105
Lynn F. Bufka and Erin F. Swedish

Chapter 5. Developing Clinical Practice Guidelines to Enhance Clinical Decision Making 125
Steven D. Hollon

Chapter 6. Using Technology to Enhance Decision Making 147
Franz Caspar, Thomas Berger, and Lukas Frei

Chapter 7. Clinical Decision Making When the Stakes Are High 175
Jeffrey J. Magnavita

Chapter 8. Use of Empirically Grounded Relational Principles to Enhance Clinical Decision Making 193
Ken L. Critchfield and Julia E. Mackaronis

Chapter 9. Integrating Ongoing Measurement Into the Clinical Decision-Making Process With Measurement Feedback Systems 223
Thomas L. Sexton and Adam R. Fisher

Chapter 10. Clinical Decision Making and Risk Management 245
Steven A. Sobelman and Jeffrey N. Younggren

Chapter 11. Teaching Clinical Decision Making 273
Gregg Henriques

Index 309

About the Editor 321

CONTRIBUTORS

Jack C. Anchin, PhD, University at Buffalo, State University of New York
Thomas Berger, PhD, University of Bern, Bern, Switzerland
Lynn F. Bufka, PhD, American Psychological Association, Washington, DC
Franz Caspar, PhD, University of Bern, Bern, Switzerland
Ken L. Critchfield, PhD, James Madison University, Harrisonburg, VA
Adam R. Fisher, MA, Indiana University, Bloomington
Lukas Frei, MSc, University of Bern, Bern, Switzerland
Gregg Henriques, PhD, James Madison University, Harrisonburg, VA
Steven D. Hollon, PhD, Vanderbilt University, Nashville, TN
Gerald P. Koocher, PhD, ABPP, DePaul University, Chicago, IL
Scott O. Lilienfeld, PhD, Emory University, Atlanta, GA
Julia E. Mackaronis, PhD, VA Puget Sound Health Care System–Seattle Division, Seattle, WA
Jeffrey J. Magnavita, PhD, ABPP, Glastonbury Psychological Associates, Glastonbury, CT
Thomas L. Sexton, PhD, ABPP, Indiana University, Bloomington
Jefferson A. Singer, PhD, Connecticut College, New London
Steven A. Sobelman, PhD, Loyola University Maryland, Baltimore
Erin F. Swedish, MA, Toledo, OH
Jeffrey N. Younggren, PhD, ABPP, Professor, UCLA David Geffen School of Medicine, Los Angeles, CA

FOREWORD

GERALD P. KOOCHER

One of my favorite quotations appears in a collection of proverbs written by Goethe in 1819: "Es ist nichts schrecklicher als eine tätige Unwissenheit." This translates roughly as, "Nothing is more dangerous than ignorance in action," or more literally, "Nothing is more dangerous than active un-knowing-ness." Sadly, this maxim too often seems overlooked in clinical decision making by psychotherapists. In many ways the complexity of influences on human behavior makes this state of affairs understandable. Our behavior flows from our biology and our life experiences in all the rich combinations that genetics, environmental influences, relationships, and the passage of time impose. Those who have sought to practice psychotherapy (i.e., to improve the behavior of people who become distressed or distressing to others) have often evidenced struggles with the same complex variability as they attempt to bring about "cures."

Ask psychotherapists about the ethics underlying their work and they tend to become philosophers. Writing on the ethics of their craft, psychotherapists have referred to the practice of therapy as a science, an art, a source of honest and nonjudgmental feedback, the systematic use of a human relationship for therapeutic purposes, and a means of exploring one's ultimate values. Less flattering descriptions from within the profession have included a house of cards, the purchase of friendship, a means of social control, and tradecraft.[1] My personal favorite definition of psychotherapy came from the secretary of the historic Boulder, Colorado, conference on the training of psychologists, who satirically noted, "We have left therapy as an undefined technique which is applied to unspecified problems with a nonpredictable outcome. For this technique we recommend rigorous training."[2]

In this context of complexity and radically different perspectives Magnavita and his colleagues have compiled an impressive guide to making sound clinical decisions in psychotherapy practice amid an array of potential distractions. The readings guide us through decision-making biases, help us base decisions on sound evidence, point us to existing guidelines, advise us on the use of technology, help us to consider risk management, and advise us in teaching. The result is a major resource to help us avoid the dangers of our own biases and blind spots in a quest to avoid acting on *Unwissenheit*.

---

[1] Koocher, G. P., & Keith-Spiegel, P. (2008). *Ethics in psychology and the mental health professions*. New York, NY: Oxford University Press.
[2] Lehner, G. F. J. (1952). Defining psychotherapy. *American Psychologist, 7*, 547.

PREFACE

Bias is inherent in just about every part of our lives and is often an unacknowledged but influential part of clinical practice. Understanding our propensity for bias will go a long way toward enhancing our clinical decision-making. Try this story, for example:

> A father and his son are in a car accident. The father is killed and the son is seriously injured. The son is taken to the hospital, where the surgeon assesses the situation and declares, "I cannot operate because this boy is my son." Why is that so?[1]

The answer to this brainteaser, which as many as 75% of those who hear it cannot solve, is that the boy's mother is the surgeon. Gender bias is deeply ingrained.

This volume represents a new and exciting area for me after more than 3 decades of clinical practice and clinical research spent viewing videotapes of psychotherapy sessions ultimately trying to decide on the optimal course of action. My efforts, which I have compiled and published in a series of

---

[1] Grant, A., & Sandberg, S. (2014, December 6). When talking about bias. *New York Times*, p. 46.

volumes and articles, involve working to distill the essential elements of psychotherapy. The latest of my books is *Unifying Psychotherapy: Principles, Methods, and Evidence From Clinical Science*,[2] written with my collaborator and friend Jack C. Anchin, who shares a passion for clinical work and the scholarly and scientific search for the unifying principles and components of clinical science and psychotherapy. My current work represents a departure from my early interests in the treatment of personality disorders, integrative and unified models of psychotherapy, and personality theory.

It was Eileen Bonetti's infectious belief in and knowledge of decision analytics that brought my awareness to this topic and sparked my curiosity and interest in decision making. Clinicians, as well as all health professionals, are involved in a continual process of decision making, basing critical decisions on various streams of information, from the microprocesses in interpersonal relationships to the results of meta-analytic studies on the efficacy of various treatment approaches. It became apparent after an extensive review of the decision-making literature that clinical practitioners can benefit from this important body of work; the result is this volume.

I was also inspired to explore this exciting field following my experience serving on the Clinical Practice Guideline Advisory Steering Committee that the American Psychological Association initiated to begin the important process of developing clinical practice guidelines. What became apparent to me is that many components of clinical practice are not supported by empirical evidence with which to guide decision making. One example is how we determine the length or frequency of sessions. We continue to use the 50-minute session as the standard unit for delivering psychotherapy, yet I am aware of no empirical evidence that examines the influence of various session lengths and formats on outcome. How, then, do you make decisions such as that one when there is no empirical evidence on which to draw? Mostly we rely on clinical lore, assuming that Freud had it right when he framed psychotherapy in sessions of 50-minute duration. I think we can improve how we respond clinically by examining our biases.

This volume would not have happened without the support and collaboration of many people. I have been actively engaged with a number of friends, scholars, and clinicians over the years who have influenced and sharpened my thinking and improved my own decision-making processes. I want to especially thank Jack C. Anchin and Steven A. Sobelman for their friendship and collaboration over the years. We have taken on a number of exciting projects and spent many hours trying to figure out how to make

---

[2]Magnavita, J. J., & Anchin, J. C. (2013). *Unifying psychotherapy: Principles, methods, and evidence from clinical science.* New York, NY: Springer.

clinical science and psychotherapy more effective. Steve has taught so many of us about the value of technology bringing us digital immigrants to the 21st century. Together we founded the Unified Psychotherapy Project. I also thank William C. Alder, Frank Knoblauch, John Santopietro, Peter Tolisano, and Anne Shapiro, all part of my core professional support and friendship group over the decades. I remember Vincent Stephens, an important member of our core group, whose loss we deeply mourn. I also express my appreciation for the collaboration and friendship over the years to Gregg Henriques, Kenneth L. Critchfield, Jay L. Lebow, Andre Marquis, Jeffrey E. Barnett, Rosie Adam-Terem, Craig N. Shealy, David M. Allen, Michael Alpert, Kristin A. R. Osborn, Lori Calabrese, and many others who have influenced my work and collaborated with me in patient care. I acknowledge the many people I have had the privilege of working with on the road to achieving more abundance in their lives who have trusted me with their concerns. Finally, I thank my partner, Anne G. Magnavita, and my daughters Elizabeth, Emily, and Caroline for more than they will ever know.

Clinical Decision Making in Mental Health Practice

1

OVERVIEW AND CHALLENGES OF CLINICAL DECISION MAKING IN MENTAL HEALTH PRACTICE

JEFFREY J. MAGNAVITA

You have made a decision to begin reading this volume, *Clinical Decision Making in Mental Health Practice*, on the basis of certain information that influenced your decision to pick up this copy, open it, and begin reading at this moment. Other decision-making processes will determine whether you become engaged in the topic and continue reading the book or lose interest and decide to redirect your valuable resources elsewhere. You will not be disappointed if you continue with the book; the contributors herein are well informed and offer useful information and wisdom as well as new ways of thinking to improve your decision making from various perspectives.

Perhaps, in the back of your mind, you have been preoccupied and perplexed by a complicated individual, couple, or family you are treating, and this may have unconsciously attracted you to the title of this volume. Maybe your challenging case didn't fit your personal internal heuristics, or "rules of thumb"—mental shortcuts on which we often base our decisions that are sometimes reliable but, unchecked, are prone to errors of thinking. Clinicians

---

http://dx.doi.org/10.1037/14711-001
Clinical Decision Making in Mental Health Practice, J. J. Magnavita (Editor)
Copyright © 2016 by the American Psychological Association. All rights reserved.

probably utilize hundreds or more of these heuristics in daily practice. For example, one that comes to mind is how I view poor eye contact as a marker of anxiety about emotional closeness and intimacy. In spite of the fact that you may be highly trained in a particular model of treatment or well versed in a number of evidence-based approaches and deem yourself a well-trained and competent or even "expert" clinician, you may be uncertain about how to proceed with treatment in certain situations. Developing expertise is not a straightforward proposition of attaining the appropriate education, training, and practice—more is required of us. We have a duty to those we treat for continuous improvement. Some of your cases may not be progressing in the manner you anticipated or expected, possibly creating a crisis of confidence. For example, a patient may have dropped out of treatment and harmed himself or someone else, showing deterioration in functioning instead of improving. None of us likes to face these disappointing outcomes. Often treatment doesn't unfold as depicted in the textbooks or manualized versions of treatment so ubiquitous these days. Treatment is often in the moment, and our responses require trust in our intuition. With certain cases, you may be perplexed, confused about how to proceed, and worried about how to make appropriate decisions when there are few empirical data to guide you. You may find yourself trying harder with a favored approach because you have already invested a lot of time and energy in pursuing a particular course of action. I found this to be a common response while in training in brief dynamic therapy and afterward as a supervisor. I noticed that it was not uncommon for trainees to increase their effort with a particular method, such as defensive restructuring, when they were not getting the desired results. Instead of trying a different method, they might resort to what is best described as "hammering"—looking for the results viewed in the master therapist's videos by doing more of the same approach. An increase in the frequency and intensity of a method all too often would lead to iatrogenic reactions and premature termination. In one of my cases, a patient walked out of the session, and there were others who never returned.

Although one psychotherapeutic strategy may work wonderfully with many patients, with others, increasing our efforts and investment in a tried-and-true strategy may prove ineffective or worse. In such a situation, trainees may fall prey to the *sunk-cost effect*, which occurs when one continues to invest in something in which he or she has already made an investment of time and energy (Kahneman, 2011). In economics and business, we can see that people often invest more money in a failing venture in an attempt to recoup their losses. This may also be true for some addictive behaviors. Those readers who treat gamblers know this narrative all too well. You have heard people say that after they lost all of their money they used their credit card to try to get back what they lost—this is the sunk-cost effect in operation. We may also witness the *sunk-cost fallacy* (Kahneman, 2011) in the treatment context. This is a type of bias that can occur after we invest our resources in pursuing a particular approach to treatment and then find ourselves trying to apply this approach to all our patients instead of using tools of differential treatment selection and finding the approach that best fits the patient and his or her situation. This may be when it is warranted to seek a consultation or to get a trusted colleague's perspective.

We are also prone to want to present our best selves to the public. This is evident when you attend treatment conferences where cases are presented. Almost everyone presenting audiovisual tapes of their therapy sessions at these conferences shows their best work. We select videotapes of patients demonstrating great process and outcome. This selection bias may have serious consequences for trainees, as it surely did when I was in training. This often leads to what decision researchers term *confirmation bias*—we honor data that support our approach and dismiss that which calls what we do into question (Kahneman, 2011). Viewing positive treatment outcomes proves the veracity of the approach being demonstrated, and ignoring treatment failures intensifies this effect. How would the field evolve if instead we presented our worst outcomes or compared our best with our worst outcomes at these conferences? Would the learning process progress more rapidly by a study of errors and mistakes instead of only ideal treatments?

You may have made assumptions about patients in your clinical practice on the basis of diagnostic labels accrued from previous therapists, resulting in an *anchoring bias*—placing too much weight on one aspect or trait, which reduces the utility of predicting (Tversky & Kahneman, 1974). What biases do you notice when a referring clinician describes a patient as "psychopathic," "borderline," "narcissistic," or "a pedophile"? Which one of these labels has greater emotional activation? I think I can predict which one does. Emotional responses can bias our judgment, compromising our decision making. Diagnostic labels serve as anchors that may color our thinking and influence our decision making on the basis of very limited information, thereby leading to reliance on a *representative heuristic* (Kahneman, 2011), whereby we prematurely arrive at conclusions without sufficient data, using too few data points. We may hastily assume that a very slender individual suffers from an eating disorder. The sheer complexity or uniqueness of some of our cases may leave us uncertain of both diagnosis and treatment approach.

Without an understanding of decision theory we are more likely to fall prey to various traps in our thinking or to biases of which we are unaware but that nevertheless influence us. Decision theory allows us to be aware of the underlying processes from which we derive our decisions. The quality of evidence from which we make decisions is essential, and efforts to remain doubtful and question our thinking are imperative. We should strive to falsify our hypotheses instead of proving them correct. Kahneman (2011) implored us in this regard to not "expect this exercise of discipline to be easy—it requires a significant effort of self-monitoring and self-control" (p. 153). Reading the remainder of this volume will enhance your awareness of potential errors in decision making as well as various perspectives to consider when making difficult clinical decisions.

Wouldn't it be nice if our patients fit the prototypes we learned in school? Clinical practice is messy and at times chaotic. Patients are not exactly like the prototypes described in our textbooks, and treatment manuals, although helpful, necessarily attempt to simplify and organize information into useful knowledge. Our patients are more likely to present us with complicated physical and emotional symptoms, relational disturbances, and challenges in their current lives, along with histories of abuse and neglect as well as other developmental challenges. Heuristics and cognitive templates are essential. We navigate the world using pattern recognition tools based on schema and theory, but we must be cognizant that these can be error prone. These sources are often useful starting points, but clinical expertise is more than just textbook knowledge; it includes the ability to use the best information available in an unbiased manner and convert this information into knowledge. Transforming data and information into knowledge and wisdom usually requires extensive practice with relevant feedback to adjust our practice. Understanding the differences among data, information, knowledge, and wisdom is helpful when one is besieged with multiple sources of information (Mayer-Schonberger & Cukier, 2013). These categories are explored in Chapter 2 in this volume.

We may at times rely on our intuitive or rapid decision-making strategies, and at other times we may seek a more deliberative approach, gathering as much data as possible first (Kahneman, 2011). You may already view yourself as an "expert" clinician and not feel the need to learn more about decision making, and if this is the case, you may have fallen prey to a common prejudice, *overconfidence bias*, which is the tendency to overestimate one's ability. Most clinicians view themselves as at least average or better in their psychotherapeutic ability even while being aware that it is statistically impossible for almost everyone to be average or above (Walfish, McAlister, O'Donnell, & Lambert, 2012). Even when psychotherapists receive feedback about patients' conditions worsening, many continue to assess themselves as effective and discount the feedback as inaccurate or inconsequential. The practice of discounting information that does not match our internal self- or worldview can be dangerous. Why are we so prone to this type of bias to the point of ignoring patients who are deteriorating as a result of our treatment, making it difficult in some cases to prevent negative outcomes (Lambert,

2010)? These questions and many others can be understood through the lens of decision analytics that are based on advances in decision theory and through empirical investigation of various ways that we make decisions and the traps we can fall into.

A certain amount of energy will be required to master the material in this volume. Some readers may consider the deliberative system of thinking "lazy" and would rather defer to their intuitive "fast" response system (Kahneman, 2011), which will have already biased readers with information regarding the stickiness of the title, status of the publisher, the names of the editor and contributors, endorsements, or even the attractiveness of the cover. Your personal biases will influence how effortfully you engage with and learn the material presented in this volume. Your hidden biases may also determine whether as a result of reading this book your clinical decision making is enhanced and clinical efficacy improved. You have made a decision to continue reading this volume, and as the volume editor, this pleases me because there is so much information in the remaining chapters that you will find useful and practical. Your decision to invest resources in this volume was made using two very different but interrelated styles of thinking—one *fast* (you may have impulsively picked the book off a shelf in a bookstore responding to some intuitive sense that it might be worthwhile) and the other *slow* (you may have carefully read an advertisement and deliberately called on an internal book-buying algorithm). You probably are unaware, or only vaguely aware, of what influenced your decision to allocate your precious resources of money and time that could be spent in other activities. Take a few minutes to consider what factors influenced you, but try to remember that I already made some suggestions that may have created a *recency effect*. Just as you made this decision for reasons of your own, I decided that the topic of decision making and its application to mental and behavioral health was worth the allocation of my resources. I am confident that it has been, although I admit I may have succumbed to *attributional bias*—justifying to myself that this is an important topic that is worth my effort (Heider, 1958). Maybe you received a brochure online or in the mail, read a book review that piqued your interest, were exploring a related topic and found this book, or were attracted to the cover at the annual convention or on the shelf in a bookstore. At some level of awareness you weighed the *cost–benefit* outcome of investing your resources, made a decision, and followed a course of action about which I am pleased. All of these responses, and many more, are heavily influenced by hidden biases associated with two main systems for decision making, one tending to be more cognitive and the other more emotionally derived. These systems exert a powerful influence on just about every aspect of clinical decision-making practice and research and more broadly on every decision you make.

THE MOST ADVANCED OF THE DECISION MAKERS

Humans are the most evolved, advanced decision-making species, and yet we are extraordinarily prone to biases and cognitive errors that result in less-than-optimal outcome. We all exercise decision-making processes from birth. Early on we orient to our mother's voice and smiling face. Our brains evolve to adapt to the decision demands of our environment and the relational matrix. Connections in our neural circuits are pruned so that those not necessary are eliminated, and resources can strengthen connections that will enhance our adaptation and capacity for decision making. We need to be able to make decisions rapidly to ensure our survival. Our limbic system, evolved to respond to danger, can easily go haywire, responding when there is no imminent threat, the result of unprocessed trauma (van der Kolk, 2014). No one has to tell us to escape a house on fire or avoid dangerous activities—we are unconsciously wired for rapid detection of and response to danger (Bargh, 2013). This is the neural foundation for rapid decision making and for our survival. These primal defensive structures are part of our reptilian and early mammillary brain development. Threat detection offers quick template matching and attention to environmental cues that are novel and unfamiliar and therefore potentially threatening. Trauma results when our limbic systems cannot process information because it has been overwhelmed and fragmented, and thus our decision making falters. We often perceive danger where none exists and live in state of hyperarousal, good for responding to threat but not so good for most decisions. This type of rapid decision making, when it does not go awry, is well suited for many situations, and when it is activated in the right circumstances is something to behold. Remember Chessey Sullenberger, the pilot who landed US Airways Flight 1549 in the Hudson River when both engines were put out of commission after the plane collided with geese? This is a truly remarkable example of someone operating with this type of intuitive, rapid response system based on many years of training and experience. He didn't have time to refer to a flight manual, nor would there be one that could tell him what he should do—he just did it. But intuition can also be dead wrong in many cases. The bleeding of patients with cholera seemed intuitive to 18th-century physicians—even though what they really needed in order to survive was hydration.

We have also developed an advanced deliberative and demanding style of decision making with the evolution of higher cortical structures. As we discussed, the process of your decision making about investing in this book began before you picked it up and opened it or read the dust jacket or viewed it online.

The goal of this volume is to provide you with a foundation in decision-making theory and offer you some critical tools to enhance the efficacy of clinical decision making, especially in situations of uncertainty, which are so common in clinical practice where our ability to predict is often so limited. This volume will introduce you to the rapidly advancing science of decision analytics and review the decision biases that affect us all. More important, this volume will explore the application of decision theory through a number of interrelated topics relevant to clinical practice, research, training, and behavioral health care administration. Decision theory is influencing just about every scientific discipline, including mathematics, sociology, behavioral economics, computer science, and many others, and yet even though psychologists have conducted most of the essential research, many psychologists are not familiar with this topic. Because mental health professionals have been slow to absorb these groundbreaking new interdisciplinary developments, it is my hope that reading this book will be a step in remedying this lack of knowledge by exposing you to the advantages of using decision theory as a framework for clinical practice. I hope that you will continue to read and absorb the concepts in this volume and that that this knowledge will provide you with a foundation in decision analytics. This deeper appreciation for the value of decision theory and related topics will help you achieve better therapeutic results by increasing your awareness of the biases that detract from optimal decision making. This volume also offers strategies and approaches that will mitigate these biases and thus enhance your decision-making skills and optimize the outcomes of all your decisions.

PILLARS OF EFFECTIVE DECISION MAKING

Five pillars of effective decision making are presented in this volume, each offering important information and perspectives to optimize decision making. These are (a) access to high-quality empirical evidence, (b) developing clinical expertise, (c) using sound theoretical constructs, (d) including ethical considerations, and (e) foundation in decision theory.

Access to High-Quality Empirical Evidence

One pillar of effective decision making rests on a foundation of evidence derived from science and clinical experience (Hollon et al., 2014). The best available evidence optimizes decisions (Gawande, 2009; Lilienfeld, 2012). Unfortunately, we do not usually have perfect information with which to make clinical decisions. Psychology is still a relatively young scientific discipline, and the complexity of the subject is enormous. It is only relatively recently in scientific time, over the past 5 decades or so, that we have established that psychosocial treatments for a variety of behavioral and mental disorders are effective. And even more recent is the beginnings of an evidence base showing the efficacy of a spectrum of approaches. Even so, the adoption of evidence-based treatments has been slow. Rosen et al. (2004) found that fewer than 10% of mental health providers at six sites surveyed provided evidence-based treatment for posttraumatic stress disorder.

> The science to practice lag for [evidence-based practices] is, in fact, longer (and in many cases, far longer) than the typical lengthy lag time of 15 to 20 years identified for medical interventions by the Institute of Medicine (2001) in the seminal report *Crossing the Quality Chasm: A New Health System for the 21st Century*. (Karlin & Cross, 2014, pp. 19–20)

Clinicians' effectiveness at decision making ranges (as one would expect) on a normal curve. Some clinicians are more expert in their decision making, whereas others tend to regularly fall prey to common biases that reduce effectiveness. Little is known about what constitutes expert clinical practice, but one thing that is essential is the knowledge and ability to make decisions in the face of uncertainty.

Developing Clinical Expertise

Another pillar of effective decision making is *expertise*, the definition of which is not straightforward (Kahneman & Klein, 2009). It has been described, for example, as "(a) reputation, (b) performance, or (c) client outcomes" (Tracey, Wampold, Lichtenberg, & Goodyear, 2014, p. 219). Behavioral and mental health professionals are consulted because of our perceived expertise based on our specialized knowledge of human behavior and methods of change. Expertise, however, goes beyond having information about the domains that encompass a scientific–professional discipline (Norcross, Hogan, & Koocher, 2008). Information by itself is available to anyone who has access to the Internet, but clinical decision-making skills are needed to distill and crystalize information into useful knowledge (Ariely, 2008). Much more is required to hone these skills. Several factors interfere with expertise, "including the cognitive and information processes of therapists, therapist' failure to engage routinely in deliberate practice, the inaccuracy of therapists' self-appraisals of their competence, and the lack of accurate feedback that affects learning" (Tracey et al., 2014, p. 220).

The public is somewhat skeptical that the study of human behavior is scientific (Lilienfeld, 2012). This skepticism should not be limited to the science of psychology. A recent issue of *The Economist* titled "How Science Goes

Wrong" (2013) challenged the assumption that science is self-correcting. Daniel Kahneman was quoted in an open letter challenging the widely accepted concept of *priming* (the notion that decisions we make are influenced by irrelevant events presented right before a choice is made) in psychological research as poorly founded, and many studies trying to replicate findings that seemingly support priming have failed to show support. Jerome Kagan (2012), in his book *Psychology's Ghosts: The Crisis in the Profession and the Way Back*, challenged many of the assumptions that serve as the basis for contemporary psychology. The assumptions that we make and may hold dear influence a cascade of treatment issues from diagnostic labels to the treatments that follow. Kagan illustrated the assumptions, often unexamined and based on limited evidence, that guide our conceptualizations and approach to treatment. He held that a biological bias may prematurely lead clinicians toward suggesting a pharmacological approach, on the basis of a belief that genetic predispositions have led to certain symptom constellations. Kagan's view is that although psychopharmacological treatment for mental disorders is fraught with biases, it continues to dominate the clinical landscape even though most psychotropic medication "can be likened to a blow on the head and resemble the cocktail of drugs used with many cancers that kill both healthy and cancerous tissues" (p. 209). American Psychological Association initiatives to develop clinical practice guidelines (Hollon et al., 2014) based on the most robust accumulated evidence should assist the public, behavioral and mental health consumers, policymakers, and other scientific disciplines in being assured that psychology is indeed a science and one that may be moving to a unifying framework (Magnavita & Anchin, 2014).

Using Sound Theoretical Concepts

A theoretical framework provides a map with which to test reality and therefore represents a fundamental pillar for decision making (Magnavita & Anchin, 2014). Theories evolve over time as new advances are made and the utility of the theory is time tested. Theoretical formulations are a type of decision-analytic process that encourages testing hypotheses and gathering data to test the validity of the construct. Theories address how the interrelated component domains of the biopsychosocial model interact and shape human behavior. Theories limited to one domain are prone to attributional biases and theories, which are too general and are difficult to test. Theories of the mind, personality, psychopathology, and behavior should be congruent and increasingly based on findings from neuroscience as well as effectiveness in the consulting room.

Ethical Considerations

An ethical framework is another pillar of effective decision making. An ethical examination of our actions and treatments can prevent us from being subject to the various types of biases that are discussed in this volume. An ethical framework serves as an important system of checks and balances when making complicated clinical decisions, and a strong ethical foundation for our decision making provides many safeguards to our patients and ourselves. Understanding how easily we are influenced by our biases can keep us from engaging in practices that are inert or, in the worst case, destructive.

Knowledge of Clinical Decision Making

Who would not like to improve their clinical outcomes or assist students and trainees in attaining the best results? The National Institute of Mental Health (1999) identified the incorporation of patient and provider decision making as an important research agenda for improving mental health interventions. In an effort to improve quality of mental health care, the Institute of Medicine (2001) suggested that the study of decision-making theory (Roberto, 2009), concepts, and preferences is imperative. Probably one reason you are reading this volume is that you want to maximize your clinical expertise or assist others in doing so by adding to your knowledge base, thus increasing your effectiveness in your own and your students' treatment of behavioral and mental health disorders. Clinical decision making is the foundation of behavioral and mental health practice, yet most clinicians receive very little formal training in this complex activity. Clinical decision making requires a depth and range of knowledge that requires years of education, training, and supervision, yet this critical activity is not systematically taught. I hope this volume serves as an agent of change by bringing decision making to the forefront of science, practice, and education. Decision making has characteristics of both intuitive and deliberative modes (Stanovich, 2010). Both are necessary, and neither can operate without the other. The most profound responsibility a clinician has is discerning which interventions are beneficial and which may prove inert or even harmful for those who seek our assistance. A series of "correct" decisions can have a potentially profound impact on improving the lives of those in our care. A series of "incorrect" decisions can have dire results: Patients may fail to improve or will deteriorate, and in extreme cases the outcome may be death. The science and theory of clinical decision making is the focus of this volume.

DECISION MAKING: THE KEY TO EVIDENCE-BASED PRACTICE

Providing a high-quality evidence-based practice informed by the best information through the lens of clinical expertise requires a foundation in how to make optimal decisions given the many choices available. Evidence-based practice represents the new era of contemporary health care: combining the best available evidence with clinical expertise. "Evidence-based practice in psychology (EBPP) is the integration of the best available research with clinical expertise in the context of patient characteristics, culture, and preferences" (APA Presidential Task Force, 2006, p. 273). All clinicians would likely agree that practice should be based on the best evidence. The evidence base for the treatment of behavioral and mental health disorders is growing, but it remains inadequate in the face of the extreme complexity and uncertainty in most domains of clinical science. We need to find and utilize the best evidence available from divergent credible sources and combine it with an appreciation of decision theory and deliberative decision analytics. We all make decisions, and we usually believe that what we decide is logical and that the consequences will be beneficial for those who seek our services. But decision theory requires us to constantly examine and challenge our beliefs and, more important, be alert for the common decision traps humans are likely to fall into. Thus we often find ourselves "down the rabbit hole" without understanding how we fell into such a state of upside-down reality.

THE BIRTH OF DECISION THEORY

The formal study of decision theory was initially applied to economic analysis. Frank Knight (1921/2006) distinguished between risk when the probability of an outcome can be calculated and uncertainty when there is no way to determine the probability of an outcome. Later, John von Neumann and Oskar Morgenstern (1944) developed game theory, which deals with how people make decisions using unknown variables. Daniel Kahneman and Amos Tversky (see Kahneman, 2011), over many decades of collaboration, researched and described many facets of decision theory.

> Decision theory has evolved since the 1950s from the fields of psychology and economics and has been applied in healthcare research since the 1960s. Theoretical perspectives in decision-making research encompass a wide variety of prescriptive approaches; for example, judgment and information processing analysis, decision analysis, and natural decision making. (Wills & Holmes-Rovner, 2006, p. 9)

The landmark work in this field that should be standard reading for all clinicians and social scientists is *Thinking Fast and Slow* by Kahneman (2011), who was awarded a Nobel Prize for his contributions in economics.

ENCODING AND DECODING OUR ENVIRONMENT: USING SCHEMATA AND PROTOTYPES FOR DECISION MAKING

I have already discussed the evolutionary basis for and some of the neural circuits involved in decision making. Our brains have evolved to perceive, filter, organize, and respond to a potentially overwhelming amount of environmental stimuli. Without strategies to organize this incoming information and develop internal patterns or templates, we would be rendered helpless. We encode information and store it for later use maintaining internal schemata, which are prototypes we use to compare current situations with past situations and look for a match. We learn by encoding and storing new information and then decode what comes in by seeing how it matches our internal representation. Most decisions are made automatically without having to strain our mental resources: This is the fast thinking mode. "The mental work that produces impressions, intuitions, and many decisions goes on in silence in our mind" (Kahneman, 2011, p. 4). This type of decision making represents what is often experienced as intuitive and real but as prone to error. We activate the slow thinking system to prevent the fast one from ruling our lives. We help patients learn how and when to apply slow thinking with respect to their therapeutic endeavors, regardless of the approach and what it is termed.

ASSESSING AND MANAGING RISK

Assessing risk in the face of uncertainty and even chaos by optimizing our choices is fundamental to decision making. In many important areas we are woefully inadequate at predicting human behavior. There is no area in which this is more visible than in the failure to predict the kinds of extreme violence that we have witnessed in schools in the United States beginning with the Columbine massacre. How could we let these events happen? If there were so many signs of trouble, how did we fail to notice? The unfortunate answer is that we are not good at predicting who will be violent. In a perfect world, where we have access to high-quality information, decision making is probabilistic. In the clinical setting, where there is often a dearth of empirical evidence, there is a need to be vigilant to the forms of biases and cognitive traps that influence our approach to making decisions. Almost every aspect of clinical practice is influenced by how we make decisions.

SHARED DECISION MAKING

Decision making in clinical practice should be shared and collaborative. There are various perspectives through which to examine clinical decision making. Much of what has been presented so far is decision making with the locus being the clinician. We may also consider shared decision making, which is dyadic or triadic in that there are interpersonal and larger system processes that are in operation, with multiple stakeholders. Various aspects of decision making are critical to improving mental and behavioral health care. Clinical decision making examines the thought processes that are incorporated by the clinician in practice. Patient decision making is a relatively new area of investigation. "How patients make decisions, the testing of interventions to support effective decision making, and the development of measures of patient decision making have only recently begun to be studied for mental health contexts" (Wills & Holmes-Rovner, 2006, p. 10). Shared decision making involves a partnership between the patient system and provider system. It requires a collaborative approach in which the patient's preferences are considered and information is shared to enhance decision making (Adams & Drake, 2006).

DECISION ANALYTICS

Most forward-thinking executives have fully adopted decision analytics as an essential tool. A recent article in the *Harvard Business Review* was titled "How to Make Smarter Decisions" (2013).

> Techniques from the field of decision analysis formalize the question of whether (provisionally) to adopt or reject an intervention. Decision analysis identifies the set of consequences of concern to the decision maker that might result from each available option (for example, the therapeutic effects and side effects associated with a drug, its direct costs, and its impact on social costs such as productivity losses) and determines their associated probabilities. Aggregating these probability-weighted consequences using an appropriate common metric yields an expected net impact for each option. (Claxton, Cohen, & Neumann 2005, p. 95)

Health care as a whole (with mental health soon to follow) will be seeing a greater reliance on the use of aggregated data to inform decision making, which will certainly have an economic impact in terms of who will get reimbursed and at what level. This trend is being fueled by computer technology, which is allowing us to mine data as never before.

BIG DATA AND DECISION MAKING

Technological advances have led to new possibilities for using big data for making decisions, which will inevitably change how behavioral and mental health care is delivered. This trend is in large part being driven by the expansion of the Internet along with powerful computer processing to change the fundamental ways we gather and process information. "The fruits of the information society are easy to see, with a cellphone in every pocket, a computer in every backpack, and big information technology systems in back offices" (Mayer-Schonberger & Cukier, 2013, p. 8). Since the beginning of the era of information technology, humans have generated more information than had been heretofore produced in the cumulative history of our species (Lehrer, 2009). "From sciences to healthcare, from banking to the Internet, the sectors may be diverse yet together they tell a similar story: the amount of data in the world is growing fast, outstripping not just our machines but our imaginations" (Mayer-Schonberger & Cukier, 2013, p. 8). This has important implications that are beyond the scope of this volume, so I suggest that those interested read *Big Data* by Viktor Mayer-Schonberger and Kenneth Cukier (2013), which presents an in-depth review of the trend and its implications.

ORGANIZATION OF THIS VOLUME

This volume offers a range of topics that will introduce the reader to the field of decision making in mental health practice. Decision making influences every aspect of clinical practice and is increasingly important for behavioral and mental health clinicians, as well as all health care providers, because of the inherent uncertainty in many aspects of clinical science. Many decisions are made that do not derive from an empirical evidence base and that necessitate a comfort with uncertainty. The topics covered in the remainder of this volume provide a sample of some of the important areas with which clinicians, researchers, and educators should be familiar. Decision theory and decisional research are far ranging and rapidly expanding into exciting areas such as big data and data mining that will influence all aspects of health care in the future. There is also an accelerating trend in all areas of health care to develop guidelines that practitioners, patients, policymakers, and others can use to optimize treatment of physical and behavioral health disorders.

The current chapter, Chapter 1, has introduced the topic of decision making in an effort to provide a brief overview of the subject of this volume and to highlight some of the essential constructs, common biases in decision making, and the five pillars of effective decision analytics. In Chapter 2

("Clinical Expertise and Decision Making: An Overview of Bias in Clinical Practice"), my coauthor Scott O. Lilienfeld and I present an overview of decision analytics and the biases and traps of which clinicians and researchers should beware. This chapter provides a solid foundation in some of the important topics related to decision making, along with a brief compendium of common traps or errors to which we are subject when making clinical decisions. Decision-making theory is included in a robust body of literature that emanates from research from many disciplines. The fundamentals of decision analytics and the biases that present danger are critical aspects of optimal clinical practice. In Chapter 3 ("A Dual Process Perspective on the Value of Theory in Psychotherapeutic Decision Making"), Jack C. Anchin and Jefferson A. Singer explore the importance of theory in decision making, an essential tool that has been evolving and becoming more sophisticated over the course of clinical science history. Theory presents a way of organizing and understanding clinical phenomena, offering a road map for decision making if used appropriately. In Chapter 4 ("Clinical Practice Guideline Development and Decision Making"), Lynn F. Bufka and Erin F. Swedish introduce the science and processes that go into the development of treatment guidelines. These cutting-edge developments include both exciting and somewhat controversial trends and the safeguards that ensure that clinical practice guideline development is as scientifically valid and transparent as humanly possible. After reading the chapter by Bufka and Swedish, the next question you might ask is what to do with this information. Clinical practice guidelines are all well and good, but we want to know how they help us treat behavioral and mental health disorders. In Chapter 5 ("Developing Clinical Practice Guidelines to Enhance Clinical Decision Making"), Steven D. Hollon explains how using an evidence base can enhance clinical decision making and how clinicians can maximize their effectiveness by referring to practice guidelines. In Chapter 6 ("Using Technology to Enhance Decision Making"), Franz Caspar and coauthors show the importance of technology in clinical decision making. Technology is fundamentally changing who we are as a species and providing us with multiple options to enhance our decision making. The number of technological developments available to us seems to steadily increase, and having knowledge of these can increase our decision making skills. In Chapter 7 ("Clinical Decision Making When the Stakes Are High"), I present a model of collaborative decision making that was developed while working in close collaboration with a psychiatrist treating complex clinical presentations. Clinical decision making is most challenging when the stakes are high, when cases may not have a simple solution and hence involve a high level of risk and potential harm. In Chapter 8 ("Use of Empirically Grounded Relational Principles to Enhance Clinical Decision Making"), Ken L. Critchfield and Julia E. Mackaronis show how relational principles offer a vital approach to clinical decision making. Having evidence for the effectiveness of a particular treatment approach is certainly important, but having an understanding of evidence-based principles adds another significant dimension. In Chapter 9 ("Integrating Ongoing Measurement Into the Clinical Decision-Making Process With Measurement Feedback Systems"), Thomas L. Sexton and Adam R. Fisher describe how client feedback can be used to improve treatment outcome. As I have discussed, decision making is about assessing probabilities and managing risk. Receiving ongoing feedback about how a patient is responding to treatment is immensely useful for monitoring treatment and altering one's approach in a responsive fashion. This is certainly going to be a part of most practice situations in the future. In Chapter 10 ("Clinical Decision Making and Risk Management"), Steven A. Sobelman and Jeffrey N. Younggren offer an important perspective on how understanding risk can enhance clinical management. Formal training in decision making is not yet part of graduate curricula in behavioral and mental health programs. Most of what is taught is done through a mentoring relationship. So the time seems right to begin to develop formal curricula and advanced training in decision analytics for behavioral and mental health professionals. In Chapter 11 ("Teaching Clinical Decision Making"), Gregg Henriques offers his novel approach to this area of the field.

The chapters in this volume are arranged in a sequence that walks the reader through a variety of interrelated topics. The wealth of information in the chapters will allows readers to see how pragmatic decision theory is and how applicable it is to just about everything we do in clinical practice and life in general. Learning to apply these tools is also very useful for financial decision making and will assist in any major decision, especially when there is uncertainty among various options.

SUMMARY

This volume, *Clinical Decision Making in Mental Health Practice*, applies the theory and research of decision analytics to the field of behavioral and mental health with a particular focus on how to improve clinical decision making. Decision theory is an exciting development that began as an attempt to deal with making decisions in situations of uncertainty, which has direct relevance to health care and mental health practice and training. There are basically two types of thinking that are called upon in making decisions. One is *fast*, intuitive, and emotional, excellent when rapid responses are vital to outcome. The other is *slow* or "lazy" in that a great deal of cognitive effort is required in order to consider the information and determine probabilities of outcomes from various choices. According to Kahneman (2011), both the fast and the slow systems of thinking must flexibly interact and can balance each other to maximize outcome. There are a number of biases that occur without our knowledge when we rely too much on the fast response system. These errors can be avoided by developing knowledge of various types of biases that are common to problem solving.

The chapters that follow will take you along a fascinating path that you will find has direct bearing on just about every aspect of your clinical practice, regardless of the setting or the types of decisions that you must make. Enhancing our decision-making skills and knowledge will advance the practice of behavioral and mental health treatment and allow us to adapt and thrive in the new era of health care that is emerging in this country and the world. Thank you for deciding to read this chapter, and I hope you will decide that this volume is worth your investment.

REFERENCES

Adams, J. R., & Drake, R. E. (2006). Shared decision-making and evidence-based practice. *Community Mental Health Journal, 42,* 87–105.

APA Presidential Task Force on Evidence-Based Practice. (2006). Evidence-based practice in psychology. *American Psychologist, 61,* 271–285. http://dx.doi.org/10.1037/0003-066X.61.4.271

Ariely, D. (2008). *Predictably irrational: The hidden forces that shape our decisions.* New York, NY: Harper Collins.

Bargh, J. A. (2013). Our unconscious mind. *Scientific American, 310,* 30–37. http://dx.doi.org/10.1038/scientificamerican0114-30

Claxton, K., Cohen, J. T., & Neumann, P. J. (2005). When is evidence sufficient? *Health Affairs, 24*(1), 93–101. http://dx.doi.org/10.1377/hlthaff.24.1.93

Gawande, A. (2009). *The checklist manifesto: How to get things right.* New York, NY: Henry Holt.

Heider, F. (1958). *The psychology of interpersonal relations.* New York, NY: Wiley. http://dx.doi.org/10.1037/10628-000

Hollon, S. D., Areán, P. A., Craske, M. G., Crawford, K. A., Kivlahan, D. R., Magnavita, J. J., . . . Kurtzman, H. (2014). Development of clinical practice guidelines. *Annual Review of Clinical Psychology, 10,* 213–241. http://dx.doi.org/10.1146/annurev-clinpsy-050212-185529

How science goes wrong. (2013, October 19). *The Economist.* Retrieved from http://www.economist.com/news/leaders/21588069-scientific-research-has-changed-world-now-it-needs-change-itself-how-science-goes-wrong

How to make smarter decisions. (2013, April). *Harvard Business Review.* Available at https://hbr.org/2013/04/innovation-risk-how-to-make-smarter-decisions

Institute of Medicine. (2001). *Crossing the quality chasm: A new health system for the 21st century.* Washington, DC: Author.

Kagan, J. (2012). *Psychology's ghosts: The crisis in the profession and the way back.* New Haven, CT: Yale University Press.

Kahneman, D. (2011). *Thinking fast and slow.* New York, NY: Farrar, Straus & Giroux.

Kahneman, D., & Klein, G. (2009). Conditions for intuitive expertise: A failure to disagree. *American Psychologist, 64,* 515–526. http://dx.doi.org/10.1037/a0016755

Karlin, B. E., & Cross, G. (2014). From the laboratory to the therapy room: National dissemination and implementation of evidence-based psychotherapies in the U.S. Department of Veterans Affairs Health Care System. *American Psychologist, 69,* 19–33. http://dx.doi.org/10.1037/a0033888

Knight, F. (2006). Risk, uncertainty and profit. Mineola, NY: Dover. (Original work published 1921)

Lambert, M. J. (2010). *Prevention of treatment failure: The use of measuring, monitoring, and feedback in clinical practice.* Washington, DC: American Psychological Association. http://dx.doi.org/10.1037/12141-000

Lehrer, J. (2009). Thinking meta. *Seed, 58*–60.

Lilienfeld, S. O. (2012). Public skepticism of psychology: Why many people perceive the study of human behavior as unscientific. *American Psychologist, 67,* 111–129. http://dx.doi.org/10.1037/a0023963

Magnavita, J. J., & Anchin, J. C. (2014). *Unifying psychotherapy.* New York, NY: Springer.

Mayer-Schonberger, V., & Cukier, K. (2013). *Big data: A revolution that will transform how we live, work, and think.* New York, NY: Houghton Mifflin Harcourt.

National Institute of Mental Health. (1999). *Bridging science and service: A report by the National Advisors Mental Health Council Clinical Treatment and Services Research Workgroup.* Washington, DC: Author.

Norcross, J. C., Hogan, T. P., & Koocher, G. P. (2008). *Clinician's guide to evidence-based practices: Mental health and the addictions.* New York, NY: Oxford University Press.

Roberto, M. A. (2009). *The art of critical decision making.* Chantilly, VA: The Great Courses—The Teaching Company.

Rosen, C. S., Chow, H. C., Finney, J. F., Greenbaum, M. A., Moos, R. H., Sheikh, J. I., & Yesavage, J. A. (2004). VA practice patterns and practice guidelines for treating posttraumatic stress disorder. *Journal of Traumatic Stress, 17,* 213–222. http://dx.doi.org/10.1023/B:JOTS.0000029264.23878.53

Stanovich, K. E. (2010). *Decision making and rationality in the modern world.* New York, NY: Oxford University Press.

Tracey, T. J., Wampold, B. E., Lichtenberg, J. W., & Goodyear, R. K. (2014). Expertise in psychotherapy: An elusive goal? *American Psychologist, 69,* 218–229. http://dx.doi.org/10.1037/a0035099

Tversky, A., & Kahneman, D. (1974). Judgment under uncertainty: Heuristics and biases. *Science, 185*, 1124–1131. http://dx.doi.org/10.1126/science.185.4157.1124

van der Kolk, B. (2014). *The body keeps the score: Brain, mind, and body in the healing of trauma.* New York, NY: Viking.

von Neumann, J., & Morgenstern, O. (1944). *Theory of games and economic behavior.* Princeton, NJ: Princeton University Press.

Walfish, S., McAlister, B., O'Donnell, P., & Lambert, M. J. (2012). An investigation of self-assessment bias in mental health providers. *Psychological Reports, 110*, 639–644.

Wills, C. E., & Holmes-Rovner, M. (2006). Integrating decision making and mental health interventions research: Research directions. *Clinical Psychology, 13*, 9–25.

2

CLINICAL EXPERTISE AND DECISION MAKING: AN OVERVIEW OF BIAS IN CLINICAL PRACTICE

JEFFREY J. MAGNAVITA AND SCOTT O. LILIENFELD

At a recent dinner party, a guest told a story about an older mentor who said, "Kid, I smoke and drink, and now the doctor who told me to stop smoking is dead, and another one after him who said to stop drinking is also dead." And so the guest mused, "Why should I stop smoking and drinking?" This is an illustrative example of flawed reasoning—in this case, the failure to follow Bayesian logic. The mentor is ignoring probability and *base rates*—the frequency of a condition or event: Smokers have a high incidence of lung cancer. The decisions we make are guided by many factors, and sometimes as in the case of the smoker, these may have dire consequences. We have excellent data on the relationship between smoking and health risk. Clinicians are continuously making decisions, some of which are also prone to biases, which also can have unfortunate consequences.

What guides clinicians in making complex decisions? Do expertise and intuition account for better treatment outcomes? What biases are we prone to

http://dx.doi.org/10.1037/14711-002
Clinical Decision Making in Mental Health Practice, J. J. Magnavita (Editor)
Copyright © 2016 by the American Psychological Association. All rights reserved.

when making decisions, and how can we avoid these? Clinicians and researchers alike routinely fall prey to errors in this type of thinking and many others that can have dire consequences, but as clinical experts we have a responsibility to avoid these cognitive traps. Clinicians have a "duty to know," which refers to an *"epistemic duty* . . . best enacted through a critical knowledge of the scientific method in psychology and the relevant scientific literature" (O'Donohue, Lilienfeld, & Fowler, 2007, p. 4). For example, we must try to avoid missing a high-risk marker for self-destructive behavior, pushing a patient too hard or fast in treatment, failing to corroborate information with other family members, selectively including and excluding certain studies in a meta-analysis, and so forth. Complex decisions are often influenced by hidden biases that can lead to faulty reasoning. These decision biases bear major implications for almost every aspect of clinical practice and research, and it is thus imperative for clinicians to be knowledgeable about them.

There are some "great" ideas and guiding principles every mental health practitioner should know (Lilienfeld & O'Donohue, 2007). Advances in clinical science over a century have led to a substantial body of information, including robust theoretical constructs, empirical evidence in a variety of domains, accumulated clinical experience, and evidence from related disciplines, which serve as the foundation for and as a guide to decision making in clinical practice (Magnavita & Anchin, 2014). However, accumulated experience or knowledge alone does not necessarily result in expertise (Tracey, Wampold, Lichtenberg, & Goodyear, 2014). "Expertise in any endeavor requires, among other things, a considerable amount of dedicated practice" (Ruscio, 2007, p. 40). The 10,000-hour rule suggests that to become expert at a complex endeavor, one must practice at least 10,000 hours to achieve mastery (Gladwell, 2008). And yet, clinical expertise requires more than this extensive knowledge base and much practice; we also must be wise enough to know how, and when, to apply what we know. "To be effective clinical scientists, we must base our actions and decisions on reliable knowledge. We should not simply guess or believe, but instead *know* how nature, in this case human nature, actually operates to influence behavior" (O'Donohue et al., 2007, p. 4). Accumulated knowledge does not necessarily determine how to proceed in the consulting room. Expertise requires training and experience in making complex decisions, which in part derives from training and clinical experience, combined with effective supervision and feedback. The empirical evidence on whether more experienced psychotherapists get better outcomes is equivocal. There is some evidence that experienced psychotherapists do have an advantage in the face of complexity over less experienced ones (Oddli & Halvorsen, 2014), but other evidence suggests that expertise does not play a role in outcome (Beutler, 1997; Okiishi, Lambert, Nielsen, & Ogles, 2003). Expertise does not arise solely from experience because there is no guarantee that we are not doing the wrong thing over and over again. Genuine expertise results from extracting the relevant information from experience and applying it in the appropriate situation (McKnight & Sechrest, 2003) as well as avoiding the biases that are common in decision making, which are reviewed later in this chapter. Regular high-quality feedback is also critical to developing expertise. In spite of extensive training, clinicians and researchers are often subject to cognitive errors or systematic sources of irrationality that impair decision making. We are all vulnerable to inherent bias-generative errors, and according to Daniel Ariely (2010), "we are not only irrational, but predictably irrational—that our irrationality happens the same way, again and again" (p. xx). The intersection of decision-making processes and clinical expertise influences all aspects of behavioral and mental health practice.

This chapter explores the relationship between expertise and decision making, with specific focus on providing an overview of the essential pragmatic aspects of decision making essential to ethical and effective practice, fulfilling our epistemic duty. We begin with a description and explanation of evidence-based practice and clinical expertise.

CLINICAL EXPERTISE: A NECESSARY COMPONENT OF EVIDENCE-BASED PRACTICE

Clinical expertise is an essential component of providing quality evidence-based mental and behavioral health care. Access to knowledge does not confer expertise. Let us first consider the meaning of *expertise*. A review of the literature on clinical expertise highlights various ways of conceptualizing expertise, including reputation, performance, and client outcomes (Tracey et al., 2014). Tracey et al. (2014) endorsed Shanteau's (1992) definition of expertise as improvement over time. Expertise is an important component of an evidence-based practice. "*Evidence-based practice in psychology* (EBPP) is the integration of the best available research with clinical expertise in the context of patient characteristics, culture, and preferences" (APA Presidential Task Force on Evidence-Based Practice, 2006, p. 273). Norcross, Hogan, and Koocher (2008), in their volume *Clinician's Guide to Evidence-Based Practices*, wrote: "We all recognize that clinical practice should be predicated on the best available research integrated with the clinician's expertise within the context of the particular patient" (p. xi). The best available information must be filtered through clinical expertise and grounded in the pragmatics of decision analytics, which are examined in this chapter and throughout this volume.

The APA Presidential Task Force on Evidence-Based Practice (2006) described *clinical expertise* "as competence attained by psychologists, through education, training, and experience that results in effective practice" (p. 275). Clinical expertise includes

> identifying and integrating the best research evidence with clinical data (e.g., information about the patient obtained over the course of treatment) in the context of the patient's characteristics, culture, and preferences to deliver services that have the highest probability of achieving the goals of therapy. (p. 275)

What is not clearly articulated in this definition is the central role of *decision analysis*. "Decision analysis identifies the set of consequences of concern to the decision maker that might result from each available option" (Claxton, Cohen, & Neumann, 2005, p. 95). Decision analytics bridge the gap between clinical practice and valid sources of information by offering heuristics to maximize the decision-making capabilities of the clinician to enhance treatment process and outcome.

Professional psychologists and other mental health clinicians must acquire an extensive knowledge base derived from various domains and related disciplines, including, but not limited to, psychopathology, neuroscience, developmental psychology, theories of personality and psychotherapy, evidence-based treatments, statistics, research methodology, and diagnostics systems as well as various modalities of treatment. This foundation of knowledge and specialized language, along with pattern recognition skills, which are not common in everyday life, confers "expertise." Effectively combining these domains of information into a useful knowledge base requires sophisticated decision-making processes that are largely free from cognitive errors. Unfortunately, we are often not cognizant of errors in thinking that bias our decisions and can easily gravitate toward a style of thinking that requires little effort and may conflate our self-perception about our competence. Clinicians are notorious for believing in the veracity of our approaches and often not questioning the clinical dogma of one approach or another. As Roberto (2009) noted, "Our cognitive limitations lead to errors in judgment—not because of a lack of intelligence, but simply because we are human. Systematic biases impair the judgment and choices that individuals make" (p. 31). "True experts, it is said, know when they don't know" (Kahneman & Klein, 2009, p. 524).

Abundant psychological research, including groundbreaking work by scholars Tversky and Kahneman (1973), Kahneman, (2011), and Stanovich (2010), has illuminated the inherent traps that arise from widely held cognitive, affective, and perceptual biases. These often useful heuristics that we draw on for rapid decision making can nevertheless become "traps" when they are misused. A controversial form of this type of flawed decision making is racial profiling. *Heuristics* are mental shortcuts or "rules of thumb"; more formally, they constitute methods of thinking that allow us to process information rapidly, which in some cases can be useful and even indispensable for making rapid decisions under conditions of uncertainty. However, when we are unaware of how these heuristic devices affect our thinking, or when we incorporate them when more systematic effort is required, our problem solving can be impaired. Even expert clinicians and researchers are prone to biases that strongly affect their clinical decision making and slide toward "lazy," less rigorous, thinking (Kahneman, 2011); indeed, the two authors of this chapter are just as susceptible to these biases! But what makes us lazy, Fiske and Taylor (1991) argued, is that we are "cognitive misers" when it comes to effortful thinking; we use heuristics to save resources. For many decisions it is not necessary to use effortful modes of analysis. As we shall see, these rules of thumb can be extremely useful for certain purposes, but require vigilance when used. Only by being aware of these biases or cognitive traps in decision making can we combat the inherently human tendencies toward thrift and minimize the risk of falling into decision-making traps.

THE PRAGMATICS OF DECISION MAKING

One of the leading figures in the scientific study of decision making, Keith Stanovich (2010), wrote, "Nothing could be more practical or useful for a person's life than the thinking processes that help him or her find out what is true and what is best to do" (p. 2). Clinicians, regardless of whether their discipline is psychology, social work, psychiatry, nursing, or medicine, must process enormous amounts of data and information, distilling them into coherent diagnostic formulations followed by a logical course of action, which are modified and corrected as new information is gleaned. Often important decisions have to be made quickly, so these heuristics can be invaluable because they allow us to implement the "thin slice"—a type of rapid pattern recognition (Ambady & Rosenthal, 1992; Gladwell, 2005). Because there will almost always be a high degree of uncertainty in human behavior, the natural world, and clinical science, we cannot always respond in an optimal manner, and at times mistakes occur. Developing an understanding of cognitive biases that may lead to faulty decision making and understanding how to minimize these errors can improve clinical expertise and increase wisdom.

In his book *How Doctors Think*, Groopman (2007) wrote, "Experts studying misguided care have recently concluded that the majority of errors are due to flaws in physician thinking, not technical mistakes" (p. 24). As the old saying goes, "The operation was a success but the patient died." In spite of endorsing an evidence-based approach, such as following a manualized treatment approach, a patient may worsen or not return, prematurely discontinuing treatment. These situations may require and capitalize on our expertise. Although most psychotherapists generally have a positive view of treatment manuals (Najavits, Weiss, Shaw, & Dierberger, 2000), research is equivocal about whether clinicians who too closely adhere to a treatment manual have better or worse outcomes (Hogue et al., 2008). It is clear that sophisticated treatment must go beyond a cookbook approach, and thoughtfully constructed therapy manuals recognize what Kendall, Gosch, Furr, and Sood (2008) termed "flexibility within fidelity." At this point in time, the preponderance of research seems to suggest that outcome is improved when adherence is maintained. Nevertheless, there are times when strict adherence to any approach is contraindicated and clinical judgment based on decision theory must supersede blindly enforcing a particular treatment approach (see also Grove & Meehl, 1996, for a discussion of the "broken leg" scenario in clinical judgment and prediction). As Groopman described the complexity of information processing, "Throughout the day we are detecting frequencies hundreds of times, using our language modules repeatedly, inferring the thoughts of others constantly, and so on—all of which are adaptive and serve personal goal satisfaction" (p. 141). Given the complexity of clinical practice, our clinical expertise can be strengthened and our results optimized by learning the basics of decision analysis and the cognitive traps to which we are prone. As we shall discuss, certain types of decision making are best suited for particular situations.

ACKNOWLEDGING THE UNCERTAINTY IN DECISION ANALYTICS

In our chaotic and unpredictable world, many of the decisions we make represent our best efforts to deal with greater or lesser degrees of uncertainty. It is important to acknowledge the uncertainty in the world and be skeptical when it comes to any evidence we analyze. We should always be asking ourselves, "What do the data say, and what is the evidence?" The more risk involved in a decision, the greater the importance of incorporating principles of decision analytics to reduce unnecessary bias in our response. It is not always prudent to "trust your gut or your judgment" when making decisions. For example, incorrectly diagnosing a patient may have severe consequences; failure to provide the appropriate diagnosis may lead to undertreatment or inappropriate treatment. Misguided interventions can in turn predispose a patient to destructive behavior; similarly, placing a patient on a potentially harmful medication that is not required would be erroneous and possibly iatrogenic.

Problems encountered in clinical practice will demand differing approaches to decision making. A patient who seems to be in a high level of limbic arousal may call for quick action as opposed to a patient with Bipolar I disorder, for example, who refuses to take a mood stabilizer. It is essential to understand how we make decisions and what types of problems are best addressed through rapid processing as opposed to a more deliberative approach. Similarly, individuals can be described as either high or low on the polarity of emotional versus rational decision makers: Some may say that they just "know in their heart" what is right, whereas others "use their heads" when making decisions.

RATIONALITY AND EMOTIONALITY: TWO APPROACHES TO DECISION MAKING

There are two basic processes we incorporate in our decision making, which Lehrer (2009) described as *rational* and *emotional* (see also Kahneman, 2011). The first, based largely on logic, uses rationality by accumulating appropriate information, weighing findings, testing hypotheses, and using feedback to modify them. This type of systematic thinking tends to be rational, language based, and linear and requires a great deal of effort. The second type tends to be based largely on unconscious emotional ("gut") reactions and intuitions and often bypasses rational thinking. This type of decision making generally requires much less effort and is used to navigate many situations in which effortful thinking may not be required (Epstein, 1994).

Each type of problem solving has an important place in clinical decision making, and when the types are properly combined they can most effectively enhance our judgments. When we fall prey to biases that are inherent to each of these systems, our clinical decision making can be hindered and our expertise compromised, resulting in less than desirable outcomes or iatrogenic effects. When this occurs, we should ideally monitor the process and then use feedback we gather to make adjustments.

For example, when formulating a treatment plan for a patient with a particular clinical presentation, we systematically weigh options, predict the benefits of each, discuss patient preferences, and determine a course of treatment. Thus, a patient who presents with suspicious features might have a paranoid personality disorder; alternatively, his or her clinical presentation may stem from other sources. Reviewing the prevalence of paranoid personality disorder in the general population, we would find the base rate to be rather low. Determining base rates for clinical phenomena is a critical aspect of psychodiagnosis and other clinical tasks, which represents a logical, rational approach. There will be times when we need to respond on a largely emotional level, which is more intuitive and rapid. This often occurs in the moment-to-moment process of clinical work. For example, we may make a suggestion to a patient or summarize what he or she is describing and notice that he or she is grimacing. Our intuitive sense is that we have created a rupture in the alliance to which we may respond before we even consciously process what occurred—for example, by asking whether we said something that offended our client. In his book *Blink*, Malcolm Gladwell (2005) wrote, "The part of our brain that leaps to conclusions like this is called the adaptive unconscious, and the study of this kind of decision making is one of the most important new fields in psychology" (p. 11). In addition, in his book *Strangers to Ourselves: Discovering the Adaptive Unconscious*, Timothy Wilson (2002) discussed how much of what occurs in our minds lies outside of conscious awareness. Hassin, Uleman, and Bargh (2005), in their volume *The New Unconscious*, also presented compelling evidence for the scope of unconscious processing and suggested that transference and countertransference phenomena are rooted partly in these ubiquitous template-matching processes. Much of what occurs in the moment-by-moment process in psychotherapy may capitalize on bringing this system to conscious awareness so that practitioners can exert greater agency over their schema-driven responses.

Objective and rational processes are valuable in clinical decision making, but sometimes even these more deliberate processes are prone to unconscious bias. Our internal state also influences our decision-making processes. "The [clinician's] internal state, his state of tension, enters into and strongly influences his clinical judgments and actions" (Groopman, 2007, p. 36). Effective decision making requires an optimal level of anxiety; too much anxiety may compromise rational thinking, but too little anxiety may not be optimal. Research has increasingly identified neurobiological correlates of the inefficiencies of effective decision making. For example, neuroscientific findings suggest that when individuals are confronted with a financial expert, regions of the brain linked to decision making become less active. Similarly, when we see the same phenomena repeatedly, our brain uses less energy to process it (Berns, 2008). When we find information that supports our decisions, we tend to experience an increase in dopamine similar to consuming chocolate, having sex, or falling in love (Hertz, 2013, p. SR6). We like it when what we believe is affirmed. "But there are moments," according to Gladwell (2005), "particularly in times of stress, when haste does not make waste, and our snap judgments and first impressions can offer a much better means of making sense in the world" (p. 14). Clinicians often report that they are at their best when their intuitive sensing is operative. This may create a state that Mihaly Csikszentmihalyi (1990) described as *flow*. There exists much folklore regarding these concepts in the clinical community. "Good" therapists are often described as working intuitively and thereby capitalizing on the information discerned through the filter of the "nonconscious" system. Recent neuroscientific research shows evidence of neural networks that allow for the rapid intuitive processing of implicit information, a process referred to as *mentalization* (van Overwalle & Vanderkerckhove, 2013). At the same time, subjective experience, although accurate in some interpersonal situations, may not be suitable for most decisions, so one must use data to substantiate these informal impressions.

ELEMENTS OF OPTIMAL DECISION MAKING: DATA, INFORMATION, KNOWLEDGE, AND WISDOM

Optimal decision making involves forecasting outcomes in the face of uncertainty. The use of intuition, a relatively rapid form of decision making, is subject to error, but it can sometimes be a useful clinical aid. Effective decision making involves gathering relevant information, considering and evaluating alternatives, making judgments that are relatively free of biases, and appraising the outcomes of our decisions. What are the basic elements of decision making? Stanovich (2010) wrote this succinct description:

> Decision situations can be broken down into three components: (a) possible actions, (b) possible events or possible states of the world, and (c) evaluations of the consequences of possible actions in each possible state of the world. Because there are almost always one or more possible future states of the world, any action can be viewed as a gamble—the consequences of the gamble are unknown because the future state of the world is unknown. (p. 9)

Clinical expertise may be viewed as a form of wisdom because having access to a plethora of information does not confer wisdom, as we now experience in the digital–Internet age. One very intelligent professional, while in treatment with the first author, reported that when she looks up her symptoms on the Internet she has almost every possible disorder described. It is therefore helpful to differentiate among the hierarchy of classes of knowledge on which we base our decisions, and it is important to differentiate among the classes of knowledge relevant to decision making. The hierarchy of knowledge, referred to as DIKW (data, information, knowledge, wisdom), is a useful framework with which to organize classes of information and has been used extensively in business, technology, and information science (Rowley, 2007; Zins, 2007). Although the originator of this system is unknown, numerous scholars have described similar constructs in the literature (Russell Ackoff was one of the leading proponents of this system; Ackoff, 1967). Each level of the system, similar to Maslow's (1954) hierarchy of needs, is posited to be a precursor for the next level. The hierarchy of knowledge includes the elements described in the following paragraphs.

Data

Data are discrete units of information that are not yet organized on the basis of observations or facts. For example, a list of names and telephone numbers and discrete observations from a research study are classified as data. There is no inherent usefulness to data because they become useful only when they are coherently and systematically organized. Computers rely on enormous quantities of nonprocessed bytes encoded as 0 or 1 units, or data, that when organized into code become useful. Never before in the history of our species have we had the capability to amass such voluminous amounts of data. These "big data" that most often comes from the Internet is a new frontier for information technology. "Today, every e-mail, instant message, phone call, line of written code and mouse-click leaves a digital signal" (Lohr, 2013, p. 4). This constitutes a revolution in data gathering that is beginning to fundamentally transform the world. Data patterns are being mined and used to enhance innovations in health care and business. "Digital technology also makes it possible to conduct and aggregate personality-based assessments, often using online quizzes or games, in far greater detail and numbers than ever before" (Lohr, 2013, p. 4). This emphasis on mining big data is leading to an ever greater reliance on data-driven decision making. The future of clinical decision making will almost certainly be shaped by innovative uses of big data.

Information

When data have been endowed with some meaning and have been organized into a useful form, they are called *information*. A phone book is an example of information because the data (names and phone numbers) are organized in a way to be easily accessed. The development of clinical practice guidelines, discussed in Chapter 4 in this volume, exemplifies what should eventually be useful information that when accessed by clinicians and the public will serve to reduce uncertainty. Anyone will be able to read the guidelines, a source of information, but applying them will require more than simply assimilating the information provided—expertise is necessary.

Knowledge

When information is synthesized, it becomes *knowledge*. For example, a knowledgeable practitioner should be able to appropriately apply the information that is provided in the form of clinical practice guidelines. In contrast, such application is unlikely to take place for those untrained in the domains discussed at the beginning of the chapter, which serve as a foundation for employing this information.

Wisdom

The ability to use knowledge to increase our effectiveness is known as *wisdom*. The highest level of clinical expertise reflects a substantial knowledge base and the ability to effectively use decision analytics to make the best choices in the face of uncertainty. Scott Miller and colleagues studied ostensible "supershrinks" and found that they worked hard at deliberate practice, which entails actively planning, considering strategies, tracking and reviewing process, and adjusting the intervention (Miller, Duncan, & Hubble, 2008). The downside of deliberate practice is that it is not inherently motivating and increases costs. Lambert (2010) has conducted extensive research showing that expert therapists are more likely than other therapists to respond to information regarding the therapeutic process and accurately self-assess compared with less effective psychotherapists, who tend to overrate their skill. When we make the effort to understand different types of decision making—one "fast" and one "slow"—we can learn how to use these modes to our advantage.

THE DUAL PROCESSORS OF DECISION MAKING: FAST AND SLOW THINKING

As suggested earlier, abundant research has accrued over many decades supporting the presence of two types of decision-making processes or styles that have evolved in humans to assure our survival and enhance adaptation (Stanovich & West, 2000). An understanding of the way we think is essential for optimizing our decision making. It is imperative to know what type of system is called for in clinical situations that require us to process information and make complex decisions. In his book *Thinking, Fast and Slow*, Nobel Prize–winning psychologist Daniel Kahneman (2011) presented two systems that are operative when we think. Keith Stanovich and Richard West (2000) classified these two modes into System 1 and System 2 thinking. In his book *Rationality and the Reflective Mind*, Stanovich (2011) argued that System 1 is rapid, intuitive, and emotional, and System 2 is slower, logical, and more deliberately algorithmic. Although Stanovich now uses the terms *Type 1* and *Type 2* when referring to these systems, we use Kahneman's more familiar System 1 and System 2 designations in this chapter. It is worthwhile to develop an understanding of the strengths and weaknesses of both systems so that we are aware of how each may be useful in clinical decision making and of the biases inherent in System 1 (Kahneman, 2011, p. 79). Fortunately, the biases have been well researched and articulated and are discussed later in this chapter. The two systems described in greater detail in the following section are interactive and can effectively work together, but awareness of how these operate is critical to avoid thinking traps.

System 1—Essential for Survival but Notorious for Bias

Operating automatically with little or no voluntary control, System 1 is the rapid processor or the *fast* thinking system (Kahneman, 2011). It is easy to be seduced by System 1 thinking, which is relatively effortless, nonconscious, and utilizes intuition. Most of us fall prey to the ease of use and overconfidence of thinking fast, and therein is the problem. This system generates complex patterns of ideas, drawing effortlessly on feelings and impressions, often responding efficiently and effectively. However, System 1 is most efficient when responding to short-term predictions and does less well with longer term predictions. This mode of thinking is essential when we have to rapidly assess the environment for threat, such as in fight–flight responses, and for falling in love, or swiftly reacting to a potentially violent patient. However, the modern world is "simply littered with Type 1 traps" (Stanovich, 2010, p. 141), which can lead to costly decisions such as buying on impulse, amassing credit card debt, and taking on predatory mortgages, to name a few. When we need to be deliberate and analyze information to make a decision, System 1 often falls short, although, as we shall note, many important aspects of clinical practice incorporate and may benefit from System 1 processing. Clinicians often refer to this type of fast thinking as intuition based on clinical expertise and gut feelings (Kahneman & Klein, 2009).

Clinical expertise is a hard-earned and valuable commodity for practitioners that is derived from extensive training and experience. It is helpful to understand how expertise often relies on intuition. We must understand the strengths and limitations of intuition and the circumstances under which it is most effectively utilized because intuition, when unchecked, can be prone to bias. Kahneman (2011) wrote,

> Expert intuition strikes us as magical, but it is not. Indeed, each of us performs feats of intuitive expertise many times each day. Most of us are pitch-perfect in detecting anger in the first word of a telephone call, recognize as we enter a room that we were the subject of the conversation, and quickly react to subtle signs that the driver in the next lane is dangerous. (p. 11)

This wisdom comes from having a sound knowledge base and relevant experience derived from seeing multiple cases in clinical practice. Emerging from this intuitive and deliberative information-processing experience are complex pattern-recognition skills and useful clinical heuristics to guide treatment (Kahneman & Klein, 2009). Clinicians often rely on intuition in the face of uncertainty. Sometimes, we may try to justify a gut feeling with a "rational veneer" (Ariely, 2010, p. 53). However, as Paul Meehl (1954) noted in his landmark volume, *Clinical Versus Statistical Prediction*,

> Four decades of research consisting of over 100 research studies have shown that, in just about every clinical prediction domain that has ever been examined (psychotherapy outcome, parole behavior, college graduation rates, response to electroshock therapy, criminal recidivism, length of psychiatric hospitalization, and many more), actuarial prediction has been found to be superior to clinical prediction. (pp. 84–85)

So does adding clinical to actuarial prediction improve our results? The answer appears to be clear: As Stanovich (2010) noted, "Clinical prediction does not work" (p. 84). Predicting human behavior is not precise and never will be, so we employ heuristics, which sometimes improve our decisions.

Nevertheless, there are rare exceptions. Meehl (1954) described "broken leg" cases, in which extremely low base rate events that are too rare to be incorporated into the formula should lead us to overrule this formula. For example, if an empirically derived actuarial formula tells us that a client is extremely unlikely to attempt suicide, but the client informs us that he is about to kill himself and has recently bought a gun, we should probably disregard the formula and act quickly. Nevertheless, these cases are rare exceptions. In the substantial majority of cases, we are better advised to trust the output of statistical prediction rules that have been derived from actual output data. As Kahneman (2011) noted,

> Most impressions and thoughts arise in your conscious experience without knowing how they got there. You cannot trace how you came to the belief that there is a lamp on the desk in front of you, or how you detected a hint of irritation in your spouse's voice on the telephone, or how you managed to avoid threat on the road before you became consciously aware of it. The mental work that produces impressions, intuitions, and many decisions goes on in the silence of your mind. (p. 4)

In *Blink*, Malcolm Gladwell (2005) popularized the term *thin slicing*, which was coined by Ambady and Rosenthal (1992) to describe this rapid, intuitive style of processing information. For example, the first 3 minutes of marital dialogue is highly predictive of whether a couple will divorce (Carrère & Gottman, 1999).Clinicians who have not developed the capacity to rapidly respond to stimuli at an unconscious level are handicapped. We call this skill *clinical intuition* and recognize it in others as a "gift," but "supershrinks" may in fact be differentiated from others by their deliberative focus on improving performance (Miller et al., 2008). We contend, however, that although clinical intuition is important for effective mental and behavioral health practice, its output must be checked continually against another more logical system.

System 2—The "Lazy" Processor

More effortful than System 1, System 2 utilizes a higher level of mental activity and requires "agency, choice, and concentration" (Kahneman, 2011, p. 21). This system draws heavily on our cognitive resources and can lead to ego depletion. In fact, more energy is used by the nervous system for System 2 processing. Nonetheless, System 2 is notoriously "lazy" and reluctant to do more than is necessary. According to Kahneman, we tend to find the cognitive effort required of System 2 unpleasant and too effortful, leading us to avoid the demands necessary and often defaulting to the less effortful System 1 style of processing information. The type of thinking outlined by Stanovich (2011) requires us to approach our decision analysis much more slowly, using computational skills that he termed *algorithmic*. As we become more skilled in a task, it is less effortful but still requires engagement. Actuarial prediction is predominantly a System 2 process, whereas clinical prediction is predominantly a System 1 process.

Relying on Both System 1 and System 2

Clinicians generally and understandably favor System 1 decision making, which is the rapid pattern recognition type necessary for navigating the often enormous multitude of decisions that are faced on a moment-to-moment basis in clinical practice. Researchers, in contrast, tend to favor System 2 decision making, which relies on using systematically derived data and well-substantiated conclusions. There is often much saber rattling and polarization among devotees of these two types of decision making. Some clinicians appear to believe that data derived from research studies are not especially useful in clinical decision making, whereas some researchers appear to believe that many clinicians ignore the fact that actuarial prediction typically outperforms clinical decision making based on expertise. Nevertheless, such polarization is largely unnecessary. In the heat of the therapy session, clinicians must of course rely on their intuitions; they must "use their heads." At the same time, such intuitions should be guided and double-checked by systematic data.

CLINICAL VERSUS ACTUARIAL PREDICTION

What we observe in the world is a complex mixture of random and systematic factors, in large part driven by the former (Stanovich, 2010). Our reluctance to acknowledge the role of chance in predicting outcomes can decrease our ability to predict events accurately. Stanovich (2010) wrote,

> Research on the issue of clinical versus actuarial prediction has been consistent. Since the publication of Paul Meehl's classic book *Clinical Versus Statistical Prediction*, four decades of research consisting of over 100 research studies have shown that, in just about every clinical prediction domain that has ever been examined (psychotherapy outcome, parole behavior, college graduation rates, response to electroshock therapy, criminal recidivism, length of psychiatric hospitalization, and many more), actuarial prediction has been found to be superior to clinical prediction. (pp. 84–85)

In a more recent meta-analytic study, the actuarial or statistical prediction was about 10% more accurate than the clinical prediction. This seems to be the case regardless of types of judgment and amount of experience. In a few studies, clinical prediction was slightly more accurate, although it is not clear whether these findings are replicable. Interestingly, when clinical interview data are included, the accuracy of prediction typically deteriorates, suggesting that such data can dilute the validity of clinicians' information appraisal (Grove, Zald, Lebow, Snitz, & Nelson, 2000). Stanovich (2010), citing Gawande (1998), noted that

> the clinicians in these studies believed their experience allowed them to make better predictions than those that can be made from quantified information in the client's file. In fact, their "insight" is nonexistent and leads them to make predictions that are worse than those they would make if they relied only on the public, actuarial information. It should be noted, though, that the superiority of actuarial prediction is not confined to psychology but extends to many other clinical sciences as well—for example, to the reading of electrocardiograms in medicine. (pp. 85–86)

Why then are many clinicians opposed to actuarial prediction? Clinicians commonly cite a number of reasons for eschewing actuarial prediction (Grove & Meehl, 1996). In many cases, it seems that we exhibit the very biases presented in this chapter. Indeed, Meehl's ideas were met with hostility and disbelief from the clinical community. Kahneman (2011) wrote that they were under the influence of "an illusion of skill" and commented, "On reflection, it is easy to see how the illusion came about and easy to sympathize with the clinicians' rejection of Meehl's research" (p. 227).

Some clinicians may assume that the quality of their judgments should override statistical evidence. Kahneman (2011) noted, "Psychologists who work with patients have many hunches during each therapy session, anticipating how the patient will respond to an intervention, guessing what will happen next" (p. 227). Much of what happens on a moment-by-moment basis in the clinical situation seems to substantiate clinician intuition. Psychotherapists practice and hone their skills over many years and develop a keen sense of what will transpire in the therapeutic process. Certain clinicians are clearly superior to others in their competence level. However, they typically are not good at making predictions about longer term future events; these are best handled by actuarial prediction.

THE BASICS OF CRITICAL DECISION MAKING: PATTERN RECOGNITION AND DECISION MAKING

Clinical decision making begins at the point of first contact with the patient, when we initiate our pattern-detection process. During the first contact, the clinician has to make multiple decisions that involve comparisons with internal schema. The clinician rapidly matches internal templates when considering decisions such as who should attend the initial session (patient, couple, family, significant others), proposed duration of the session, how much should be discussed on the phone, and many other issues that immediately must be contemplated and decided on. Science in large part is about finding patterns in nature. One way we make clinical decisions is to draw from the depth and range of information and clinical experience we have amassed and compare external reality with internal patterns that we have constructed.

Specifically, clinicians utilize *prototypes* as a form of template to help compare cases and organize decision making. Essentially, we use these heuristics to make predictions. When we make a diagnostic formulation, we do so in part to predict the course of a disorder, the client's response to treatment, and therapeutic strategies that optimize outcome. Each strategy we employ in treatment is based on an implicit or explicit decision to achieve a therapeutic goal. For example, the regulation of anxiety is a central aspect of the treatment process (Faust, 2007). We are continually matching patterns derived from past experience with our current ones, and thereby comparing and evolving our mental maps. If anxiety is too high, a patient may be flooded, whereas if it is too low, there may be little motivation to change and treatment may stagnate. This process of anxiety management often occurs with the fast processing of System 1, but anxiety regulation should be based on extensive knowledge and drawn from clinical experience. Groopman (2007) described this as occurring "within seconds, largely without any conscious analysis; it draws most heavily on the doctor's visual appraisal of the patient" (pp. 34–35). This is not a "linear, step-by-step combining of cues" but the mind acting like a magnet, assimilating data from many domains of the patient (pp. 34–35).

Intuition is fundamentally a complex pattern-recognition process whereby we use cues from a situation that we match to these internalized patterns or schemas (Roberto, 2009). In using intuition, we must guard against our tendency to find nonexistent patterns in the world and thus impose them on everything. Our propensity to perceive order in disorder and sense in nonsense is basically adaptive because it is an attempt to reduce the chaos and randomness of the world (Stanovich, 2010, p. 81). At the same time, we may falsely assume a pattern in events that are random. This sometimes leads to false positives, in which we perceive a pattern (e.g., a connection between certain ineffective intervention techniques and outcomes in our clinical practice) that does not exist. Prototypes, although an essential element of clinical decision making, can also lead to errors in thinking. We may ignore or selectively reinterpret information that does not fit our prototype and thereby increase the probability of clinical errors.

TYPES OF ERRORS THAT INFLUENCE DECISION MAKING

Heuristics are essentially rules of thumb or shortcuts in thinking that allow us to reduce the complexity in our world and reduce the effort of constantly attending to and responding to every detail in our environment (Groopman, 2007, p. 35). They can be useful but are notoriously error prone. In their classic work, Tversky and Kahneman (1973) explored the topic of heuristics, which enable us to respond rapidly to uncertainty but also have associated dangers. Developing our awareness of the dangers will serve as an important check and balance to System 1 thinking. Familiarizing ourselves with the most common types of cognitive biases optimizes our decision making by helping us avoid common errors. The following sections offer a basic overview of many of these heuristics and their associated biases (we refer the reader to the references provided to attain a deeper appreciation).

Anchoring Bias

Anchoring bias refers to a tendency to allow an initial reference point to unduly influence or distort our estimates. Anchoring is often based on an arbitrary reference point (Ariely, 2010). This anchoring phenomenon is prevalent in economics and can lead to arbitrary coherence, whereby arbitrary anchor points can nevertheless influence our future decisions. Ariely's (2010) research in behavioral economics showed "that our first decisions resonate over a long sequence of decisions" (p. 38). In this way, random anchoring effects may have sway on the way we make future decisions.

This effect can exert a strong influence on our clinical conceptualization and interfere with proper decision analysis. This bias is often present when someone presents a patient or a case and uses a powerful anchoring label, such as *borderline* or *narcissistic*. Receiving a new referral from a colleague along with his or her case formulation may result in falling into a trap whereby we fail to perform our own systematic investigation of the case. When a diagnosis is communicated before we form our own opinion, it is too easy to heavily weight one piece of evidence such as "the patient engages in parasuicidal behavior" when she merely scratched her arm lightly with a pin.

Attributional Bias

Attributional bias refers to people's tendency to minimize their errors and maximize the errors of others (Heider, 1958). Gottman (1999) reported on this phenomenon in couples, in which negative traits in a partner are frequently exaggerated. When working with a team of other providers, we may inaccurately assess our contribution as a positive component of the treatment process and that of other providers as a lesser and/or more negative component.

Availability

Availability is a heuristic whereby we estimate the likelihood of an event or phenomenon using the ease with which relevant examples are recalled (Tversky & Kahneman, 1973). A clinician who has recently seen a number of patients with posttraumatic stress disorder (PTSD) might diagnose a troubled patient with PTSD even in the absence of an identified traumatic event. He or she may further miss the fact that the patient suffers from hyperthyroidism, given that this medical condition is often not readily accessible in memory (Schildkrout, 2011). Availability, if misused, can lead to distorted pattern recognition (Groopman, 2007). We generally have easy access to memories of occurrences that are especially vivid, rare, and emotionally activating (Nisbett & Ross, 1980). For example, many clinicians have formed a schema for multiple personality disorder (now termed *dissociative identity disorder*) based on the sensational and now largely discredited (see Nathan, 2011) case of Sybil (Schreiber, 1973). Cases such as Sybil's can adversely affect the judgment of clinicians by heightening the ease of recall, resulting in biased judgments (Ruscio, 2007).

Confirmation Bias

In *confirmation bias*, we look for information that supports our beliefs and affirms our perspective while neglecting or selectively reinterpreting evidence that contradicts this perspective. In a sense, this tendency reduces cognitive dissonance (Festinger, 1957; Tavris & Aronson, 2007). An example of this type of bias is implicit in a report that I have heard many times from patients in alcohol treatment. Patients are asked whether they are alcoholic, and if they say no, the clinician may inform them that this "denial" confirms the diagnosis. Such "confirmation bias" is probably a variant of the anchoring bias we discussed earlier because it leads us to be overly influenced by initial information. We tend to avoid integrating information that challenges our beliefs and also cherry-pick features that fit our prototype (Groopman, 2007, p. 65). Selectively gathering data that support our initial views and interpreting data in a manner that confirms our beliefs tends to reduce the accuracy of our decision making.

Magnavita and Anchin (2014) gave an example of a troubling trend in psychotherapy. In certain cases, a psychotherapist who held a belief that most women had endured sexual abuse would frequently ask leading questions when a particular constellation of symptoms was present, with the assumption that these symptoms were the result of childhood sexual trauma. If a patient responded by saying that she had not experienced sexual abuse, the clinician would often take this as a sign of repression, which he or she felt provided strong corroborating evidence for the assumption of abuse. Confirmation bias may also explain my friend's thinking about smoking and drinking, discussed in this chapter's opening paragraph. Hertz (2013) wrote,

> Smokers often persist with smoking despite the overwhelming evidence that it's bad for them. If their unconscious belief is that they won't get cancer, for every warning from an antismoking campaigner, their brain is giving a lot more weight to that story of the 99-year-old lady who smokes 50 cigarettes a day but is still going strong. (p. SR6)

Clinicians are often subject to confirmation bias when they have strong allegiance to a particular approach to psychotherapy. One can observe this phenomenon at psychotherapy conferences in which presenters show videotapes of patients' treatment, most of which depict impressive results. However, it is well known that many of these psychotherapists have also experienced many treatment failures, which are very rarely shown. This bias is not limited to clinicians; researchers are more likely to publish and advertise their positive findings than their negative findings (Rosenthal, 1979).

Gambler's Fallacy

Gambler's fallacy refers to our tendency to see a link between past and present events when in fact they are independent (Stanovich, 2010). For example, if you flip a coin once and get heads, the chance that you will flip the coin and get tails is independent of the first flip because the probability of outcome remains the same. In other words, random events don't have memories. "Two outcomes are independent when the occurrence of one does not affect the probability of the other" (Stanovich, 2010, p. 79). Much to the delight of casino owners, those who play games of chance are often taken in by the faulty assumption that the probability of a number coming up at a particular time is based on the previous occurrence. As Stanovich (2010) observed,

> Psychologists, physicians, and marriage counselors often see couples who, after having two female children, are planning a third child because, "We want a boy, and it's bound to be a boy this time." This of course, is the gambler's fallacy. The probability of having a boy (approximately 50%) is exactly the same after having two girls as it was in the beginning (roughly 50%). The two previous girls make it no more likely that the third baby will be a boy. (p. 80)

Clinicians often inaccurately perceive patterns in random events and are likely to develop narratives to explain the occurrence of these events, a tendency that should be vigilantly guarded against. It is often very tempting to forget that even though two events are occurring together on a regular basis, this does not imply causality. Other unknown factors may be at play.

Endowment Effect

People have a tendency to be biased toward the status quo, a phenomenon termed the *endowment effect* (Stanovich, 2010). "Endowment effects result from loss aversion and are a special case of even more generic status quo biases, where the disadvantages of giving up a situation are valued more highly than the advantages of an alternative situation" (Stanovich, 2010, p. 37). Clinical science has been notorious for reifying orthodoxy that often emerges from the beliefs and practices of charismatic psychotherapists. Psychoanalysis, among many other paradigms, has long been criticized for its orthodoxy (Masson, 1984, 1990). An example in psychotherapy of the endowment effect is that for almost a century the length of a session was based on the 50-minute psychoanalytic hour. Interestingly, the authors of this chapter are aware of no research support for this treatment frame. Not only have psychotherapists continued this tradition without much critical scrutiny, but it also became the unit of time (plus or minus 5 minutes) preferred by insurance companies. Of course, a few psychotherapists have experimented with adjusting the length of a session, but most clinicians rely on the status quo without consideration of alternatives.

Egocentrism

We have a propensity to attribute credit to ourselves for an outcome that is perceived as deserving less credit than we would receive from an outside party. Clinicians fall into the trap when they believe that a particular intervention produces a positive result, which may be better explained by extraneous factors such as passage of time or extratherapeutic experiences. One empirical investigation revealed that 25% of clinicians rated themselves in the top 10%, and none viewed themselves as below average (Walfish, McAlister, O'Donnell, & Lambert, 2012). We psychotherapists can potentially ward off falling into this thinking bias, clinically referred to as *narcissism*, which results when egocentrism is excessive, if we keep in mind that we are notorious for overestimating our effectiveness.

Failure to Attempt to Falsify Hypotheses

Consistent with the literature on confirmation bias that we have already reviewed, more than 4 decades of research have demonstrated that we tend not to acknowledge data that falsify our focal hypotheses (Stanovich, 2010). We have difficulty assessing information that points to alternative hypotheses. Stanovich (2010) wrote,

> Thus, the bad news is that people have a difficult time thinking about the evidence that would falsify their focal hypothesis. The good news is that this thinking skill is teachable. All scientists go through training that includes much practice at trying to falsify their focal hypothesis, and they automatize the verbal query "What alternative hypothesis should I consider?" (p. 90)

This bias in thinking may explain why practitioners often strongly advocate and employ a specific approach to treatment, even if this treatment is not compellingly supported by research.

Fixed Frames

We rely on mental models or metaphors to map our world. In her book *Of Two Minds: An Anthropologist Looks at American Psychiatry*, Luhrmann (2000) explored the gulf between psychological and biological psychiatry. Each of these perspectives represents a powerful frame that drives case conceptualization and treatment decisions. The preferred frame of the psychiatrist selected would heavily influence the outcome of a patient who consulted that psychiatrist. One patient would leave with a prescription for medication and the other five-times-a-week psychoanalysis. Most clinicians are aware of the power of reframing, such as describing phenomena in a more positive or negative way. The manner in which we frame an event may affect the outcome. As F. Scott Fitzgerald (1936/1993) wrote, "The test of a first-rate intelligence is the ability to hold two opposite ideas in mind at the same time and still retain the ability to function" (p. 69).

Often the clinical process requires a holding of dialectic polarities. Physicians as well as psychologists frame cases all the time and are susceptible to the influence of this bias (Groopman, 2007). We often receive referrals using this shorthand way of communicating: A referring clinician might say that he or she is referring a patient with a borderline personality disorder, attention-deficit/hyperactivity disorder, or posttraumatic stress disorder to another clinician. The clinician looks through the lens of his or her own expertise and, on this basis or his or her experience, communicates that a given patient is alcoholic. This bias may limit our desire to look at the patient and his or her presentation through a different lens. In Chapter 3 in this volume, Anchin and Singer examine the importance of theory in decision making. Our theory of the world, of change, and of psychotherapy has tremendous influence on our decision making.

Mental health clinicians, even those who are extensively medically trained, can succumb to a number of errors in thinking arising from framing. For example, mental health clinicians are generally biased to see symptoms through a psychological frame. But consider that Graves' disease, a variant of hyperthyroidism, may cause anxiety and depression and may be related to Parkinson's disease as well as many other physical conditions (Schildkrout, 2011). Being overly attached to a frame may not allow us to consider alternatives. The manner in which we frame a problem is rooted in part in our attitudes and beliefs. Patients viewed as having a biologically as opposed to psychologically based disorder are more likely to be treated psychopharmacologically (Ahn, Proctor, & Flanagan, 2009). This reflexive decision may have serious consequences for unified treatment because it may lead to an artificial division between mind and brain, which are merely different levels of analysis of the same phenomenon. The attitudes and beliefs we hold must be thoughtfully examined and considered. For example, data show that when a clinician perceives that a mental disorder has a biological basis as opposed to a psychological one, there is likely to be less stigma attributed to the patient with the perceived biologically based mental disorder (Ahn et al., 2009). If persons with behavioral or mental disorders are held accountable for their disturbances, they are more likely to be referred to psychotherapy than medication. It is also interesting that emotions lead to differential appraisals of violence—fear increases pessimism, and anger optimism (Lerner, Gonzalez, Small, & Fischhoff, 2003).

Hindsight Bias

Hindsight bias is well known to sports fans as "Monday-morning quarterbacking." More formally, hindsight bias leads us to believe that we could have successfully predicted an outcome even when we would not have been able to do so. When looking back, we tend to erroneously judge events as being more predictable than they were. This error can result in overconfidence. For example, a practitioner might persuade himself after a client attempts suicide that he "saw it coming" or "knew it all along." As a consequence, he may overestimate his capacity to successfully forecast suicide attempts, which could be dangerous to his clients.

Ignoring Alternative Hypotheses

Stanovich (2010) described a famous psychology study that exemplifies the problems that can emerge when we ignore alternative hypotheses. The *Barnum effect*, a term coined by psychologist Paul Meehl, is based on the famous circus entrepreneur P. T. Barnum's observation that "there's a sucker born every minute." In an introductory psychology class demonstration (conducted on many occasions by this chapter's second author), the students are given an individualized report of their personality with highly generalized statements such as "At times you are extraverted, affable, and sociable, but at other times you are wary and reserved" based (for example) on a graphological analysis of their handwriting. The students then rate the accuracy of the description on a scale of 1 to 10. More than 50 years of studies have yielded average ratings from 7 to 9. Following the ratings, students are instructed to compare their descriptions with those of their classmates and to discover, much to their chagrin, that the descriptions are all identical (see Furnham & Schofield, 1987, for a review).

It is easy to be misled in this regard as a clinician and important to be cognizant of these influences. For example, most clinicians have to use extensive resources to attain training in various approaches to treatment; this process can be daunting. Deciding whether to seek advanced training in the variety of approaches can be overwhelming because the claims made by the progenitors of the interventions tend to be seductively appealing. We may attend a seminar in which a prominent therapist presents videotape demonstrating what appears to be a genuine transformation in the patient. This may lead to entering a costly training program to advance one's expertise, even though there may be limited evidence to support such an approach. Many of the biases that we have reviewed may come into play and enhance a clinician's allegiance to a particular approach to psychotherapy in which much investment has been made and beliefs become self-perpetuating.

Illusory Correlation

We often assume statistical associations between statistically unrelated variables, especially when these associations are intuitively plausible (Chapman & Chapman, 1967). For example, we might falsely assume a correlation between highly conflictual parental subsystems and the likelihood of certain psychological symptoms in children. Recent evidence, however, has failed to document a consistent link between levels of marital adjustment and behavior problems in children (Hindman, Riggs, & Hook, 2013).

Inverting Conditional Probabilities

Another form of faulty decision making results from our tendency to invert probabilities. As Stanovich (2010) stated,

> It has been found that both patients and medical practitioners can sometimes invert probabilities, thinking mistakenly, that the probability of disease, given a particular symptom is the same as the probability of the symptom, given the disease (as a patient you are concerned with the former). (p. 75)

For example, an inexperienced clinician may erroneously believe that a client with an elevated Scale 2 (Depression) on the Minnesota Multiphasic Personality Inventory—2 (MMPI–2) is likely to meet criteria for major depression. In fact, although many or most patients in the throes of major depression exhibit elevated MMPI–2 Scale 2 scores, the substantial majority of patients with elevated Scale 2 scores are not clinically depressed.

Narrative Fallacy

We humans are marked by a tendency to weave together facts and observations into what seems to be a coherent narrative, even when the facts are not meaningfully related. Storytelling is a powerful device that can make events appear more plausible by adding details (Tversky & Kahneman, 1983). We may become seduced by a story if it appears to explain seemingly unconnected details; in turn, we may not sufficiently explore rival explanations. We may have many useful narratives that can be explanatory. In fact, the ultimate narrative that we use is theory, which is discussed in Chapter 3 in this volume.

Overconfidence Bias

It is well known that most professionals (e.g., physicians, psychotherapists, economists, lawyers) tend to overestimate their knowledge and ability, especially with respect to difficult tasks. Research shows that clinicians also tend to be overly confident about the accuracy of their decision making and expertise, although researchers are by no means immune to this tendency either. Overconfidence among clinicians has been substantiated by Lambert's (2010) research, which demonstrated that clinicians frequently underestimate the proportion of negative outcomes among clients in their caseloads. Following other authors, Lambert described this phenomenon as the *Lake Woebegone effect*, from Garrison Keillor's fictional town described on his program *A Prairie Home Companion*, in which all the children are above average. Again, the results from Walfish et al. (2012) are revealing in that when a group of therapists was asked to rate their skill level, 25% assessed themselves at the 90% level compared with their peers; none rated himself as below average. Attending to patient feedback is critical to reducing overconfidence. Even if we believe that psychotherapy is progressing well, we need to consider that our patients' perceptions might be different.

Recall Bias

Memory is not always a sound source of reliable information. Wheelan (2013), the best-selling author of *Naked Statistics: Stripping the Dread From the Data*, wrote,

> We have a natural human impulse to understand the present as a logical consequence of things that happened in the past—cause and effect. The problem is that our memories turn out to be "systematically fragile" when we are trying to explain some particularly good or bad outcome in the present. (p. 122)

For example, psychoanalysis has been widely criticized for its tendency to look to the past for causal explanations of current disorders. Part of the challenge here is that patients in treatment may erroneously "recall" events that seem to confirm the psychoanalyst's hypotheses, thereby reinforcing potentially mistaken lines of inquiry.

Recency Effect

We tend to place too much emphasis on evidence that we have recently encountered. This *recency effect* results from an overuse of the availability heuristic. For example, if our psychotherapy client has been distressed but largely emotionally stable over the course of the past few months, yet was angry and affectively labile in her most recent session, we may overestimate the likelihood that she has borderline personality disorder.

Representative Heuristic

This mental shortcut operates by the rule of "like goes with like" (Tversky & Kahneman, 1974). There are "virtues" to judging information on the basis of our impressions. In many cases, reliance on stereotypes (e.g., the extent to which a client reminds us of our prototype of the modal patient with schizophrenia) is more accurate than sheer guessing (Kahneman, 2011, p. 151). Nevertheless, this tendency can lead to errors in the clinical context. We may assume that a client with bipolar disorder who reminds us of a previous client with borderline personality disorder has the latter condition; as a consequence, the client may receive inappropriate or inadequate treatment. However, it is tempting to predict unlikely events even when the base rates are low. This error can lead to the phenomenon of *base rate neglect*, a corollary of the overuse of the representativeness heuristic. For example, if a client who acts differently on different occasions reminds us of our prototype of dissociative identity disorder, we may jump too readily to assign this diagnosis, forgetting that the prevalence of this condition in the general population is probably extremely low.

Sunk-Cost Effect

We tend to escalate our commitment to a course of action in which we have made a substantial prior investment of resources. Instead of considering another approach or modality of treatment when the patient is not progressing adequately, we might suggest that he or she continue with the same approach but come more frequently. The therapeutic process can be susceptible to this form of escalating commitment. For example, trainees in various approaches to psychotherapy often persist and escalate their effort using a favored method of psychotherapy, such as cognitive, affective, or defense restructuring (Magnavita, 2005). They believe in the efficacy of their interventions and have put a lot of effort into learning them. Unfortunately, following a course of action without attention to patient feedback often results in poor outcome or premature termination. In some cases, patients have walked out of sessions when the therapist relentlessly persists with a particular method.

Selection Bias

Where and from whom we gather our data influences our analyses. Most psychologists have been trained to recognize the inherent problems when samples are not obtained by random selection. This bias can be introduced in many ways. For example,

> A survey of consumers in an airport is going to be biased by the fact that people who fly are likely to be wealthier than the general public; a survey

at a rest stop on Interstate 90 may have the opposite problem. (Wheelan, 2013, p. 118)

Clinicians in forensic (prison) settings, for example, must remain cognizant of the fact that their clients have higher rates of childhood physical abuse than do individuals in the general population. If they do not, they may overestimate the extent to which physical abuse causes criminal behavior in the general population.

Survivorship Bias

Another factor that can bias our thinking is the fact that in datasets from clinical and research settings, dropout rates are often high. Those who remain in treatment may not be representative of the population. Wheelan (2013) wrote, "If you have a room of people with varying heights, forcing the short people to leave will raise the average height in the room, but it doesn't make anyone taller" (p. 123). In psychotherapy, the clients who remain in treatment are typically those who are benefiting from it. If we do not take survivorship bias into account, we may overestimate our effectiveness as therapists.

Publication Bias

There is general agreement that there is a crisis in science, including psychological science. A recent edition of *The Economist* examined "How Science Goes Wrong" (2013) in a front-page article. One major source of concern is publication bias (Rosenthal, 1979), which seems to be rampant in a number of disciplines. In psychiatry, especially in the subfield of psychopharmacology, the results of studies in many instances have been biased by the pharmaceutical industry, which has often overstated the efficacy of certain medications for psychological disorders (Whitaker, 2010). Publication bias assumes various forms; the most common is a tendency for journals to publish only research that shows novel findings, positive findings, or both. The pharmaceutical industry has been accused of publishing research that supports the efficacy of their products and squelching findings that are less flattering. This tendency can exert a negative downstream effect. For example, when meta-analytic studies eventually challenged many of the accepted findings regarding the efficacy of selective serotonin reuptake inhibitors, the results were very different when unpublished negative results were included (see Chapter 5 in this volume). Researchers are under so much pressure to produce groundbreaking results that few are interested in replicating studies that have yielded significant effects, which results in a lack of replication of many key findings (Pashler & Wagenmakers, 2012). Unfortunately, psychology is not immune from similar problems with careerism and publication bias (Kagan, 2012).

ENHANCING CLINICAL DECISION MAKING

All clinical practice involves explicit and implicit prediction (Faust, 2007, p. 51). Much of what is decided in clinical practice cannot be derived directly from research evidence. However, Kahneman (2011) observed that when we have doubts about the veracity of evidence, we must not let judgment stray too far from the base rates. He cautioned, "Don't expect this exercise of discipline to be easy—it requires a significant effort in self-monitoring and self-control" (p. 153).

Balancing the two primary systems of thinking is essential to effective clinical decision making, as Gladwell (2005) wrote: "Truly successful decision making relies on a balance between deliberate and instinctive thinking" (p. 141). We should write down and compare what is known with what is unknown (Roberto, 2009, p. 87). It is important to keep in mind epistemology, or the nature of knowledge, given that we have a limited understanding of the mind and how it goes wrong. As a consequence, we should continually be striving to combat confirmation bias and allied biases by questioning the veracity of everything we consider to be true. In the final section of this chapter we conclude by presenting some of the safeguards that can be used to avoid cognitive traps and enhance our clinical decisions.

Tracey et al. (2014) summarized some important ways to enhance clinical decision making:

> (a) adopting a Bayesian approach by looking at base rates, (b) obtaining quality information (e.g., relying on valid measures rather than impressions), (c) relying less on memory, (d) recognizing personal biases and their effects, (e) being aware of regression to the mean where less extreme behavior follows extreme behavior, and (f) adopting a disconfirming, scientific approach to practice. (p. 224)

In the following, we elaborate on the first two of these recommendations, followed by an additional recommendation: tolerating uncertainty.

Adopting a Bayesian Approach

Probabilistic thinking offers rules to follow, which provide a basis for decision making (Stanovich, 2010). "Decision-making is a very complex endeavor, something that we engage in all the time, some decisions more high stakes than others, but oftentimes decision-making can perplex us"

(Roberto, 2009, p. 9). Intuition can lead us astray by drawing from outdated patterns or challenging our relied-on rules of thumb. Bayesian analysis uses a mathematical approach to making decisions based on the numerical probability of various potential outcomes. A basic understanding and incorporation of Bayesian reasoning is crucial to accurate decision making. Bayes's rule states that the "diagnosticity of evidence must be weighted by the base rate" (Stanovich, 2010, p. 59). *Diagnosticity* refers to the validity of the information, which in studies of psychiatric diagnosis is obtained by drawing on conditional probabilities (true positive rate, false positive rate, true negative rate, false negative rate). Stanovich (2010) wrote that

> when the case evidence gives the illusion of concreteness—people combine information in the wrong way. The right way is to use Bayes' rule, or, more specifically, insight from Bayes' rule. . . . It is enough that people learn to "think Bayesian" in a qualitative sense—that they have what might be called "Bayesian instincts," not that they have necessarily memorized the rule. (p. 59)

For example, if a test is known to have a high percentage of false positive results, and is applied to a group with a low base rate, there is a low likelihood that the test will overdiagnose psychopathology in that sample. Stanovich (2010) wrote that if nothing else is understood about Bayesian reasoning, the acknowledgement of base rates is all that is essential but "of course, greater depth of understanding would be an additional plus" (p. 59). He believes that this type of "qualitative understanding" affords us the opportunity to make "guesstimates," which are approximate and close enough to prevent serious errors in practice (p. 59). The importance of a Bayesian approach to decision making is to remind us not to ignore the statistical influence of base rates when calculating probabilistic decisions.

Mining Quality Information

The access to information that is available with the Internet and search engines is fundamentally changing human social memories and transcending some of the limitations of human cognition (Wegner & Ward, 2013). Most clinicians now have access to high-quality information that has never been so readily available and can be easily used to enhance decision making by using Boolean operators—search commands—to access relevant databases (Norcross et al., 2008). In Chapter 5 in this volume, Hollon discusses the steps involved in generating structured questions in the development of clinical practice guidelines. These are called PICOTS, a mnemonic that stands for populations, interventions, comparisons, outcomes, time, and settings.

Clinical science has advanced to the stage at which we now have a number of treatment approaches that have been substantiated as effective for a range of mental and behavioral disturbances. As Karlin and Cross (2014) noted,

> Over the past 30 years, psychotherapeutic interventions have been developed and empirically validated for a wide range of psychological conditions, including conditions that not too long ago were considered untreatable, such as posttraumatic stress disorder. (p. 19)

However, a serious problem with dissemination remains. The science-to-practice lag time for evidence-based practices is, in fact, longer (and in many cases, far longer) than the typical lengthy lag time of 15 to 20 years identified for medical interventions by the Institute of Medicine (2001) in its seminal report *Crossing the Quality Chasm: A New Health System for the 21st Century* (pp. 20–21).

Where possible, rely on established empirically based algorithms. As computer technology and the capacity to effectively mine big data advances, there will be an increasing trend to rely on algorithms. It is well documented that even experts are typically inferior to algorithms, so the hostility that many hold needs to be addressed through education. Kahneman (2011), summarizing the work of Paul Meehl, noted that some clinicians have a natural antipathy to algorithmic thinking because it goes against many of the beliefs that clinicians hold dear. "The research suggests a surprising conclusion: to maximize predictive accuracy, final decisions should be left for formulas, especially in low-validity environments" (p. 225). An example of a classic algorithm developed by the pediatrician Virginia Apgar in 1953 is still used today to assess newborns' health using a rating of five variables (heart rate, respiration, reflex, muscle tone, and color). This simple rating is credited for significantly reducing infant mortality (Kahneman, 2011). A very pragmatic algorithm identified by John Gottman (1999), called the Four Horsemen of the Apocalypse, is highly predictive of the demise of a marital relationship. The "four horsemen" are partners' criticism, defensiveness, contempt, and stonewalling. When these warning signs are observed in a couple, on average they divorce following 5.6 years, much sooner than other couples. Clinical algorithms such as Gottman's are easy to use and helpful, not only as predictive tools but as educational tools for clients in treatment.

Tolerating Uncertainty: Assuming a Reflective Stance

As we have discussed, uncertainty in the face of complexity is an unavoidable part of clinical practice. We encounter three types of uncertainty in clinical practice. The first concerns not having mastered the material necessary to guide our decision making—continuous learning is essential as the field of clinical science is rapidly advancing. The second concerns acknowledging the limitations of the evidence base on which we rely to inform our decision making. In terms of the exponential number of variables and their interrelationships, it is highly unlikely that the field will ever have perfect knowledge or anything close to it. Therefore, many clinical questions will remain murky because of lack of information—we must be able to effectively function in situations of less than perfect knowledge. In fact, clinical advances often emerge from these states of unknowing. The third type of uncertainty concerns a combination of the first two, whereby clinicians cannot distinguish between their lack of mastery or ineptitude and limitations of their knowledge (Groopman, 2007, p. 152). Groopman (2007) argued that a tendency for many practitioners to deny uncertainty often leads to a closed mind and suboptimal decision making.

There are many aspects of decision-making theory and research that we can incorporate into our clinical processes with the goal of increasing mindfulness and thereby honing our clinical decision-making skills. Assuming a "mindful" stance when making decisions and acknowledging our feelings can be like an "emotional thermostat" recalibrating our decision analysis (Hertz, 2013, p. SR6). Kahneman (2011) suggested that "continuous vigilance" when making all decisions is not practical and that "the best we can do is a compromise: learn to recognize situations in which mistakes are likely and try harder to avoid significant mistakes when the stakes are high" (p. 28). The more aware we are of our cognitive biases, including those discussed in this chapter and this volume, the greater chance we have of guarding against these cognitive and perceptual traps. Actively identifying the biases present in our work enhances the value of our expertise by balancing System 1 and System 2 processes inherent in most decision making. It is important to keep in mind that "conscious doubt is not in the repertoire of System 1; it requires maintaining incompatible interpretations in mine at the same time, which demands mental effort. Uncertainty and doubt are the domain of System 2" (Kahneman, 2011, p. 80).

There may be a partial antidote, however. Kahneman (2011) wrote, "To derive the most useful information from multiple sources of evidence, you should always try to make these sources independent of each other" (p. 84). Hence, we should remember to try to minimize redundancy from information sources. In some cases crowds make better decisions than individuals, especially when the crowds consist of independent opinions (Surowiecki, 2004). This may be an important and unexamined way to shed light on what the public finds useful. As the general public's level of sophistication concerning behavioral and mental health treatments rises, new patients increasingly request certain types of treatment. This may be similar to the trend that physicians have witnessed with the rise of direct-to-consumer advertising by the pharmaceutical industry, which has resulted in more patients requesting specific drugs. The industry's heavy advertising, often promising a quick fix to their distress, may have influenced them.

SUMMARY

In the absence of perfect information, compounded by the complexity of human nature, which to a large degree is unpredictable, uncertainty is an inherent element of clinical practice. Such uncertainty must be addressed using a pragmatic approach to decision making. Clinical expertise requires an understanding of decision analytics to guard against common decision-making traps. Effectiveness in behavioral and mental health practice requires not only an extensive knowledge base and experience but also the ability to understand the ways in which our fast and slow approaches to processing information influence our decision making. Decision making, which often relies unduly on intuition, can be influenced by a host of documented cognitive biases with which clinicians should be conversant. It is imperative that we seek to minimize bias in clinical practice by increasing awareness of decision analytics, providing training in decision making for all clinicians regardless of their experience, and developing decision aids such as clinical practice guidelines. We are duty-bound to ensure the best care by reducing biases, which are inherent in human thinking.

We can distill several crucial pieces of advice from the literature on clinical decision making. In aggregate, these principles can enhance clinical outcomes. These include the following:

1. Familiarize yourself with the field of decision analytics and use it to enhance your awareness of decision-making traps.
2. When making clinical decisions, be sure to "conceptualize problems in multiple ways" (Ruscio, 2007, p. 44).
3. Always consider using existing algorithms when making clinical decisions by referring to the extant literature. Moreover, as clinical practice guidelines become the state of the science, refer to them frequently to keep current.
4. "Recognize that personal experience is anecdotal evidence" (Ruscio, 2007, p. 4) and, as substantial research has shown, that anecdotal evidence is not sufficient to ensure optimal decision making. As a wise person once said, the plural of anecdote is not data. Anecdotes can be enormously helpful for generating hypotheses in treatment, but they are rarely useful for testing or corroborating them.

5. Always rely on principles of probability for complex decision analytics. Keep in mind that clinical judgment must be based on a solid evidence base.
6. When there are cases that do not fit the statistical trends, proceed with caution and keep in mind the cognitive traps to which one may easily resort.
7. In your practice, refer to the extant literature on a regular basis. This is becoming much easier with the development of information technology, clinical practice guidelines, and systems that make patient feedback much easier to incorporate.
8. Develop formats that provide feedback about one's work, such as videotape review of sessions, a consultation group, incorporating patient feedback systems, and using metrics to monitor outcome.
9. Carefully examine and be aware of attitudes and beliefs that influence your conceptualization of the mind, treatment, and human change processes.

The remaining chapters in this volume explore many facets of decision making relevant to clinical practice. We hope you find these illuminating and useful to your daily work.

REFERENCES

Ackoff, R. L. (1967). Management information systems. *Management Sciences, 14,* 147–156.

Ahn, W. K., Proctor, C. C., & Flanagan, E. H. (2009). Mental health clinicians' beliefs about the biological, psychological, and environmental bases of mental disorders. *Cognitive Science, 33,* 147–182. http://dx.doi.org/10.1111/j.1551-6709.2009.01008.x

Ambady, N., & Rosenthal, R. (1992). Thin slicing of expressive behavior as predictors of interpersonal consequences: A meta-analysis. *Psychological Bulletin, 111,* 256–274. http://dx.doi.org/10.1037/0033-2909.111.2.256

APA Presidential Task Force on Evidence-Based Practice. (2006). Evidence-based practice in psychology. *American Psychologist, 61,* 271–285.

Ariely, D. (2010). *Predictably irrational: The hidden forces that shape our decisions* (Rev. ed.). New York, NY: Harper Perennial.

Berns, G. (2008). *Iconoclast: A neuroscientist reveals how to think differently.* Boston, MA: Harvard Business Press.

Beutler, L. E. (1997). The psychotherapist as a neglected variable in psychotherapy: An illustration by reference to the role of therapist experience and training. *Clinical Psychology: Science and Practice, 4,* 44–52. http://dx.doi.org/10.1111/j.1468-2850.1997.tb00098.x

Carrère, S., & Gottman, J. M. (1999). Predicting divorce among newlyweds from the first three minutes of a marital conflict discussion. *Family Process, 38,* 293–301. http://dx.doi.org/10.1111/j.1545-5300.1999.00293.x

Chapman, L. J., & Chapman, J. P. (1967). Genesis of popular but erroneous psychodiagnostic observations. *Journal of Abnormal Psychology, 72,* 193–204. http://dx.doi.org/10.1037/h0024670

Claxton, K., Cohen, J. T., & Neumann, P. J. (2005). When is evidence sufficient? *Health Affairs, 24*(1), 93–101. http://dx.doi.org/10.1377/hlthaff.24.1.93

Csikszentmihalyi, M. (1990). *The psychology of optimal experience.* New York, NY: Harper Row.

Epstein, S. (1994). Integration of the cognitive and the psychodynamic unconscious. *American Psychologist, 49,* 709–724. http://dx.doi.org/10.1037/0003-066X.49.8.709

Faust, D. (2007). Decision research can increase the accuracy of clinical judgment and thereby improve patient care. In S. O. Lilienfeld & W. T. O'Donohue (Eds.), *The great ideas of clinical science: 17 principles that every mental health professional should understand* (pp. 49–76). New York, NY: Routledge.

Festinger, L. (1957). *A theory of cognitive dissonance.* Palo Alto, CA: Stanford University Press.

Fiske, S. T., & Taylor, S. E. (1991). *Social cognition* (2nd ed.). New York, NY: McGraw Hill.

Fitzgerald, F. S. (1993). *The crack-up.* New York, NY: New Directions. (Original work published 1936)

Furnham, A., & Schofield, S. (1987). Accepting personality test feedback: A review of the Barnum effect. *Current Psychological Research & Reviews, 6,* 162–178. http://dx.doi.org/10.1007/BF02686623

Gawande, A. (1998, February 8). No mistake. *The New Yorker,* pp. 74–81.

Gladwell, M. (2005). *Blink: The power of thinking without thinking.* New York, NY: Little, Brown.

Gladwell, M. (2008). *Outliers: The story of success.* New York, NY: Little, Brown.

Gottman, J. M. (1999). *The marriage clinic: A scientifically based marital therapy.* New York, NY: Norton.

Groopman, J. (2007). *How doctors think.* New York, NY: Houghton Mifflin.

Grove, W. M., & Meehl, P. E. (1996). Comparative efficiency of informal (subjective, impressionistic) and formal (mechanical, algorithmic) prediction procedures: The clinical-statistical controversy. *Psychology, Public Policy, and Law, 2,* 293–323. http://dx.doi.org/10.1037/1076-8971.2.2.293

Grove, W. M., Zald, D. H., Lebow, B. S., Snitz, B. E., & Nelson, C. (2000). Clinical versus mechanical prediction: A meta-analysis. *Psychological Assessment, 12*, 19–30. http://dx.doi.org/10.1037/1040-3590.12.1.19

Hassin, R. R., Uleman, J. S., & Bargh, J. A. (Eds.). (2005). *The new unconscious.* New York, NY: Oxford University Press.

Heider, F. (1958). *The psychology of interpersonal relations.* New York, NY: Wiley. http://dx.doi.org/10.1037/10628-000

Hertz, N. (2013, October 20). Why we make bad decisions. *The New York Times,* p. SR6.

Hindman, J. M., Riggs, S. A., & Hook, J. (2013). Contributions of executive, parent–child, and sibling subsystems to children's psychological functioning. *Couple and Family Psychology: Research and Practice, 2,* 294–308. http://dx.doi.org/10.1037/a0034419

Hogue, A., Henderson, C. E., Dauber, S., Barajas, P. C., Fried, A., & Liddle, H. A. (2008). Treatment adherence, competence, and outcome in individual and family therapy for adolescent behavior problems. *Journal of Consulting and Clinical Psychology, 76,* 544–555. http://dx.doi.org/10.1037/0022-006X.76.4.544

How science goes wrong. (2013, October 19). *The Economist.* Retrieved from http://www.economist.com/news/leaders/21588069-scientific-research-has-changed-world-now-it-needs-change-itself-how-science-goes-wrong

Institute of Medicine. (2001). *Crossing the quality chasm: A new health system for the 21st century.* Washington, DC: National Academies Press.

Kagan, J. (2012). *Psychology's ghosts: The crisis in the profession and the way back.* New Haven, CT: Yale University Press.

Kahneman, D. (2011). *Thinking fast and slow.* New York, NY: Farrar, Straus & Giroux.

Kahneman, D., & Klein, G. (2009). Conditions for intuitive expertise: A failure to disagree. *American Psychologist, 64,* 515–526. http://dx.doi.org/10.1037/a0016755

Karlin, B. E., & Cross, G. (2014). From the laboratory to the therapy room: National dissemination and implementation of evidence-based psychotherapies in the U.S. Department of Veterans Affairs Health Care System. *American Psychologist, 69,* 19–33. http://dx.doi.org/10.1037/a0033888

Kendall, P. C., Gosch, E., Furr, J. M., & Sood, E. (2008). Flexibility within fidelity. *Journal of the American Academy of Child & Adolescent Psychiatry, 47,* 987–993. http://dx.doi.org/10.1097/CHI.0b013e31817eed2f

Lambert, M. J. (2010). *Prevention of treatment failure: The use of measuring, monitoring, and feedback in clinical practice.* Washington, DC: American Psychological Association. http://dx.doi.org/10.1037/12141-000

Lehrer, J. (2009). *How we decide.* New York, NY: Houghton Mifflin Harcourt.

Lerner, J. S., Gonzalez, R. M., Small, D. A., & Fischhoff, B. (2003). Effects of fear and anger on perceived risks of terrorism: A national field experiment. *Psychological Science, 14,* 144–150. http://dx.doi.org/10.1111/1467-9280.01433

Lilienfeld, S. O., & O'Donohue, W. T. (Eds.). (2007). *The great ideas of clinical science: 17 principles that every mental health professional should understand.* New York, NY: Routledge.

Lohr, S. (2013, April 21). Big data, trying to build better works. *The New York Times,* p. 4.

Luhrmann, T. M. (2000). *Of two minds: An anthropologist looks at American psychiatry.* New York, NY: Knopf.

Magnavita, J. J. (2005). *Personality-guided therapy: A unified approach.* Washington, DC: American Psychological Association. http://dx.doi.org/10.1037/10959-000

Magnavita, J. J., & Anchin, J. C. (2014). *Unifying psychotherapy: Principles, methods, and evidence from clinical science.* New York, NY: Springer.

Maslow, A. H. (1954). *Motivation and personality.* New York, NY: Harper.

Masson, J. M. (1984). *The assault on truth: Freud's suppression of the seduction theory.* New York, NY: Farrar, Straus & Giroux.

Masson, J. M. (1990). *Final analysis: The making and unmaking of a psychoanalyst.* New York, NY: Addison-Wesley.

McKnight, P., & Sechrest, L. (2003). The use and misuse of the term "experience" in contemporary psychology: A reanalysis of the experience–performance relationship. *Philosophical Psychology, 16,* 431–460. http://dx.doi.org/10.1080/0951508032000121814

Meehl, P. E. (1954). *Clinical versus statistical prediction: A theoretical analysis and review of the literature.* Minneapolis: University of Minnesota Press. http://dx.doi.org/10.1037/11281-000

Miller, S. D., Duncan, B., & Hubble, M. (2008). Supershrinks: What is the secret of their success? *Psychotherapy in Australia, 14*(4), 14–22.

Najavits, L. M., Weiss, R. D., Shaw, S. R., & Dierberger, A. E. (2000). Psychotherapists' views of treatment manuals. *Professional Psychology, Research and Practice, 31,* 404–408. http://dx.doi.org/10.1037/0735-7028.31.4.404

Nathan, D. (2011). *Sybil exposed: The extraordinary story behind the famous multiple personality case.* New York, NY: Free Press.

Nisbett, R. E., & Ross, L. (1980). *Human interference: Strategies and shortcomings of social judgment.* Englewood Cliffs, NJ: Prentice-Hall.

Norcross, J. C., Hogan, T. P., & Koocher, G. P. (2008). *Clinician's guide to evidence-based practices: Mental health and the addictions.* New York, NY: Oxford University Press.

Oddli, H. W., & Halvorsen, M. S. (2014). Experienced psychotherapists' reports of their assessments, predictions, and decision making in the early phase of psychotherapy. *Psychotherapy, 51,* 295–307. http://dx.doi.org/10.1037/a0029843

O'Donohue, W. T., Lilienfeld, S. O., & Fowler, K. A. (2007). Science is an essential safeguard against human error. In S. O. Lilienfeld & W. T. O'Donohue (Eds.), *The great ideas of clinical science: 17 principles that every mental health professional should understand* (pp. 3–27). New York, NY: Routledge.

Okiishi, J., Lambert, M. J., Nielsen, S. L., & Ogles, B. M. (2003). Waiting for supershrink: An empirical analysis of therapist effects. *Clinical Psychology & Psychotherapy, 10,* 361–373. http://dx.doi.org/10.1002/cpp.383

Pashler, H., & Wagenmakers, E. J. (2012). Editors' introduction to the Special Section on Replicability in Psychological Science: A crisis of confidence? *Perspectives on Psychological Science, 7,* 528–530. http://dx.doi.org/10.1177/1745691612465253

Roberto, M. A. (2009). *The art of critical decision making.* Chantilly, VA: The Teaching Company.

Rosenthal, R. (1979). The file drawer problem and tolerance for null results. *Psychological Bulletin, 86,* 638–641. http://dx.doi.org/10.1037/0033-2909.86.3.638

Rowley, J. (2007). The wisdom hierarchy: Representation of the DIKW hierarchy. *Journal of Information Science, 33,* 163–180. http://dx.doi.org/10.1177/0165551506070706

Ruscio, J. (2007). The clinician as subject: Practitioners are prone to the same judgment errors as everyone else. In S. O. Lilienfeld & W. T. O'Donohue (Eds.), *The great ideas of clinical science: 17 principles that every mental health professional should understand* (pp. 29–47). New York, NY: Routledge.

Schildkrout, B. (2011). *Unmasking psychological symptoms: How therapists can learn to recognize the psychological presentation of medical disorders.* Hoboken, NJ: Wiley. http://dx.doi.org/10.1002/9781118083598

Schreiber, F. R. (1973). *Sybil.* Chicago, IL: Henry Regnery.

Shanteau, J. (1992). Competence in experts: The role of task characteristics. *Organizational Behavior and Human Decision Processes, 53,* 252–266. http://dx.doi.org/10.1016/0749-5978(92)90064-E

Stanovich, K. E. (2010). *Decision making and rationality in the modern world.* New York, NY: Oxford University Press.

Stanovich, K. E. (2011). *Rationality and the reflective mind.* New York, NY: Oxford University Press.

Stanovich, K. E., & West, R. F. (2000). Advancing the rationality debate. *Behavioral and Brain Sciences, 23,* 701–717. http://dx.doi.org/10.1017/S0140525X00623439

Surowiecki, J. (2004). *The wisdom of crowds: Why the many are smarter than the few and how collective wisdom shapes business, economics, societies, and nations.* New York, NY: Anchor Books.

Tavris, C., & Aronson, E. (2007). *Mistakes were made (but not by me).* New York, NY: Harcourt.

Tracey, T. J. G., Wampold, B. E., Lichtenberg, J. W., & Goodyear, R. K. (2014). Expertise in psychotherapy: An elusive goal? *American Psychologist, 69,* 218–229. http://dx.doi.org/10.1037/a0035099

Tversky, A., & Kahneman, D. (1973). Availability: A heuristic for judging frequency and probability. *Cognitive Psychology, 5,* 207–232. http://dx.doi.org/10.1016/0010-0285(73)90033-9

Tversky, A., & Kahneman, D. (1974, September). Judgment under uncertainty: Heuristics and biases. *Science, 185,* 1124–1131.

Tversky, A., & Kahneman, D. (1983). Extensional versus intuitive reasoning: Conjunction fallacy in probability judgment. *Psychological Review, 90,* 293–315. http://dx.doi.org/10.1037/0033-295X.90.4.293

van Overwalle, F., & Vandekerckhove, M. (2013). Implicit and explicit social mentalizing: Dual processes driven by a shared neural network. *Frontiers in Human Neuroscience, 7,* 560. http://dx.doi.org/10.3389/fnhum.2013.00560

Walfish, S., McAlister, B., O'Donnell, P., & Lambert, M. J. (2012). An investigation of self-assessment bias in mental health providers. *Psychological Reports, 110,* 639–644. http://dx.doi.org/10.2466/02.07.17.PR0.110.2.639-644

Wegner, D. M., & Ward, A. F. (2013). How Google is changing your brain. *Scientific American, 309*(6), 58–61. http://dx.doi.org/10.1038/scientificamerican1213-58

Wheelan, C. (2013). *Naked statistics: Stripping the dread from the data.* New York, NY: Norton.

Whitaker, R. (2010). *The anatomy of an epidemic: Magic bullets, psychiatric drugs, and the astonishing rise of mental illness in America.* New York, NY: Crown.

Wilson, T. D. (2002). *Strangers to ourselves: Discovering the adaptive unconscious.* Cambridge, MA: Harvard University Press.

Zins, C. (2007). Conceptual approaches for defining data, information, and knowledge. *Journal of the American Society for Information Science and Technology, 58,* 479–493. http://dx.doi.org/10.1002/asi.20508

3

A DUAL PROCESS PERSPECTIVE ON THE VALUE OF THEORY IN PSYCHOTHERAPEUTIC DECISION MAKING

JACK C. ANCHIN AND JEFFERSON A. SINGER

Over the entire course of a patient's psychotherapy, within any given session and across sessions, the practicing clinician is confronted with the highly responsible task of making countless judgments and decisions. For example, during initial assessment and evaluation, what kinds of information about the patient are essential to acquire, in what sequence, and how should this information be gathered? During initial case conceptualization, what formulation best organizes and integrates these data from the standpoint of maximizing understanding of the patient and his or her difficulties? And based on this understanding, what treatment plan is indicated? In this respect, what are appropriate and realistic treatment goals? In pursuing the latter, is brief or longer term therapy most warranted? And what specific treatment strategies, interventions, and techniques should be used to foster attainment of the established goals?

The clinician is also confronted with decisions pertaining to the process of psychotherapy. For example, as treatment unfolds, what ways of relationally responding to and interacting with the patient will best establish, build, and maintain the therapeutic alliance? At any given point when engaging in inquiry, should an open-ended or a closed-ended question be used? How long should silence be maintained before the therapist intercedes with a statement or question? At a particular juncture in treatment, what degree of balance between support and confrontation is most responsive to the patient's current treatment needs and clinical status? And what are the indicators that it is appropriate to begin addressing treatment termination, and what is the best way to implement termination with this specific patient?

Although these and innumerable other questions operate as decision choice points for the psychotherapist, one facet of psychotherapy about which the therapist does not need to make a decision is the overarching purpose of the enterprise: Psychotherapy is an intrinsically goal-directed process intended to help the patient move toward greater mental health and self-understanding in his or her day-to-day functioning and subjective experience. This metagoal frames the entire endeavor, and therefore the practice of psychotherapy presupposes that the therapist's judgments and decisions throughout the treatment process are motivated by this prevailing desire. This motivation is of course crucial, but it is not sufficient. The therapist must also have actual tools that, yoked to this essential motivation to help, facilitate and guide his or her specific decisions in therapeutic directions.

In this chapter we discuss the centrality of theory as one such tool—as vital to the psychotherapist as an architect's blueprints are to builders or a musical score is to musicians in a symphony orchestra. Just as blueprints or a musical score stipulate the components of their ultimate product, they also presuppose a particular endpoint—a skyscraper or a symphony. They are created with a teleological purpose—to yield a particular "good outcome." Theory for psychotherapists works in the same way. It stipulates not only the working parts of the process that will unfold but also the particular endpoint of "good health" that is being pursued. Psychotherapy is always promoting a particular vision of the good life, and theory is the medium through which this message is constructed.

Theory contributes to psychotherapeutic decision making, and its utilization can be maximized for the good. In the chapter's first section we crystallize key features of theory in psychotherapy, emphasizing that both explicit and implicit theories inhabit the mind of the psychotherapist. In the second section we elucidate the centrality of dual process conceptions of the human mind by describing attributes of automatic and deliberative processing, their differential approaches to decision making, and their interactivity. We then integrate these two lines of discussion in the third section by presenting and analyzing a clinical vignette to illustrate how the judgments and decision making of a psychotherapist are guided by both the automatic and deliberate use of implicit and explicit theory. We conclude by translating our analysis into specific recommendations for optimizing clinical applications of this dual process perspective on theory's value in therapeutic judgment and decision making.

THE NATURE OF THEORY IN PSYCHOTHERAPY

The psychotherapeutic endeavor abounds with astonishing complexity, rendering theory essential—indeed, unavoidable. Over a half-century ago, Shoben (1962) enduringly captured the indispensable organizing and meaning-making functions served by theory in psychotherapy:

> The world of the counselor confronted by a client is closely analogous to the world of the baby as William James characterized it: a big, buzzing, booming confusion. The counselee reports events from his own history, considers his present and past experience, reacts directly to the counselor and the counseling relationship, responds to tests, and otherwise provides a welter of raw data about himself. The counselor, if he is to understand the person to whom he is professionally responsible, must discover (or create) some order in this chaos of impressions. In short, he must make some fruitful sense out of what his client says or does. . . . To say these things is to indulge in truisms, of course, but reminding ourselves of them leads to the proposition that theory is inevitable and inescapable in the counseling process and in the counselor's professional behavior. (p. 617)

In significantly facilitating a therapist's navigation of psychotherapy's multiple concurrent, sequential, and nonlinear complexities, theory is akin to a map (Hechter & Horne, 2003). A map provides an abstract visual representation of a geographical territory and helps a traveler to physically traverse this territory with accuracy and effectiveness. It does so in part through labeling diverse features of the territory with different symbols, such as nonlinguistic representations (e.g., lines of different thickness denoting different-sized roads; colors for indicating physical objects—blue for lakes, green for forests), words (e.g., the names of towns and streets), and numbers (e.g., the number 33 at various points on a particular line, denoting "Highway 33"). These nonlinguistic, verbal, and numeric symbols not only signify different aspects of the territory, but crucially, they also visually depict how these different aspects are organized in relation to one another. Yet maps of the same geographical territory can be very different. For example, one may include certain features but not others, but these excluded features may be depicted on a second map of the same territory, and a third may contain elements from the first two while adding still additional features absent in these but present in the actual physical geography.

A psychotherapy theory, understood metaphorically as a map, is similarly an abstract representation, but in this case the terrain of interest encompasses human personality development and functioning; psychological health and disorder; and psychotherapeutic principles, procedures, and processes (Anchin, 2006). As will be elaborated momentarily, different theories provide different maps of these same clinical domains. Each deploys its own specific set of concepts to designate what are viewed as these domains' key features as well as propositions that specify how these concepts and the features they signify are related to one another. However, this matter is not as straightforward as it may seem, in that therapists characteristically—and necessarily—navigate the complexities of psychotherapy's regions of interest with two types of maps: an explicit theory and an implicit theory (Jones-Smith, 2012; Najavits, 1997; Sandler, 1983; Shoben, 1962). Each type of theory is composed of different components, although in real time they are highly interactive.

Explicit Theory

As concisely defined by Jones-Smith (2012), a therapist's "explicit theory of psychotherapy usually represents a theoretical orientation of some school of thought" (p. 601). Principal contemporary schools of thought are exemplified by the cognitive–behavioral, psychoanalytic–psychodynamic, humanistic–experiential, family systems, and integrative paradigms. Each such paradigm is characterized by "a set of assumptions [that are] foundational, general belief statements" (Kim, 2010, p. 32) about personality, maladjustment, and the aims of psychotherapy. These assumptions are "implicit philosophies" (Elliott, 2008, p. 41), "first principles of thought" (Miller, 1992, p. 6), that cannot be proven or disproven but are nevertheless taken to be fundamental truths. And if these days they are not taken as truths with a capital T, they are still held as essential working premises that give meaning and narrative structure to what otherwise might often seem inchoate and overwhelming (Spence, 1982). Each such explicit theory of psychotherapy is a multicomponent knowledge structure composed of specific concepts that delineate and define distinctively important elements in the realms of personality, psychopathology, psychological health, and psychotherapy; explanatory propositions that explain and predict operative relationships between these elements; and specific intervention techniques for promoting change that are intimately tied to the understanding of the patient and his or her psychopathology enabled by these concepts and propositions.

It is essential to note that explicit theories of psychotherapy are nomothetic in that they are formulated to apply to patients in general. Even in the case of a theory of psychotherapy developed for a delimited class of disorders—for example, interpersonal psychotherapy of depression (Klerman, Weissman, Rousansville, & Chevron, 1984)—the concepts, propositions, and techniques are abstractions that do not provide guidance for how to tailor treatment to the particularities and vicissitudes of the individual case. As Shoben (1962) astutely pointed out,

> Thus, we are confronted with a paradox. Theories in counseling are inevitable as necessary tools to bring orderliness into the chaotic world of the counseling interchange and to promote the counselor's understanding of his client. But theories are destined, by virtue of their abstract nature, to leave out of the account the special and unique qualities of a particular counselee's behavior and history, and theories can contain the danger of luring the counselor into conceiving the case before him as a representation of abstract ideas and formal relationships rather than as a highly distinctive and individual human being. (p. 618)

Shoben's (1962) observations are a call for the necessity of bringing to the therapeutic situation not only nomothetically based knowledge of personality, psychopathology, and psychotherapy provided by explicit theory but also the willingness and capacity to blend applications of this knowledge with an evolving idiographic understanding of the patient. More than 50 years later, Shoben's caution is mirrored by the attentiveness to specificity strongly encouraged by today's evidence-based practice movement in psychology. The APA Presidential Task Force on Evidence-Based Practice (2006) suggested that "psychological services are most likely to be effective when they are responsive to the patient's specific problems, strengths, personality, sociocultural context, and preferences (Norcross, 2002)" and "that sensitivity and flexibility in the administration of therapeutic interventions produces better outcomes than rigid application of manuals or principles (Castonguay, Goldfried, Wiser, Raue, & Hayes, 1996; Henry, Schacht, Strupp, Butler, & Binder, 1993; Huppert et al., 2001)" (p. 278). Requisite to idiographic specificity, sensitivity, and flexibility is attunement to and responsiveness within the relational matrix that unfolds with the specific patient at hand—considerations that point to the important role of a therapist's implicit theory of psychotherapy.

Implicit Theory

Providing propositions that can guide a therapist's handling of every contingency or nuance that arises during the treatment process is beyond the scope of any explicit theory of psychotherapy. A therapist's implicit theory is instrumental in filling this sizeable gap. Najavits (1997) defined an implicit theory of psychotherapy "as therapists' private assumptions or 'working model' about how to conduct psychotherapy that is distinct from, but co-exists with, normal theoretical orientations" (p. 2). Moreover, as she discerningly pointed out, these assumptions and beliefs "may be conscious, preconscious, or unconscious to the therapist; 'implicit' simply refers to *ad hoc*, tacit assumptions of therapists, as distinct from the formal propositions of orientations" (p. 4). Indeed, similar to the therapist's explicit theory, implicit theory is a knowledge structure, but whereas the former can be conceived of as a formal knowledge structure, the latter is more informal in its structure. Drawing on clinical and empirical literature, Najavits provided an illuminatingly useful sampling of domains, presented in Table 3.1 (along with an example that we provide for each), in which a therapist's implicit assumptions and beliefs may operate.

The contents of specific tacit assumptions and beliefs composing a therapist's implicit theory develop in part through experience gained in practicing the craft—products of a learning process that to no small extent is itself implicit. As Patterson, Pierce, Bell, and Klein (2010) explained, "'Implicit learning' refers to the process of learning without intention and without being able to verbalize easily what has been learned" (pp. 291–292). Less-than-conscious acquisition of this clinically relevant knowledge is consistent with empirical evidence that implicit learning occurs through associative learning mechanisms that "pick up statistical dependencies encountered in the environment and generate highly specific knowledge representations" (Frensch & Rünger, 2003, p. 17). Patterson et al. characterized these statistical dependencies as "dynamical statistical patterns and features in the environment" (p. 290), and they presented evidence that among statistical patterns tacitly learned are joint probabilities (the probability that an event A and an event B will co-occur; e.g., "When I lose a sense of time passing in the session, it is likely that the patient and I have become engaged in emotionally meaningful work") and conditional probabilities (the probability that if event A occurs, then event B will follow; e.g., "If a patient with a substance disorder starts therapy highly ambivalent about change, then it is likely that his initial treatment motivation will be low"). Moreover, Patterson et al. pointed out that this kind of learning "is a ubiquitous, robust phenomenon that likely occurs in most, if not all, tasks in which individuals engage throughout their lives" (p. 299). As such, implicit associative learning significantly contributes to the development of expertise in a given content domain, and its product—tacit knowledge (Patterson et al., 2010)—informs the expert's judgments and decisions in his or her domain of expertise.

Although derived in part from experientially based associative learning of regularities, a therapist's implicit assumptions about how to conduct

TABLE 3.1
Sampling of Domains in Which Implicit Assumptions
and Beliefs May Operate

Domain	Example
Personal strategies of what to do during sessions	Keep the patient focused on material that is emotionally charged, since the charged nature of this content indicates that it contains important meanings that will be valuable to collaboratively cull out.
Views about what processes are actually occurring during therapy	Apart from the session-to-session content being dealt with, over time how the patient experiences the therapist and their interactions impacts the patient's view of and feelings about self in mutative ways.
Views about what not to do in therapy	Don't try to convince the patient to see things the way I do.
Assumptions that hinder treatment	Do not stray from the agenda that I have for the session, even if the patient wishes to focus on a different topic.
Metaphors for the therapy process	Psychotherapy is sometimes like arm wrestling with the patient's psychopathology.
Personal axioms therapists tell themselves during sessions	Be in the here-and-now.
Views on what to do when particular problem situations arise	If the patient is an acute state of crisis and despair, be willing to provide direct advice.
Ideas of what makes therapy difficult to do well	Despite assigning between-session homework that has the potential to advance therapeutic progress, patients do not always follow through with implementing assignments, and the amount of control the therapist has for getting them to do so is limited.
Subjective criteria by which therapists measure their success	The patient is experiencing meaningful changes in his or her life that on a day-to-day basis are accompanied by more frequent positive affectivity.

Note. Adapted from "Psychotherapists' Implicit Theories of Therapy," by L. M. Najavits, 1997, *Journal of Psychotherapy Integration, 7*, pp. 1–16. Copyright 1997 by the American Psychological Association.

psychotherapy develop from still additional sources. Shoben (1962) suggested that therapists, on the basis of their own life experiences, develop ideas about how people "do and should behave" (p. 619) and that these "value-laden attitudes about the nature of man [sic] may have something to do with the ideas that we regard as 'right' and fruitful" (p. 619). These ideas may in turn influence a therapist's preferences in the direction of theories that validate his or her tacit conceptions about personality and the relative importance of different classes of human behavior. In truth, how could it be any other way, given that cognitive consistency would demand that the theories we espouse be congruent with our underlying values and beliefs about human nature? Clinical supervision provides still another source of a therapist's evolving implicit beliefs about how to conduct psychotherapy. In the course of such pedagogical exercises as case discussions, analysis of segments of videotaped sessions, and providing feedback, clinical supervisors invariably not only educate supervisees about formal theoretical concepts, principles, and techniques but also communicate their own informal and tacit beliefs about the practice and processes of psychotherapy, not to mention their conceptions of what good health and a good life are.

Although the structure and content of explicit and implicit theories in psychotherapy differ considerably, they share a significant commonality: When all is said and done, both forms of theory fundamentally reside and function in the mind of the psychotherapist. As such, explicating how a psychotherapist draws on theory in making clinical judgments and decisions must incorporate an understanding of how the human mind itself operates. This knowledge is contained within a remarkably copious body of theory and research centering on the view that the mind operates through two types of "thinking, knowing, and information processing" (Slovic, Finucane, Peters, & MacGregor, 2004, p. 313), a conception embodied by dual process theories of mental functioning, to which we turn our attention in the next section.

DUAL PROCESSING IN JUDGMENT AND DECISION MAKING

Over the past 3 decades, an array of dual process models of the human mind have been developed in cognitive and social psychology. These models and their associated cross-disciplinary research programs have extended their reach to the study of judgment and decision making. Illustrating the value of these concepts through their application to medical diagnostic reasoning and decision making, Croskerry (2009b) suggested that "a variety of lines of evidence from philosophy, psychology, neurology, neuroanatomy, neurophysiology, and genetics in recent years provides support for the view that decision making might best be represented by dual process theory" (p. 29). Lying at the heart of this body of formulations is the view that the human mind is characterized by two "qualitatively distinct forms of processing" (Evans & Stanovich, 2013, p. 226), one characterized by automatic and the other by deliberative processing.[1] Comprehensive and incisive analyses by Evans (2008), Evans and Stanovich (2013), and Gawronski and Creighton (2013) make clear that dual process models are far from homogeneous, but these scholars also agree that amid this diversity sufficient commonalities exist to enable identification of generic properties and attributes characterizing dual process formulations of the mind. Here, space limitations allow only brief synopses highlighting frequently cited attributes of these two types of processing; sources informing this discussion provide more extensive detail (see Bargh, Schwader, Hailey, Dyer, & Boothby, 2012; Beevers, 2005; Bodenhausen & Todd, 2010; Croskerry, 2009a, 2009b; Evans, 2008; Evans & Stanovich, 2013; Gawronski & Creighton, 2013; Sinclair, Sadler-Smith, & Hodgkinson, 2009; Slovic et al., 2004; Smith & DeCoster, 2000). Following Evans and Stanovich (2013), we emphasize that for processing to be characterized as automatic or deliberative, it is not necessary for the entire set of attributes within each form of processing to occur together. Rather, within each type of processing, "there is a clear basis for predicting a strongly *correlated* set of features, [but] very few need be regarded as essential and *defining* characteristics" (p. 228, italics added).

Automatic Processing and Decision Making

Automatic processing accounts for information processing, including judgment and decision making, that is relatively effortless, rapid, and efficient. It transpires without conscious awareness (and thus is variously referred to as *nonconscious* and as *unconscious*), is triggered spontaneously and unintentionally by features of the immediate context, is parallel (i.e., multiple processing tasks and operations are simultaneously engaged), and occurs without necessitating working memory. Automatic processing also tends to be associative; holistic, in the sense of "process[ing] separate features as a single unified whole" (Richler, Wong, & Gauthier, 2011, p. 129); and affect laden. Knowledge structures retrieved from memory and quickly drawn on during automatic processing form slowly through experience-based

---

[1]Other theorists and researchers have characterized the distinction between these two forms of information processing as, for example, *automatic* and *controlled* (Schneider & Chein, 2003), *associative* and *reflective* (Beevers, 2005), *experiential/intuitive* and *rational/analytic* (Epstein, 2010), *reflexive* and *reflective* (Lieberman, 2007), *System 1* and *System 2* (Kahneman & Frederick, 2002), and *Type 1* and *Type 2* (Evans & Stanovich, 2013). Each such dualistic characterization captures major differentiating features encompassed by dual process theories. For present purposes, the *automatic–deliberative* terminology has been chosen to descriptively highlight a core distinguishing feature of each type of processing on which other features of each system seem to conceptually load, as it were. It must also be noted that whatever terminology is used, the dual process distinction is not without controversy (see, e.g., Keren & Schul, 2009; Newell & Shanks, 2014).

learning and skill acquisition. However, there is emerging evidence that in certain realms (e.g., social–cognitive processes) automatic processing is not exclusively dependent on the acquired products of experience but also draws on innate motivational and emotional processes (see Bargh et al., 2012; for a cognitive neuroscience perspective, see Singer & Conway, 2011).

In the realm of judgment and decision making, many of these features of automaticity are akin to a form of intuition. Although in point of fact "there are multiple kinds of intuition" (Glöckner & Witteman, 2010, p. 5), Sinclair et al. (2009) provided an action-oriented definition that is pragmatically valuable in the present context:

> "Intuiting" [is] . . . a process leading to a recognition or judgment that is arrived at rapidly, without deliberative rational thought, is difficult to articulate verbally, is based on a broad constellation of prior learning and past experiences, is accompanied by a feeling of confidence or certitude, and is affectively charged (Davis and Davis, 2003; Dane and Pratt, 2007). (p. 393)

This definition concurs with the conceptualization of intuition adopted in naturalistic decision making (NDM; see Schraagen, Militello, Ormerod, & Lipshitz, 2008), a rich paradigm for understanding and improving decision making that studies experts' in situ decisional processes in dynamic, highly taxing settings (e.g., firefighting, intensive care units, aviation, combat). Characteristic of these naturalistic situations are "uncertainty, time pressure, risk, and multiple and changing goals" (Schraagen, Militello, et al., 2008, p. xxv). The applicability of these parameters—and NDM's conceptions more generally—to psychotherapy is striking, yet this paradigm has yet to be deployed in the effort to study and understand psychotherapeutic decision making. This is slightly ironic given how often therapists are confronted with highly charged emotional interactions and on-the-spot decisions with regard to suicidality, heightened family conflict, and recruitment of additional support and/or legal authorities.

Klein's (1998) model of recognition-primed decision making (RPD), one of NDM's flagship models (Keller, Cokely, Katsikopoulos, & Wegwarth, 2010), highlights intuition in explaining how experts in complex, exacting situations rapidly identify and implement an effective course of action with minimal deliberation. As Klein (1998) explained, "intuition depends on the use of experience to recognize key patterns that indicate the dynamics of the situation" (p. 31). In this pattern-recognition process, the expert decision maker tunes in to certain situational cues and features and their configuration on the basis of experientially based situational awareness. Through matching this information to previously stored pattern exemplars or prototypes the decision maker recognizes this to be a pattern of a certain kind (detects typicality; Klein, 1998, p. 149). On the basis of this similarity, the decision maker draws automatic inferences about what to expect, what goal is plausible, and what course of action is likely to successfully achieve that goal in the context at hand. Crucial to this process's rapidity is circumvention of the time-consuming process of generating and comparing response options. Rather, intuition in RPD derives from fast, unconscious pattern matching and recognition; the decision maker consciously experiences only the output of this process—that is, the decision as to what action to take, reflected in cognitions and/or images characteristically interwoven with affect, for example the feeling of rightness (Thompson, Prowse Turner, & Pennycook, 2011). Empirical studies of experts' decision making strongly support RPD's success in yielding effective decisions (e.g., Kahneman & Klein, 2009).

An alternative to the RPD perspective on intuition is the heuristics and biases (HB) approach pioneered by Tversky and Kahneman (1974). Whereas the RPD approach focuses on "Intuitive judgments that arise from experience and manifest skill. . . . HB researchers have been mainly concerned with intuitive judgments that arise from simplifying heuristics, not from specific experience" (Kahneman & Klein, 2009, p. 519). Heuristics simplify judgment and decision making in that they entail "mental shortcuts, rules of thumb" (Croskerry, 2009b, p.1025) that enable a rapid decision to be made in the midst of time constraints and uncertainty through applying what are essentially "simple decision algorithms" (Keller et al., 2010, p. 256). Although heuristics necessarily ignore some of the information in the decision situation, they "do not try to optimize (i.e., find the best solution), but rather satisfice (i.e., find a good-enough solution)" (Gigerenzer, 2008, p. 20), and in this respect they are highly practical and efficient. More than 40 heuristics have been identified (see Shah & Oppenheimer, 2008, Table 1); representative exemplars include the representativeness heuristic (e.g., per Garb, 1996, a clinician diagnoses a patient with a particular psychological disorder because her presentation includes features that resemble—i.e., are representative of—the clinician's personal prototype of that disorder rather than on the basis of attending to the specific *Diagnostic and Statistical Manual of Mental Disorders* criteria for that disorder), the anchoring heuristic (e.g., per Harding, 2004, a case worker makes a conclusive disability decision based on initially reviewed case information and adheres—i.e., remains anchored to— that decision rather than adjusting it in light of additionally gathered information that points to a different, more reasonable decision), and the take-the-best heuristic (Todd & Gigerenzer, 2007; e.g., a person in extreme crisis with an urgent need to see a psychotherapist begins calling therapists and makes an appointment with the first therapist who can see him that day). As in RPD, the decision maker is consciously aware of the intuitive choice that results from employing a heuristic, but application of the latter is itself an unconscious process. Comparing these two perspectives does raise the question of the degree or level of awareness engaged. For RPD, the pattern matching may have a deeper level of automaticity—the match occurs and the response ensues. With the heuristic perspective, the reasoning is below the surface, but perhaps not fully out of awareness.

The accuracy and effectiveness of decisions based on the application of heuristics has been and remains a controversial issue (Evans, 2010). On the one hand, sizeable bodies of evidence, instrumental to the enduring influence of the HB approach, leave no doubt that the use of heuristics can lead to highly flawed and deficient decision making (Croskerry, 2002). On the other hand, an alternative approach to the conception and investigation of heuristics, the fast-and-frugal heuristics program developed by Gigerenzer and his colleagues (see Gigerenzer, 2008), demonstrates that heuristics are capable of rendering quite accurate, successful decisions. A key factor moderating a heuristic's effectiveness is its ecological rationality (Todd & Gigerenzer, 2007)—that is, the fit between the decision maker's objective within the environmental situation at hand and the decision heuristic deployed. A heuristic is adaptive when it yields a decision sufficient for meeting the decision maker's situational objective and flawed when it is inadequate in doing so. Croskerry's (2002) perspective is noteworthy in this context; he pointed out that the shortcuts heuristics provide for making decisions "for the majority of cases, work well. When they succeed, we describe them as economical, resourceful, and effective, and when they fail, we refer to them as cognitive biases" (p. 1201).

The study of intuition specifically and of automatic decision making more generally have also been marked by increasing interest in the role played by affective reactions. This work provides mounting evidence that not only is affect characteristically experienced as an essential output component of automatic–intuitive processes (Glöckner & Witteman, 2010), but it also operates as input to decision making (Han & Lerner, 2009), "enter[ing] the decision stream earlier than do conscious considerations" (Lodge, Taber, & Weber, 2006, p. 12). Highly pertinent in this regard is the distinction between incidental and integral affect, both of which are characterized as immediate emotions in that they "are experienced at the time of decision making" (Lowenstein & Lerner, 2003, p. 620). As Mosier and Fischer (2010) explained, incidental affect stems from sources extraneous to the decision at hand (e.g., an emotion aroused by an experience just prior to but then carried into the decision situation); it precedes the latter and is thus potentially task irrelevant. In contrast to incidental affect, integral affect is task relevant in that it is triggered by features integral to the decision making situation itself. This affect-triggering process occurs within milliseconds of the activating stimulus (Lodge et al., 2006); as Bodenhausen and Todd (2010) underscored,

"Affective reactions typically carry many of the features of automaticity, including rapidity, spontaneity, and efficiency" (p. 282).

An emerging consensus is that contrary to previous views that decision making is a purely rational process and that therefore affect only disrupts an optimal decision, "without emotional involvement, decision making might not even be possible or might be far from optimal (Damasio, 1994)" (Pfister & Bohm, 2008, p. 8; cf. Rosenbloom, Schmahmann, & Price, 2012). Slovic et al. (2004) placed affect at the center of judgment and decision making, postulating and providing supportive evidence for an affect heuristic—a shortcut in which individuals use readily available affect (feelings of goodness or badness) as the basis for their judgments and decisions. As Slovic et al. put it, "Although analysis is certainly important in some decision-making circumstances, reliance on affect and emotion is a quicker, easier, and more efficient way to navigate in a complex, uncertain, and sometimes dangerous world" (p. 313).

Bearing in mind the importance of situational and contextual considerations (Magnavita & Anchin, 2014), automatically evoked affect can help or harm optimal decision making (see Exhibit 3.1). However, one important constant remains: "The rapidity of automatic processes means that they start to unfold well before any deliberation has occurred" (Bodenhausen & Morales, 2013, p. 231). Whether reflective deliberation is brought into play during the decision stream initiated by automatic processes depends on a number of factors, a consideration to which we return after highlighting central features of deliberative information processing.

Deliberative Processing and Decision Making

Deliberative processing entails information processing that is intentionally initiated, that is relatively slower and more effortful than automatic processing, and that occurs largely within conscious awareness. It requires working memory as well as more of other cognitive resources—such as attention and declarative knowledge (e.g., knowledge of facts and concepts)—than are necessitated by automatic processing, occurs serially in that it "follows a series of steps rather than performing multiple actions at once" (Beevers, 2005, p. 978), and is rule governed. Deliberative processing prizes analysis, rational reasoning, and logic. Moreover, in contrast to the relatively slow, experience-based acquisition of knowledge that supports automatic processing, information incorporated into knowledge structures by deliberative processing can be learned rapidly, including on the basis of a single experience. This feature facilitates adaptive flexibility in both covert and overt responding to a given situation.

Within the realm of judgment and decision making, the framework of subjective expected utility theory (SEUT) and its quantified methodology

EXHIBIT 3.1
Ways in Which Automatically Evoked Affect Can Benefit and Impede Optimal Judgment and Decision Making

Task-relevant (integral) affect can benefit judgment and decision making by
- rapidly directing or heightening attention to information (e.g., external cues, internal knowledge structures) pertinent to the decision-making task at hand (Peters, Vastfjall, Garling, & Slovic, 2006; Pfister & Bohm, 2008);
- facilitating the setting of a particular situational goal (Zeelenberg, Nelissen, Breugelmans, & Pieters, 2008) and facilitating goal-directed behavior following choice (Bagozzi, Dholakia, & Basuroy, 2003);
- speeding up choice making under time constraints (Pfister & Bohm, 2008);
- guiding estimation of risk associated with different choice options (Slovic et al., 2004);
- influencing moral judgments (Bargh et al., 2012) and enhancing commitment to moral choices (Pfister & Bohm, 2008); and
- impacting whether in the course of making a decision deliberative processing is initiated (Mosier & Fischer, 2010).

Task-relevant (integral) affect can impede judgment and decision-making by
- inducing the decision maker to search for or focus on only information consistent with his or her particular affective state, thereby neglecting or distorting inconsistent information (Mosier & Fischer, 2010);
- constraining appraisal of the situation as a function of the affect's valence (i.e., positive or negative), distinct subjective–experiential quality (e.g., anger, fear, happiness), or intensity—this potentially limited and therefore biased interpretation can in turn reflexively result in an action choice that may actually be less than optimal for the context (see, e.g., Lerner & Tiedens, 2006); and
- limiting the range of options that the decision maker considers (Schottenbauer, Glass, & Arnkoff, 2007).[a]

Task-irrelevant (incidental) affect can impede judgment and decision-making by
- influencing judgments rendered and choices made without the individual knowing that this incidental emotion is biasing his or her decisional processes (Bodenhausen & Todd, 2010).

[a]An important caveat is that these narrowing effects on generating options may be distinctly more associated with negative as opposed to positive affective states. Fredrickson's (2004) broaden-and-build theory of positive affect holds that the latter is expansive and leads to more creative and open decision making. Thus, it may be the case that if and when positive affect constrains decision making, moderating variables in the specific context at hand are at play.

of decision analysis quintessentially represent deliberative processing. This approach, promulgated as the optimal way in which decisions should be made (Shaban, 2005), necessitates cognitive resources (e.g., working memory; attention) and is carried out within conscious awareness. It also requires the analytic process of identifying at the outset of the decision task all available options and each option's set of possible outcomes relative to achieving a given goal (e.g., solving a particular problem, attaining a desired state); in turn, each possible outcome is assigned a utility value (a number representing its relative desirability) and a probability value (indicating its relative likelihood of occurrence). Drawing on one of several possible mathematical algorithms, the decision maker calculates an expected utility value (EUV) for each option, and the option with the highest EUV score is considered the best choice (Jain, Aggarwal, & Rana, 2010–2011, p. 276).

Decision analysis has been successfully applied in clinical (characteristically medical) and nonclinical contexts (Chapman & Sonnenberg, 2000; Edwards, Miles, & von Winterfeldt, 2007; Parnell, Bresnick, Tani, & Johnson, 2013), demonstrating how conscious, effortful deliberation that combines such components as analysis, cognitive resources, and logic enables highly rational decision making. Yet the highly rigorous and resource-intensive requirements demanded by decision analysis (Croskerry, 2003) renders its practical feasibility nearly untenable, especially given how significantly automatic processes mediate everyday judgments and decisions (Bargh & Williams, 2006). Moreover, the decision making approach represented by SEUT and decision analysis

> fail[s] to capture the reality of most decision situations in health-care . . . that are characterized by incomplete knowledge of all available alternatives, a lack of reliable probabilistic data of the consequences of these alternatives, and few readily acceptable techniques for reliably gauging patient utility. (Shaban, 2005, p. 4)

These circumstances certainly seem to apply to psychotherapy (cf. Schottenbauer, Glass, & Arnkoff, 2007).

It is therefore not surprising that deliberative decision making focused on choosing an option for achieving a particular goal is far more likely to be implemented through the relatively less rigorous method of "option generation and comparison" (Schraagen, Klein, & Hoffman, 2008, p. 4). In this familiar method, the decision maker generates options for achieving the particular goal at hand, systematically evaluates the reasons for and against each option relative to attaining the desired goal (Hastie, 2001, p. 663), and chooses the option offering the best ratio of pros to cons.[2] Considerations about possible outcomes may consciously enter the equation, but they do so in ways less precise than assigning specific numerical values as occurs in decision analysis. An alternative approach to weighing options entails use of the previously alluded to method of satisficing, wherein the decision maker evaluates one option at a time and selects the first one judged as satisfying a subjectively set criterion level—in essence, "looking for the first workable option rather than trying to find the best possible option" (Klein, 2008, p. 458).

Whatever the degree of rigor and precision used, consciously evaluating options in order to choose one as the best course of action for pursuing

---

[2]Indeed, it is important to note that among major responsibilities of institutional review boards in evaluating proposed research is identifying and weighing the possible risks and benefits posed to participants in the proposed study (a risk–benefit analysis).

a goal epitomizes deliberative processing in judgment and decision making. Other instantiations of conscious deliberation that can enter the decision stream at different points include hypothesis generation and testing (Caspar, 1997), mental simulation (Evans & Stanovich, 2013; Klein, 1998), hypothetical thinking (Evans, 2007; Stanovich & Toplak, 2012), and metacognition (Thompson et al., 2011).

As Evans (2010) has pointed out, there has been a tendency to view deliberative processing as superior to automatic processing. In point of fact, however, deliberative processing is not necessarily a royal road to producing higher quality decisions. A decision arrived at through conscious deliberation is not immune to bias and to that extent may be erroneous; illustrative sources of bias and error in deliberative decision making are presented in Exhibit 3.2. Despite these flaws and potential pitfalls, most therapies do privilege the process of making the unconscious conscious and encouraging deliberation and rational consideration before action.

Automatic and Deliberative Processing: Independent but Interactive

Clearly, automatic and deliberative processing are "qualitatively distinct" (Evans & Stanovich, 2013), with each type of processing bringing advantages and limitations to the challenges of adapting to biopsychosocial complexities and changes over the human life course (Epstein, 2010). Lieberman and his colleagues (Lieberman, 2003; Satpute & Lieberman, 2006; Spunt & Lieberman, 2013) have strengthened the case for the dual process distinction by linking it to findings in social cognitive neuroscience (cf. Evans, 2008, p. 270). The evidence amassed by these scholars indicates that automatic and deliberative processing systems are independent; each

EXHIBIT 3.2
Sources of Bias and Error in Deliberative Decision Making

- Selective attention to or overfocus on particular stimulus characteristics of the decision situation (e.g., those that are most accessible or easily articulated) at the expense of other information more relevant to the decision (Evans, 2007; Bodenhausen & Todd, 2010)
- Gaps in the "mindware" (Stanovich, 2011) necessary to engage in rational thinking (e.g., missing declarative knowledge in a particular domain pertinent to the decision situation)
- Incorrect information (Hammond, Hamm, Grassia, & Pearson, 1987)
- Premature closure on considering alternative causal hypotheses by virtue of assuming an initial hypothesis is accurate (Croskerry, 2002)
- Reasoning that is quick and sloppy (Stanovich, 2011)
- Distraction (Croskerry, 2009b)
- Fatigue (Croskerry, 2002)

recruits distinctly different neuroanatomical structures. Crucially, however, "the systems are independent in the sense that they rely on different neural structures, but they are not independent in the sense that there is no interaction between them" (Lieberman, 2007, p. 305).

Facets of this interaction are captured in the default-interventionism model advanced by Evans and Stanovich (2013). In this view, intuitive decisions yielded by rapid automatic processing provide the default response in many decision situations and will not be modulated if accompanied by a feeling of rightness and confidence. However, when the decision maker experiences dissatisfaction or discomfort with an intuitive decision, deliberative processing may be brought to bear on this default intuition through reflection on the judgments or decision at hand; this may or may not lead to an override of the intuitive decision, a point to which we will return in the last section of this chapter. Other factors that can prompt consciously reflective intervention into a decision stream kick-started by automatic processing include violations of the decision maker's expectations (Lieberman, 2003); difficulty in pattern recognition (Klein, 1998); novel, ambiguous, or unusual features in the problem to be decided about (Croskerry, 2009b; Evans, 2010; Evans & Stanovich, 2013); availability of time and/or cognitive resources (Bodenhausen & Todd, 2010; Evans, 2010); and motivation to engage in more systematic processing to ensure accuracy in the service of decisional effectiveness (Beevers, 2005; Smith & DeCoster, 2000).

The default-interventionism model suggests a sequential interaction in which deliberation follows on the heels of automatic processing. However, we hypothesize, following Hammond's (2010) cognitive continuum theory, that in the flow of real time there is a "continuous oscillation" (Croskerry, 2009a) between automatic and deliberative processing. As Hammond (2010) explained,

> The normal form of cognition [entails] human judgment that is neither purely analytical [deliberative] nor purely intuitive [automatic] but involves *differing proportions of each*, depending on which attributes [of each type of processing] are present in our normal activities. The properties of the task move our judgments over this continuum back and forth as task conditions change (as more and different information comes in) as we try to cope with our various tasks, or various aspects of the same task; different information will make different demands. Therefore the specific attributes of intuition and analysis involved in any judgment—at any one time—will depend on the momentary location of cognition on this continuum. (p. 330, italics added)

Thus, automatic processing and its intuitive outputs are effective in choosing a course of action in many situations and tasks (see, e.g., Epstein,

2010; Evans, 2010; Gigerenzer, 2008), and in others deliberative processing is the most appropriate pathway (see, e.g., Stanovich, 2009). However, judgment and decision making not infrequently entail a variegated interplay between both types of processing and their distinct attributes (Bodenhausen & Todd, 2010; Croskerry, 2009a, 2009b; Hastie, 2001; Slovic et al., 2004).

Different scholars provide different insights into features of this interaction. For example, Bargh et al. (2012) pointed out that conscious (i.e., deliberative) and automatic processes each play a causal role vis-à-vis the other and underscore their interdependent relationship: "These two fundamental forms of human information processing work together, hand in glove, and indeed one would not be able to function without the support and guidance of the other" (p. 601). Epstein (2010) illuminated the circularity that can characterize this interplay:

> Any response (including a conscious thought) in the rational/analytic [deliberative processing] system can evoke an association in the experiential/intuitive [automatic processing] system, which can then influence conscious thoughts and behavior in the rational/analytic system, which can produce further associations in the experiential system, and so on. Thus, rather than just an interaction between single responses in the two systems, the two systems can interact in the manner of a dance, in which a step in one of the systems elicits a step in the other system. (p. 300)

Slovic et al. (2004) also used the instructive metaphor of dance, homing in on the respective identity of each of the partners: "We now recognize that the experiential mode of thinking and the analytic mode of thinking are continually active, interacting in what we have characterized as 'the dance of affect and reason' (Finucane, Peters, & Slovic, in press)" (p. 314). On the integration of the two modes of processing, Singer and Conway (2011) wrote, "Receptive to both sense and sensibility, we achieve an affectionate and clarifying unity. In this unity, we realize a kind of psychological wisdom that honors both unconscious and conscious, image and word, emotion and reason" (p. 1203). And Bodenhausen and Todd (2010) specifically drew attention to the critical issue of how diverse variations in the way these two forms of processing interact to influence the caliber of the resulting decision: "We need to work toward a conceptual synthesis that carefully delineates the multiple ways that automatic processes interact with conscious thinking to produce human decision making in all of its gradations of quality" (p. 290). We now turn to how these two types of thought processes inform an analysis of psychotherapists' use of theory to guide their decision making.

A DUAL PROCESSING ACCOUNT OF THE ROLE OF EXPLICIT AND IMPLICIT THEORY IN PSYCHOTHERAPEUTIC DECISION MAKING

Considering their conceptual richness and empirical robustness, the limited extent to which dual process theories have been explicitly applied to psychotherapy is striking. The significant exception lies in dual process formulations and investigations of selected forms of psychopathology, most notably addictive behaviors (Wiers, Gladwin, Hofmann, Salemink, & Ridderinkhof, 2013), mood disorders (Beevers, 2005; Creemers, Scholte, Engels, Pieters, & Wiers, 2013; Phillips, Ladouceur, & Drevets, 2008), and anxiety disorders (de Jong, 2014; Etkin, Prater, Hoeft, Menon, & Schatzberg, 2010). However, applications of dual process conceptions for understanding the in situ functioning of psychotherapists per se have been minimal (see, e.g., Caspar, 1997; Magnavita & Anchin, 2014, Chapter 10; Shilling, 2012). And yet, over the course of even a single therapeutic hour, the volume and heterogeneity of stimuli that the therapist must process in the service of engaging in multiple therapeutic tasks—amid circumstances that are uncertain, constrained by time, and infused with risks large and small—are enormous. Dual processing grounded in psychotherapeutic theory provides a parsimonious and internally consistent explanation for how a therapist meets these challenging demands in a way that is efficient, organized, and therapeutic.

To illustrate, we draw on a clinical vignette presented in greater detail elsewhere (Anchin & Pincus, 2010, pp. 129–135) and essentially slow down the process, taking the reader inside the psychotherapist's mind to demonstrate how his judgments and decisions are intricately tied to ongoing oscillation between automatic and deliberative applications of both explicit and implicit theory. The vignette entails an extended prototypic therapist–patient dialogue designed to illustrate assimilative integration (Messer, 2001) of interpersonal psychotherapy with elements of cognitive, experiential, constructivist, and solution-focused treatment approaches in therapeutically addressing a specific in-session event that occurs within the patient–therapist relationship.[3] Though divided into segments for purposes of analysis and discussion, the

---

[3]This approach to interpersonal psychotherapy, also characterized as the *interpersonal tradition, interpersonal paradigm, interpersonal system,* and *interpersonal nexus* (Pincus, 2010), is rooted in Sullivan's (1953) seminal interpersonal psychiatry and ensuing elaborations by such notables as Leary (1957), Carson (1969, 1982), Wiggins (1979), Benjamin (1996), and Kiesler (1996). It is also important to note that Sullivanian interpersonalism, synthesized with British object relations theory and self-psychologies rooted in Kohutian theory, has been integral to the development of relational psychoanalysis (Aron, 1996; Mitchell, 1988; Singer, 2005; Wachtel, 1997), and hence, not surprisingly, conceptual and technical–procedural parallels between the interpersonal approach described in this section and relational psychoanalysis are considerable (see Anchin, 2002).

dialogue presented in the following is quoted verbatim from the material that appears in Anchin and Pincus (2010).

The vignette begins at the point where the patient has seen the therapist glancing at his desk clock and reacts by abruptly ceasing description of an argument he had had with his wife earlier in the day and shifting into a different affective state and mode of dialogue vis-à-vis the therapist. The therapist responds in the following manner:

> *Therapist:* [*Pinpointing overt, observable behavior, focusing inward, and pinpointing affect*] Bob, you just stopped talking about the argument you and your wife had this morning and stared at me; then you looked away, shook your head, and gave this deep sigh. What are you feeling?

This two-sentence response is underpinned by processes of both automatic and deliberative judgment and decision making that fundamentally originate out of the interpersonal core of the therapist's explicit theory of psychotherapy. Whatever its specific content, a therapist's explicit theory automatically orients him or her toward certain stimulus features of the situation and away from others. These shifts in orientation are vitally important from a decisional perspective because the data selectively attended to serve as the determinative foundation for ensuing therapist processing, including subsequent data attended to, inferences drawn, and judgments rendered. Here, the therapist's theoretical perspective heightens his attentiveness to the distinct shift in the patient's interactional behavior and its negative emotional tone and leads him to automatically infer that a significant negative event has occurred in the therapeutic relationship.

This intuitive clinical judgment sparks feelings of uneasiness and concern, exemplifying integral affect in action. These emotions enter the therapist's decision stream and, integrated with his conscious attunement to their immediate relational context and meanings, prompt his engaging in a rapid deliberative process about how best to respond. He momentarily considers remaining silent but then overrides this option, deciding instead to actively intervene through initiating therapeutic *metacommunication* (literally, communication about communication), a multicomponent intervention originally defined by Kiesler (1988) that centers on the therapist and patient stepping back to examine and learn from the process that is taking place between them (cf. Anchin, 2002; Anchin & Pincus, 2010, Muran, Eubanks-Carter, & Safran, 2010). The decision to go in this direction reflects "the dance of affect and reason" (Slovic et al., 2004) alluded to above: The therapist chooses this option not only because it is logically consistent with formal interpersonal principles, which stipulate the importance of collaboratively processing a negative in-session relational event both for reparative purposes and for insights it may yield about the patient's maladaptive interpersonal behavior (Anchin & Pincus, 2010; Kiesler, 1996; Safran & Muran, 2000), but also because—by virtue of this very consistency with his core theory—this decision "feels right." The affect heuristic has thus combined with the rule-based logic of his theory to influence the therapist's decision. Although not the primary focus of our current analysis, we might also explore why the therapist looked at the clock when he did and ask what was happening in the "analytic third" or the intersubjective space shared by both participants that might have influenced the therapist's action (Ogden, 2004).

The patient provides an unambiguous response to the therapist's question as to what he is feeling, and the therapist's response is automatic; no deliberation is needed:

Client: To be honest, I'm pissed off!

Therapist: [*Encouraging the client to elaborate*] About?

Although overtly this is a simple one-word question by the therapist, it is still theory driven. In this instance, it reflects the combination of the therapist's implicit theory of psychotherapy on the one hand, which holds that depending on context it can be essential to unpack feelings expressed by the patient, and the continued operation of his explicit theory on the other hand, which, translated into technique, specifies that during metacommunication the therapist encourage the patient to express his feelings—and as will be demonstrated in the following, subsequently engage him in collaborative processing of those feelings.

The overarching therapeutic strategy of metacommunication remains in force as the dialogue continues, but as the exchange proceeds, the patient's material and the reactions it evokes in the therapist necessitate that the latter make further automatic and deliberative judgments and decisions—based on both additional facets of his explicit theory and a belief tied to his implicit theory—about ways of responding that will keep the process moving forward therapeutically. Thus, asked what he is "pissed off" about, the following exchange occurs:

Client: You; what you just did. I'm telling you about something that was very upsetting and you're looking at your clock.

Therapist: [*Not getting hooked by the client's anger; instead validating his observation*] You're right; I did. [*Preparing the way for explaining the link between meaning given to the other's behavior and consequent feeling*] How are you interpreting that?

The therapist has thus learned what it is that has precipitated the patient's anger, but he is also aware of experiencing some anxiety in response to the intensity of the patient's anger. Nevertheless, two additional interpersonal principles of therapeutic metacommunication, in tandem, have virtually automatically guided the therapist's reaction to his own anxiety and the nature of his verbal response. One such principle (Kiesler, 1988) centers on the inevitability of experiencing aversive feelings evoked by the patient but not allowing oneself to remain "hooked" (caught up in and thereby constrained) by them, which could impede the therapist's capacity to respond therapeutically. The second principle specifies the importance of the therapist providing the patient with appropriately focused validation in the course of the metacommunicative process, which characteristically includes the therapist explicitly owning his contribution to what has transpired (Muran et al., 2010). Crucially, the therapist does not have to stop and take time to access these two guiding principles; they are already deeply embedded in his theoretical knowledge structures and are automatically activated by the specific therapeutic context. Of course, the more experienced and the better trained the therapist, the more likely that such principles are embedded. To the extent that their guiding effects enter awareness, they do so in the form of the therapist experiencing his anxiety as background and concurrently, more at the foreground, the flash of an affectively tinged thought as to the importance of validating the patient's observation, reflected in his first statement ("You're right; I did.").

The therapist's immediately ensuing question ("How are you interpreting that?") demonstrates pattern recognition in action: In response to an interpersonal trigger, the patient has experienced an intense negative emotional reaction, and in the therapist's experience, this sequence characteristically signifies the activation of a mediating relational (self–other) schema (Anchin & Pincus, 2010; Muran et al., 2010). A key concept in cognitive theory of psychotherapy (e.g., Clark & Beck, 2010), a *schema* is a psychological structure composed of an interconnected set of affect-laden core beliefs about self and others that, when activated, automatically guides interpretation of and thereby meanings ascribed to another's actions (Anchin, 2002). Underpinned by this cognitive theory, the therapist automatically intuits that the pattern of interpersonal trigger → relational schema → emotional reaction is at play, and by virtue of this intuitive judgment he immediately follows up his validation of the patient's observation by asking him how he interpreted his clock-glancing behavior.

Reflecting parallel-processing facets of automatic processing, this clinical strategy is tied to multiple, overlapping, and simultaneously operating goals: to move the therapeutic process forward in a constructive direction, to elicit the specific contents of the patient's interpretation, and to "set the table" for bringing a cognitive perspective and associated interventions into the metacommunicative process. Operating from this cognitive perspective, the therapist "hears" the patient's response as an automatic thought[4] and checks to see if this cognition is indeed what went through the patient's mind; the patient confirms this while restating his automatic thought in terms that hint at features of the underlying core belief:

> Client: What interpretation?! It's obvious that you can't wait for me to leave.
>
> Therapist: [*Probing for automatic thoughts*] Is that what went through your head when you just saw me look at the clock?
>
> Client: Yeah, like, "He's not really interested; he doesn't really give a shit about me."

The therapist follows with an empathy-based response:

> Therapist: [*Empathy-based pinpointing of additional affects*] It sounds like you feel like I'm not taking you seriously—that you felt dismissed, rejected.

This empathic response is underpinned by the confluence of the therapist's feeling for the immediate context, formal principles of metacommunication (explicit theory), and knowledge acquired from previous experience (implicit theory). With lightning speed, these coalesce in his automatic judgment that at this immediate juncture it is crucial that the patient feel understood, supported, and accepted. Reflecting the extraordinary rapidity of the continuous fluctuation between automatic and deliberative processing, the therapist holds the patient's words—"Yeah, like, 'He's not really interested; he doesn't really give a shit about me'"—in working memory and seamlessly shifts from his automatic judgment about the immediate importance of empathy into consciously "trying on" what the patient has said, sparking the feelings he empathically experiences and verbally expresses. The velocity of this oscillation is further evidenced by the fact that although the therapist has intentionally—and thus consciously—engaged in and expressed empathic understanding, he does not need to consciously figure out what these feelings *feel* like or the words that capture them; on the basis of stored experiential learning, the subjective experience of these feelings and their verbal labeling kick in automatically. Just as crucial to consider is what the therapist has not said. He implicitly senses that to deny his action would be to invalidate the patient's legitimate read of the situation and understandable emotional response to his action. Similarly, the therapist automatically understands that precipitously apologizing for his behavior would interfere

---

[4] In cognitive therapy theory, automatic thoughts are immediate cognitions that consciously run through a person's mind in response to a situation and arise from the core belief activated in that situation (Clark & Beck, 2010).

with the opportunity to allow the full emotional significance and meaning of the event to be captured in their work together.

A critical sequence immediately follows and becomes the springboard for intentionally moving the metacommunicative process an essential next step, as explained momentarily:

>Client: Absolutely! Hopefully, you can see why I'd feel that way!
>
>Therapist: [Conveying acceptance of the client's subjective affective state while continuing to set the ground for explaining the relationship between interpretations and feelings] Yes; I can—interpreting what I did as meaning that I don't care about you, it makes sense that you'd feel dismissed, rejected, angry. I understand. [Beginning to engage client in the metacommunicative process of stepping back and collaboratively reflecting on the interaction in order to turn this intrasession incident to therapeutic advantage] But can we step back and look at this? Because maybe we can both learn something from what just happened.
>
>Client: It just really hit me wrong. But, yeah, go ahead, I'm listening.

In this exchange, the patient has confirmed the accuracy of the therapist's empathy, and the therapist, continuing in an empathic and supportive mode, without hesitation reciprocally responds in a manner predicated on his reflexive judgment that continued validation and acceptance is essential. However, the therapist's response to the patient's emphatic confirmatory statements is grounded in further judgments and decisions that continue to tap into explicit and implicit theory, automatically and deliberatively. Thus, although the therapist provides validation, his customary strategy of integrating cognitive intervention into metacommunication is also operating concurrently through parallel processing in that he simultaneously frames the patient's feelings as making sense within the context of the patient's interpretation. In addition, although up to this point the exchange encompasses necessary components of metacommunication—for example, the therapist owning his behavior, the patient openly expressing his feelings, and the therapist validating the patient's reactions—it is by no means sufficient for maximizing the therapeutic yield of this significant in-session relational event. Per the therapist's explicit theory, doing so requires that the therapist and patient also join together to examine the how and why of what transpired in order to attain insight into the patient's interpersonal processes and in turn draw out implications for change.

When to invite the patient to engage in this "collaborative inquiry" (Muran et al., 2010, p. 174) involves a judgment about timing, strongly suggesting that among the multiple simultaneous tasks enabled by automatic parallel processing, the therapist must necessarily also be monitoring and integrating data (e.g., not only the patient's verbal responses but also his ongoing nonverbal behavior, the emotional tenor of the exchange, his own comfort level) as bases for this judgment. Here, the therapist, on the basis of the emerging data and his explicit judgment of what the patient can tolerate and how much good will has been generated, decides that the moment is right to issue this invitation and does so in the question-and-statement sequence "But can we step back and look at this? Because maybe we can both learn something from what just happened." Highly rapid deliberative thought has also informed the therapist's judgment as to phraseology, stemming from his implicit theory-based belief that illocution and wording powerfully influence the effectiveness of verbal communication in achieving desired aims during therapeutic discourse. Thus, through the way in which this invitation has been issued, the therapist is attempting to achieve several aims—which, parenthetically, again reflect the shifting nature of multiple immediate goals. These objectives include (a) creating "a collaborative, egalitarian environment" (Muran et al., 2010, p. 175) both through intentionally requesting the patient's participation, as opposed to dominatingly imposing this agenda, and choosing phrasing that highlights the conjoint nature of the endeavor (i.e., "But can we . . ."; "Because maybe we can both . . ."); (b) specifying the task he and the patient need to engage in to move the process forward ("step back and look at this"); and (c) explicitly indicating the purpose of this process through suggesting that they can "learn something from what just happened." The effectiveness of the therapist's automatic judgment about the timing of this invitation and its conscious verbal translation is suggested by the nature of the patient's response; his first sentence, in its past-tense wording ("It just really hit me wrong"), connotes a subtle shift in his emotional tone, and his second sentence ("But, yeah, go ahead, I'm listening") suggests that at this immediate moment, he is on board for the proposed collaborative inquiry.

From here, the therapist provides brief psychoeducation explaining that how we interpret things people say and do strongly influences how we emotionally react to these things and that "different interpretations of the same situation can create very different feelings." The patient conveys understanding of this basic cognitive proposition, which prompts another virtually automatic judgment that the moment is opportune to have the patient begin the process of considering alternative interpretations of the therapist's clock-glancing behavior. Moreover, reflecting the simultaneity of implicit theory, the initial wording he uses to initiate this process reflects his tacit belief that the patient's partnership can be facilitated through actively tapping into the therapeutic relationship:

Therapist: [*Fostering collaboration, encouraging the search for alternative interpretations*] So—go with me on this—could there be other ways to interpret my looking at my clock while you were talking?

Client: I suppose; maybe you're hungry and you can't wait for the session to end so you can get something to eat.

The therapist's ensuing response is once again grounded in a fusion between components of his formal, explicit theory and his more personal implicit theory—in the case of the former, the therapeutic value experiential psychotherapy places on immediate experiencing in enhancing insight (Pascual-Leone & Greenberg, 2007), and in the case of the latter, the therapist's belief that tasting experiential consequences of an insight increases the latter's impact:

Therapist: [Fostering experiential understanding of the cognitive–affective link] And if it was that, how do you think that would make you feel?

Client: Maybe a little less pissed, but you'd still be thinking about how hungry you are, like it's more important than me.

The therapist consciously notes that in considering this alternative interpretation, the patient experiences some lessening of anger; however, he is more attuned to the fact that the patient continues to believe that he lacks importance to the therapist and that this alternative interpretation, though different from that initially rendered, is still inaccurate. Consequently, he quickly decides to persist in this line of inquiry. The patient articulates an accurate interpretation of the therapist's behavior, activating within the latter a positive feeling (another instance of integral affect), which, in conjunction with the cognitive tenets of his explicit theory, prompts automatic validation and further elaboration:

Therapist: [Encouraging the search for additional alternative interpretations] OK; but are there other possible reasons why I looked at the clock, other possible interpretations?

Client: Hmm . . . I suppose; maybe you just wanted to see what time it was so that you knew how much time we had left in the session to deal with what I was talking about.

Therapist: [Confirming the client's interpretation] Exactly; that's exactly why I looked at my clock. [Explaining the intent behind his actions] I know that this was a very upsetting situation between you and your wife, and I wanted to be sure we'd have time to hone in on what was happening there.

Client: I suppose [nods head]; that makes sense.

With the patient appearing to accept this honest explanation for the therapist's clock-glancing behavior, the latter attempts to solidify the impact of this more accurate understanding by intentionally following with the strategy, used moments earlier, of having the patient get in touch with experiential consequences:

Therapist: [*Using immediacy to further enhance interpersonal–experiential change*] Understanding it that way, do you experience at this moment a change in how you feel?

Client: I guess not really pissed off. I guess I appreciate that you understand this was an extremely upsetting situation [this morning] and that you wanted to make sure we had time to figure it out.

Hearing this, the therapist experiences a mixture of positive affect and heightened connectedness to the patient; consistent with the prescribed importance of honest therapist self-disclosure during metacommunication and his own sense of genuineness—and consciously mindful of the opportunity to provide corrective input vis-à-vis the patient's maladaptive self-other schema—the therapist deliberately chooses to share his thoughts and feelings:

Therapist: [*Reciprocating the expression of appreciation*] Good; I appreciate that you're willing to rethink this. [*Refuting the client's misconstrual of the therapist's behavior with honest self-disclosure of nurturing feelings*] And can you see, too, that in wanting to make sure we had enough time, that I do care, that I'm genuinely interested in what's happening in your life—that I care about you, that you do matter?

Client: Yes, I can see where you're also kind of saying that, too.

Therapist: [*Further honest therapist self-disclosure to underscore his genuine interest*] Good—because the last thing I would want you to feel is dismissed or rejected by me.

Client: [*Listening, nodding head*]

The therapist experiences the patient's nonverbal response as indicating that they are in synch and thus, automatically judging that it is safe, consciously decides to push forward with educative intent anchored in explicit cognitive theory. Accordingly, against the backdrop of the patient's more accurate understanding of the therapist's behavior, the latter—retrieving from short-term memory and inserting into working memory the patient's initial inaccurate interpretation—crystallizes for the patient both the cognitive distortions he engaged in and how these led to his emotional reaction:

> *Therapist:* [*Identifying cognitive distortions—selective abstraction, magnification, and jumping to conclusions*] So if we go back to what just happened, it's like you tuned in on that one piece of behavior on my part, magnified it, and then jumped to a conclusion—and a negative one, at that! And given that conclusion, you got really angry with me.

The patient resonates to this interpretive feedback and offers a significant self-observation:

> *Client:* Yeah, I guess it's true, I definitely do that . . . somebody says or does something and I lose it; it's like a switch goes off.

Automatically perceiving the patient's engagement in the exploration process and judging this resonant insight to be highly valuable by virtue of the opportunity it offers to deepen and expand understanding, the therapist experiences a sense of excited optimism and consciously chooses to seize on the patient's analogy—a decision also grounded in the dovetailing between his own implicit belief and solution-focused components of his explicit theory as to the value of analogy and metaphor as tools for promoting insight (e.g., Anchin, 2003; de Shazer, 1985):

> *Therapist:* [*Applying this analogy to the immediate context to advance the client's social–cognitive learning*] Bob, if we use what just happened here between us, what do you think flipped that switch?

The therapist's question bears fruit in advancing insight: Like a dart hitting the bull's eye of a target, the patient articulates fundamental beliefs about himself and others that the therapist immediately hears as central ingredients of a core maladaptive relational schema:

> *Client:* I guess at some level I think that people don't really care about me, that I'm insignificant, I don't matter . . . it's like this feeling is in the background; it nags at me!

Consciously perceiving this to be a critical point in the exploration, and still guided by cognitive components of his explicit theory, the therapist, in his response, intentionally chooses wording intended to crystallize the beliefs embedded in the patient's insight and to convey to the patient their centrality; the therapist's implicit beliefs about the importance of tending to the therapeutic alliance and actively fostering collaboration also come into play:

> *Therapist:* So it sounds like there's these two central beliefs—maybe core beliefs—that you have. One is that "I'm insignificant"

and the other sounds like you believe "People don't care about me." [*With an eye on maintaining the alliance, promotes collaborative exploration*] Does that feel like it fits?

Client: Yeah, definitely... I've always felt... "haunted" is the best word... by this terrifying feeling, deep down, that I'm completely insignificant, that I really mean nothing... nothing!—and that that's also what I mean to people who know me: nothing; that deep down they don't care about me.

IMPLICATIONS AND RECOMMENDATIONS

In analyzing this vignette, our goal has been to demonstrate ways in which a therapist's moment-to-moment judgments and decisions derive from continual oscillation between automatic and deliberative processing drawing on both explicit and implicit theory. The content of our illustration has centered on addressing a specific event within the therapeutic relationship through the fluctuating coupling of an integrative interpersonal approach with implicit beliefs activated by the unfolding situation at hand; however, we believe that the *types* of automatic and deliberative therapist mental processes illustrated in the preceding section continuously mediate and moderate a therapist's judgments and decisions irrespective of a therapist's theoretical orientation and the particular implicit beliefs at play. With this consideration in mind, we seek here to facilitate the reader's application of this knowledge in order to enhance his or her psychotherapeutic judgments and decision making. To do so, we extract key implications from this example and the material preceding it and translate these lessons into specific recommendations:

1. Within any given psychotherapy session, an essential metagoal is to keep the therapeutic process moving forward in a constructive direction. In this light, be aware that you are indeed continuously making rapid clinical judgments and decisions and that these play a vital role in achieving this supraordinate goal as therapeutic discourse unfolds. Awareness of these ineluctable facets of your functioning as a therapist can sharpen your attunement to thoughts and feelings associated specifically with judgments and decisions being made. Sensitivity to the ebb and flow of your dual processing should also alert you more acutely to the products of the intersubjective field and your own countertransference responses.

2. On the one hand, know that over the course of a given session many of your clinical judgments and decisions are being made automatically and that given the multiplicity of stimuli that must be processed and tasks that must be carried out under conditions of uncertainty and limited time, it can be no other way. Moreover, not only are automatically rendered judgments and decisions unavoidable, but as discussed in the preceding, they are also integral to effective psychotherapy. On the other hand, remain ever mindful of an equally critical fact concisely captured by Croskerry and Norman (2008), who—drawing on Stanovich's (2005) depiction of automatic processes as "the autonomous set of systems" (TASS)—remind us that "although TASS operates at an unconscious level, their output, once seen, can be consciously modulated by adding a System 2 [i.e., deliberative] approach" (p. S26).
3. The immediately preceding point made by Croskerry and Norman (2008) speaks to the deliberative processing system's "monitoring capacity" (Croskerry, 2009b, p. 1025) over automatic-processing system output. Consciously appraising a given automatic initial judgment or decision does not in and of itself signify that the latter needs to be overridden by a different decision or even slightly adjusted. For example, a general statement made by the patient about "the problems in my life" may prompt your automatic judgment that a moderately confrontive question, the content of which instantaneously appears in conscious awareness, needs to be posed. Rapid, deliberate consideration of the patient's nonverbal behavior, the context in which the statement was made, and the strength of the alliance may result in an appraisal that posing this question, at this moment, is minimally risky and can beneficially advance the therapeutic process, and so the decision is made to go forth with the question. However, if the patient's nonverbal behavior (e.g., tone of voice and facial expression) conveys that he is in a brittle state, the judgment may instead be made that confronting the patient at this moment is ill timed. Hence a deliberate override occurs: The decision is made not to confront the patient and instead to ask him gently what he was experiencing when he made that statement. Time constraints preclude deliberatively evaluating every automatically rendered judgment and decision whose output appears in consciousness, but be aware that your

deliberative processing system provides this capacity. When such monitoring and appraisal can and/or does occur and you experience such cognitive–affective mixtures as hesitance, discomfort, confusion, conflict, uneasiness, or dissatisfaction vis-à-vis the judgment or decision that rapidly appears in mind, consider that these negatively valenced subjective states are signaling the need to modulate the judgment or decision at hand.

4. Against the backdrop of the preceding recommendations, we note Croskerry and Norman's (2008) hypothesis that "perhaps the mark of good decision makers is their ability to match Systems 1 [automatic processing] and 2 [deliberative processing] to their respective optimal contexts and to consciously blend them into their overall decision making" (p. S26). However, whatever the proportion of automatic and deliberative processing underlying a given judgment or decision, the shifting array of patient-generated cues and stimuli serves as ongoing input to your dual processing systems. Consequently, be keenly present in the here and now of the session, studiously observe the patient's nonverbal behavior, and listen very closely to what the patient is saying lest you miss important information that might otherwise significantly bear on the judgments and decisions being made. At the same time (and this is why what we do is extraordinarily complex), you must be attuned to your own internal associative world of thoughts, fantasies, wishes, emotions, and sensations because your parallel inner world is also influencing both automatic and deliberative processing.

5. Building on this last point, be cognizant of the fact that your affective states in particular can play a powerful role in influencing your judgments and decisions. Indeed, by definition the affect heuristic can operate as the chief determinant of certain decisions that you make. However, a therapist's subjective affect can enter the decision stream at multiple points in the decision-making process. For example, in the course of a specific line of clinical inquiry intended to foster insight, in reaction to the patient's specific verbal responses during this inquiry, and/or in the context of appraising the in-session impact of this intervention, you may decide whether to continue with the exploration or to shift gears. Moreover, these affective states can be valenced positively to negatively and, depending on context, can beneficially contribute to or disadvantageously hinder the

accuracy and effectiveness of your decision making. Thus, to the extent feasible, seek to be aware of your affective states as a given session unfolds, be mindful of the fact that they can affect your judgments and decisions for better or for worse and, in this light, seek to harness and handle your emotional states in ways that work to the patient's good.

6. Given that affect unrelated to the decision task at hand can influence and thereby bias your judgments and decisions (i.e., incidental or countertransferential affect), be keenly aware of the mood state you are experiencing before beginning a given session. It is essential, especially to the extent that you are experiencing acutely positive or negative feelings stemming from extraneous circumstances, that you consciously down-regulate these feelings before the session starts. Engage in "appropriate adjustment of . . . [your] mindset" (Dumont, 1993, p. 200) through self-regulatory processes to eliminate, to the fullest extent possible, the risk of these feelings contaminating your clinical judgments and decisions in the ensuing session. As Dumont (1993) pointed out,

> As we all have our ups and downs, vigilance must be exercised, whether we are veterans or "rookies," in the measure that we sense ourselves under the influence of intense moods. This is especially important when we share the same mood as our client and thereby run the risk of potentiating the biases to which each of us is inclined. (p. 200)

Put in current parlance, the practice of "mindfulness" with regard to registering and letting go of potentially biasing emotional states prior to beginning sessions is a critical preparation for our work.

7. As the previous example demonstrates, explicit theory's impact on clinical judgments and decisions is extensive and profound. Automatically and deliberatively, it influences data selectively attended to; specific kinds of data we seek to gather and learn more about when working with the patient; meanings attributed to these data; interpretations of the patient's immediate in-session actions and verbalizations; our clinical hypotheses and formulations; and, of course, the techniques and interventions we utilize (cf. Dumont, 1993). Arguably, explicit theory thus functions as the very scaffolding of psychotherapy as the therapist and patient collaboratively seek to develop and build the latter's mental health and self-understanding. Thus, whether your explicit theory of psychotherapy is single school,

integrative, or unifying, learn, know, and understand it well; the importance of being thoroughly and intimately conversant with its evolving constructs, propositions, and techniques cannot be overestimated. In this light, being willing to revisit and open your theoretical assumptions to additional scrutiny, modification, and growth is likely to enhance the flexibility and acuity of your decision-making processes.

8. Following from the previous implication, the constructs, propositions, and techniques composing your preferred explicit theory are likely to be "tagged" (Slovic et al., 2004) with positive affect, predisposing formulations, inferences, and techniques deriving from this theory to "feel right" and hence automatically adhered to during the "doing" of psychotherapy. This begs the question of whether there may be times when one's judgments and decisions are guided more by feelings stemming from intrinsic positive valuation of one's preferred theory than by considerations about what may be best for the patient. Particularly in bogged-down cases, it may be useful to deliberatively reflect on this question between sessions and to consider the potential impact that complementing one's preferred theory with one or more alternative theoretical perspectives may have on one's clinical judgments and decisions in treating the patient.

9. Seek to explicitly articulate the beliefs composing your implicit theory of psychotherapy. Over the course of a given session these tacit beliefs interact with the concepts and propositions of your explicit theory in guiding clinical judgments and decisions and, like the latter, are drawn on consciously and unconsciously, deliberatively and automatically. Although at a given juncture their role may be more or less prominent than explicit theory, to the extent that they exert impact on judgments and decisions, they affect the process and thereby the outcome of a patient's therapy. In this respect, Najavits (1997, p. 12) astutely speculated that various kinds of inconsistency between implicit and explicit theory may play a distinct role in negative treatment outcomes. More generally, as she suggested, explicitly knowing the content of your implicit beliefs about how to do psychotherapy, compared with the level of understanding that can be derived from focusing solely on your explicit theory, can only enhance your understanding of how you work—and it would seem that this "sophisticated, richer understanding" (Najavits, 1997, p. 13) can benefit therapeutic

process and outcome. To do so, you would be advised to avail yourself of peer supervision and shared case conferences that allow you to engage in supportive but reflexive examination of particular session interactions. What you may not see with regard to implicit processing, your peers may help you to track and articulate.

10. As a pervasively goal-directed process that unfolds over time, a patient's treatment at any given moment is likely to encompass multiple goals—that is, one or more immediate goals are nested within short-term goals, which in turn are nested within the therapy's long-term goals. For example, at the outset of the vignette shown earlier, the therapist's immediate goal of understanding how the patient interpreted his clock-glancing behavior was nested within short-term goals that included engaging the patient in metacommunication and helping him understand how his interpretive processes influenced his emotional reaction and how the contents of his interpretation were driven by core beliefs about self and others. In turn, these and other short-terms goals were nested within long-term treatment goals that include fostering development of a healthy sense of self and effective patterns of interpersonal relating (see Magnavita & Anchin, 2014, Chapter 3). With any given patient, maintaining mindfulness of the therapy's long-term goals, being explicitly cognizant of your short-term goals, and striving for clarity about your immediate objectives at any given moment of the therapy are essential to accurate, effective decision making; the more aware you are of what you are aiming to accomplish, the better the judgments and decisions you can make about how to get there.

SUMMARY

To conclude this chapter, we might draw on a brief nautical analogy. A good sailor begins with a charted course (the explicit psychological theory of personality and change that guides the therapy). Influenced by this metadestination, the navigator responds both intuitively and deliberatively to the vagaries of the current, the tides, and the wind (the particular interactions of a given session). Drawing on previous knowledge of the particular waters, or ones that are similar, some adjustments come readily with a minimum of reflection. On the other hand, sudden unexpected changes in the atmospheric conditions or the introduction of uncharted obstructions can lead to heightened vigilance and arousal (moments of conflict, resistance, and elevated emotion in the therapeutic interaction), calling much more deliberative and explicit decision making into play. Good sailors and good therapists are acutely attuned to the rhythm of this navigational interplay—moments when one's hand rests gently on the tiller and other moments when an intentional tact must be implemented and more overt activity is required. This decision-making dance—shifting continuously among flow, thought, and action—is the work and art of therapy.

REFERENCES

Anchin, J. C. (2002). Relational psychoanalytic enactments and psychotherapy integration: Dualities, dialectics, and directions: Comment on Frank (2002). *Journal of Psychotherapy Integration, 12*, 302–346. http://dx.doi.org/10.1037/1053-0479.12.3.302

Anchin, J. C. (2003). Cybernetic systems, existential phenomenology, and solution-focused narrative: Therapeutic transformation of negative affect states through integratively oriented brief psychotherapy. *Journal of Psychotherapy Integration, 13*, 334–442. http://dx.doi.org/10.1037/1053-0479.13.3-4.334

Anchin, J. C. (2006). A hermeneutically informed approach to psychotherapy integration. In G. Stricker & J. Gold (Eds.), *A casebook of psychotherapy integration* (pp. 261–280). Washington, DC: American Psychological Association. http://dx.doi.org/10.1037/11436-020

Anchin, J. C., & Pincus, A. L. (2010). Evidence-based interpersonal psychotherapy with personality disorders: Theory, components, and strategies. In J. J. Magnavita (Ed.), *Evidence-based treatment of personality dysfunction: Principles, methods, and processes* (pp. 113–166). Washington, DC: American Psychological Association. http://dx.doi.org/10.1037/12130-005

APA Presidential Task Force on Evidence-Based Practice. (2006). Evidence-based practice in psychology. *American Psychologist, 61*, 271–285. http://dx.doi.org/10.1037/0003-066X.61.4.271

Aron, L. (1996). *A meeting of minds: Mutuality in psychoanalysis*. Hillsdale, NJ: Analytic Press.

Bagozzi, R. P., Dholakia, U. M., & Basuroy, S. (2003). How effortful decisions get enacted: The motivating role of decision processes, desires, and anticipated emotions. *Journal of Behavioral Decision Making, 16*, 273–295. http://dx.doi.org/10.1002/bdm.446

Bargh, J. A., Schwader, K. L., Hailey, S. E., Dyer, R. L., & Boothby, E. J. (2012). Automaticity in social–cognitive processes. *Trends in Cognitive Sciences, 16*, 593–605. http://dx.doi.org/10.1016/j.tics.2012.10.002

Bargh, J. A., & Williams, E. L. (2006). The automaticity of social life. *Current Directions in Psychological Science, 15,* 1–4. http://dx.doi.org/10.1111/j.0963-7214.2006.00395.x

Beevers, C. G. (2005). Cognitive vulnerability to depression: A dual process model. *Clinical Psychology Review, 25,* 975–1002. http://dx.doi.org/10.1016/j.cpr.2005.03.003

Benjamin, L. S. (1996). *Interpersonal diagnosis and treatment of personality disorders* (2nd ed.). New York, NY: Guilford Press.

Bodenhausen, G. V., & Morales, J. R. (2013). Social cognition and perception. In I. Weiner (Ed.), *Handbook of psychology* (2nd ed., Vol. 5, pp. 225–246). Hoboken, NJ: Wiley.

Bodenhausen, G. V., & Todd, A. R. (2010). Automatic aspects of judgment and decision making. In B. Gawronski & B. K. Payne (Eds.), *Handbook of implicit social cognition* (pp. 278–294). New York, NY: Guilford Press.

Carson, R. C. (1969). *Interaction concepts of personality.* Chicago, IL: Aldine.

Carson, R. C. (1982). Self-fulfilling prophecy, maladaptive behavior, and psychotherapy. In J. C. Anchin & D. J. Kiesler (Eds.), *Handbook of interpersonal psychotherapy* (pp. 64–77). New York, NY: Pergamon Press.

Caspar, F. (1997). What goes on in a psychotherapist's mind? *Psychotherapy Research, 7,* 105–125. http://dx.doi.org/10.1080/10503309712331331913

Chapman, G. B., & Sonnenberg, F. W. (Eds.). (2000). *Decision making in health care: Theory, psychology, and applications.* New York, NY: Cambridge University Press.

Clark, D. A., & Beck, A. T. (2010). *Cognitive therapy of anxiety disorders: Science and practice.* New York, NY: Guilford Press.

Creemers, D. H. M., Scholte, R. H. J., Engels, R. C. M. E., Pieters, S., & Wiers, R. W. (2013). Acute stress increases implicit depression and decreases implicit self-esteem. *Journal of Experimental Psychopathology, 4,* 118–132.http://dx.doi.org/10.5127/jep.025411

Croskerry, P. (2002). Achieving quality in clinical decision making: Cognitive strategies and detection of bias. *Academic Emergency Medicine, 9,* 1184–1204. http://dx.doi.org/10.1197/aemj.9.11.1184/pdf

Croskerry, P. (2003). The importance of cognitive errors in diagnosis and strategies to minimize them. *Academic Medicine, 78,* 775–780.

Croskerry, P. (2009a). Clinical cognition and diagnostic error: Applications of a dual process model of reasoning. *Advances in Health Sciences Education, 14*(Suppl. 1), 27–35. http://dx.doi.org/10.1007/s10459-009-9182-2

Croskerry, P. (2009b). A universal model of diagnostic reasoning. *Academic Medicine, 84,* 1022–1028. http://dx.doi.org/10.1097/ACM.0b013e3181ace703

Croskerry, P., & Norman, G. (2008). Overconfidence in clinical decision making. *The American Journal of Medicine, 121*(Suppl.), S24–S29. http://dx.doi.org/10.1016/j.amjmed.2008.02.001

de Jong, P. J. (2014). Information processing. In P. Emmelkamp & T. Ehring (Eds.), *The Wiley handbook of anxiety disorders*. Malden, MA: Wiley Blackwell. http://dx.doi.org/10.1002/9781118775349.ch9

de Shazer, S. (1985). *Keys to solution in brief therapy*. New York, NY: Norton.

Dumont, F. (1993). Inferential heuristics in clinical problem formulation: Selective review of their strengths and weaknesses. *Professional Psychology: Research and Practice, 24*, 196–205. http://dx.doi.org/10.1037/0735-7028.24.2.196

Edwards, W., Miles, R. F., & von Winterfeldt, D. (Eds.). (2007). *Advances in decision analysis: From foundations to applications*. New York, NY: Cambridge University Press. http://dx.doi.org/10.1017/CBO9780511611308

Elliott, R. (2008). A linguistic phenomenology of ways of knowing and its implications for psychotherapy research and psychotherapy integration. *Journal of Psychotherapy Integration, 18*, 40–65. http://dx.doi.org/10.1037/1053-0479.18.1.40

Epstein, S. (2010). Demystifying intuition: What it is, what it does, and how it does it. *Psychological Inquiry, 21*, 295–312. http://dx.doi.org/10.1080/1047840X.2010.523875

Etkin, A., Prater, K. E., Hoeft, F., Menon, V., & Schatzberg, A. F. (2010). Failure of anterior cingulate activation and connectivity with the amygdala during implicit regulation of emotional processing in generalized anxiety disorder. *The American Journal of Psychiatry, 167*, 545–554. http://dx.doi.org/10.1176/appi.ajp.2009.09070931

Evans, J. St. B. T. (2007). *Hypothetical thinking: Dual processes in reasoning and judgement*. Hove, England: Psychology Press.

Evans, J. St. B. T. (2008). Dual-processing accounts of reasoning, judgment, and social cognition. *Annual Review of Psychology, 59*, 255–278. http://dx.doi.org/10.1146/annurev.psych.59.103006.093629

Evans, J. St. B. T. (2010). Intuition and reasoning: A dual-process perspective. *Psychological Inquiry, 21*, 313–326. http://dx.doi.org/10.1080/1047840X.2010.521057

Evans, J. St. B. T., & Stanovich, K. E. (2013). Dual-process theories of higher cognition: Advancing the debate. *Perspectives on Psychological Science, 8*, 223–241. http://dx.doi.org/10.1177/1745691612460685

Fredrickson, B. L. (2004). The broaden-and-build theory of positive emotions. *Philosophical Transactions of the Royal Society of London. Series B, Biological Sciences, 359*, 1367–1377. http://dx.doi.org/10.1098/rstb.2004.1512

Frensch, P. A., & Rünger, D. (2003). Implicit learning. *Current Directions in Psychological Science, 12*, 13–18. http://dx.doi.org/10.1111/1467-8721.01213

Garb, H. N. (1996). The representativeness and past-behavior heuristics in clinical judgment. *Professional Psychology: Research and Practice, 27*, 272–277. http://dx.doi.org/10.1037/0735-7028.27.3.272

Gawronski, B., & Creighton, L. A. (2013). Dual-process theories. In D. E. Carlston (Ed.), *The Oxford handbook of social cognition* (pp. 282–312). New York, NY: Oxford University Press.

Gigerenzer, G. (2008). Why heuristics work. *Perspectives on Psychological Science, 3,* 20–29. http://dx.doi.org/10.1111/j.1745-6916.2008.00058.x

Glöckner, A., & Witteman, C. (2010). Beyond dual-process models: A categorization of processes underlying intuitive judgment and decision making. *Thinking & Reasoning, 16,* 1–25. http://dx.doi.org/10.1080/13546780903395748

Hammond, K. R. (2010). Intuition, no! . . . Quasirationality, yes! *Psychological Inquiry, 21,* 327–337. http://dx.doi.org/10.1080/1047840X.2010.521483

Hammond, K. R., Hamm, R. M., Grassia, J., & Pearson, T. (1987). Direct comparison of the efficacy of intuitive and analytical cognition in expert judgment. *IEEE Transactions on Systems, Man, & Cybernetics, 17,* 753–770. http://dx.doi.org/10.1109/TSMC.1987.6499282

Han, S., & Lerner, J. S. (2009). Decision making. In D. Sander & K. Scherer (Eds.), *The Oxford companion to emotion and the affective sciences* (pp. 111–113). New York, NY: Oxford University Press.

Harding, T. P. (2004). Psychiatric disability and clinical decision making: The impact of judgment error and bias. *Clinical Psychology Review, 24,* 707–729. http://dx.doi.org/10.1016/j.cpr.2004.06.003

Hastie, R. (2001). Problems for judgment and decision making. *Annual Review of Psychology, 52,* 653–683. http://dx.doi.org/10.1146/annurev.psych.52.1.653

Hechter, M., & Horne, C. (2003). What is theory? In M. Hechter & C. Horne (Eds.), *Theories of social order: A reader* (pp. 1–8). Stanford, CA: Stanford University Press.

Jain, T. R., Aggarwal, S. C., & Rana, R. K. (2010–2011). *Basic statistics for economists.* New Delhi, India: VK Enterprises.

Jones-Smith, E. (2012). *Theories of counseling and psychotherapy: An integrative approach.* Thousand Oaks, CA: Sage.

Kahneman, D., & Frederick, S. (2002). Representativeness revisited: Attribute substitution in intuitive judgment. In T. Gilovich, D. Griffin, & D. Kahneman (Eds.), *Heuristics and biases: The psychology of intuitive judgment* (pp. 49–81). Cambridge, MA: Cambridge University Press. http://dx.doi.org/10.1017/CBO9780511808098.004

Kahneman, D., & Klein, G. (2009). Conditions for intuitive expertise: A failure to disagree. *American Psychologist, 64,* 515–526. http://dx.doi.org/10.1037/a0016755

Keller, N., Cokely, E. T., Katsikopoulos, K. V., & Wegwarth, O. (2010). Natural heuristics for decision making. *Journal of Cognitive Engineering and Decision Making, 4,* 256–274. http://dx.doi.org/10.1518/155534310X12844000801168

Keren, G., & Schul, Y. (2009). Two is not always better than one: A critical evaluation of two-system theories. *Perspectives on Psychological Science, 4,* 533–550. http://dx.doi.org/10.1111/j.1745-6924.2009.01164.x

Kiesler, D. J. (1988). *Therapeutic metacommunication: Therapist impact disclosure as feedback in psychotherapy.* Palo Alto, CA: Consulting Psychologists Press.

Kiesler, D. J. (1996). *Contemporary interpersonal theory and research: Personality, psychopathology, and psychotherapy.* New York, NY: Wiley.

Kim, H. S. (2010). *The nature of theoretical thinking in nursing* (3rd ed.). New York, NY: Springer.

Klein, G. (1998). *Sources of power: How people make decisions.* Cambridge, MA: MIT Press.

Klein, G. (2008). Naturalistic decision making. *Human Factors, 50,* 456–460. http://dx.doi.org/10.1518/001872008X288385

Klerman, G. L., Weissman, M. M., Rousansville, B. J., & Chevron, E. S. (1984). *Interpersonal psychotherapy of depression.* New York, NY: Basic Books.

Leary, T. F. (1957). *Interpersonal diagnosis of personality.* New York, NY: Ronald.

Lerner, J. S., & Tiedens, L. Z. (2006). Portrait of the angry decision maker: How appraisal tendencies shape anger's influence on cognition. *Journal of Behavioral Decision Making, 19,* 115–137. http://dx.doi.org/10.1002/bdm.515

Lieberman, M. D. (2003). Reflective and reflexive judgment processes: A social cognitive neuroscience approach. In J. P. Forgas, K. R. Williams, & W. von Hippel (Eds.), *Social judgments: Implicit and explicit processes* (pp. 44–67). New York, NY: Cambridge University Press.

Lieberman, M. D. (2007). The X- and C-systems: The neural basis of automatic and controlled social cognition. In E. Harmon-Jones & P. Winkelman (Eds.), *Fundamentals of social neuroscience* (pp. 290–315). New York, NY: Guilford Press.

Lodge, M., Taber, C. S., & Weber, C. (2006). First steps toward a dual process model of political beliefs, attitudes, and behavior. In D. P. Redlawsk (Ed.), *Feeling politics: Emotion in political information processing* (pp. 11–30). New York, NY: Palgrave Macmillan.

Lowenstein, G., & Lerner, J. S. (2003). The role of affect in decision making. In R. Davidson, K. Scherer, & H. Goldsmith (Eds.), *Handbook of affective science* (pp. 619–642). New York, NY: Oxford University Press.

Magnavita, J. J., & Anchin, J. C. (2014). *Unifying psychotherapy: Principles, methods, and evidence from clinical science.* New York, NY: Springer.

Messer, S. B. (2001). Introduction to the special issue on assimilative integration. *Journal of Psychotherapy Integration, 11,* 1–4. http://dx.doi.org/10.1023/A:1026619423048

Miller, R. B. (1992). Introduction: Philosophical problems of clinical research. In R. B. Miller (Ed.), *The restoration of dialogue: Readings in the philosophy of clinical psychology* (pp. 1–27). Washington, DC: American Psychological Association. http://dx.doi.org/10.1037/10112-010

Mitchell, S. A. (1988). *Relational concepts in psychoanalysis*. Cambridge, MA: Harvard University Press.

Mosier, K. L., & Fischer, U. (2010). The role of affect in naturalistic decision making. *Journal of Cognitive Engineering and Decision Making, 4*, 240–255. http://dx.doi.org/10.1518/155534310X12844000801122

Muran, J. C., Eubanks-Carter, C., & Safran, J. D. (2010). A relational approach to the treatment of personality dysfunction. In J. J. Magnavita (Ed.), *Evidence-based treatment of personality dysfunction: Principles, methods, and processes* (pp. 167–192). Washington, DC: American Psychological Association. http://dx.doi.org/10.1037/12130-006

Najavits, L. M. (1997). Psychotherapists' implicit theories of therapy. *Journal of Psychotherapy Integration, 7*, 1–16.

Newell, B. R., & Shanks, D. R. (2014). Unconscious influences on decision making: A critical review. *Behavioral and Brain Sciences, 37*, 1–19. http://dx.doi.org/10.1017/S0140525X12003214

Ogden, T. H. (2004). The analytic third: Implications for psychoanalytic theory and technique. *The Psychoanalytic Quarterly, 73*, 167–195. http://dx.doi.org/10.1002/j.2167-4086.2004.tb00156.x

Parnell, G. S., Bresnick, T. A., Tani, S. N., & Johnson, E. R. (Eds.). (2013). *Handbook of decision analysis*. Hoboken, NJ: Wiley. http://dx.doi.org/10.1002/9781118515853

Pascual-Leone, A., & Greenberg, L. S. (2007). Insight and awareness in experiential therapy. In L. G. Castonguay & C. Hill (Eds.), *Insight in psychotherapy* (pp. 31–56). Washington, DC: American Psychological Association.

Patterson, R. E., Pierce, B. J., Bell, H. H., & Klein, G. (2010). Implicit learning, tacit knowledge, expertise development, and naturalistic decision making. *Journal of Cognitive Engineering and Decision Making, 4*, 289–303.

Peters, E., Vastfjall, D., Garling, T., & Slovic, P. (2006). Affect and decision making: A "hot" topic. *Journal of Behavioral Decision Making, 19*, 79–85. http://dx.doi.org/10.1002/bdm.528

Pfister, H.-R., & Bohm, G. (2008). The multiplicity of emotions: A framework of emotional functions in decision making. *Judgment and Decision Making, 3*, 5–17.

Phillips, M. L., Ladouceur, C. D., & Drevets, W. C. (2008). A neural model of voluntary and automatic emotion regulation: Implications for understanding the pathophysiology and neurodevelopment of bipolar disorder. *Molecular Psychiatry, 13*, 829, 833–857. http://dx.doi.org/10.1038/mp.2008.65

Pincus, A. L. (2010). Introduction to the special series on integrating personality, psychopathology, and psychotherapy using interpersonal assessment. *Journal of Personality Assessment, 92*, 467–470. http://dx.doi.org/10.1080/00223891.2010.513706

Richler, J. J., Wong, Y. K., & Gauthier, I. (2011). Perceptual expertise as a shift from strategic interference to automatic holistic processing. *Current Directions in Psychological Science, 20*, 129–134. http://dx.doi.org/10.1177/0963721411402472

Rosenbloom, M. H., Schmahmann, J. D., & Price, B. H. (2012). The functional neuroanatomy of decision-making. *The Journal of Neuropsychiatry and Clinical Neurosciences, 24*, 266–277. http://dx.doi.org/10.1176/appi.neuropsych.11060139

Safran, J. D., & Muran, J. C. (2000). *Negotiating the therapeutic alliance: A relational treatment guide*. New York, NY: Guilford Press.

Sandler, J. (1983). Reflections on some relations between psychoanalytic concepts and psychoanalytic practice. *The International Journal of Psychoanalysis, 64*, 35–45.

Satpute, A. B., & Lieberman, M. D. (2006). Integrating automatic and controlled processes into neurocognitive models of social cognition. *Brain Research, 1079*, 86–97. http://dx.doi.org/10.1016/j.brainres.2006.01.005

Schneider, W., & Chein, J. M. (2003). Controlled & automatic processing: Behavior, theory, and biological mechanisms. *Cognitive Science, 27*, 525–559. http://dx.doi.org/10.1207/s15516709cog2703_8

Schottenbauer, M. A., Glass, C. R., & Arnkoff, D. B. (2007). Decision making and psychotherapy integration: Theoretical considerations, preliminary data, and implications for future research. *Journal of Psychotherapy Integration, 17*, 225–250. http://dx.doi.org/10.1037/1053-0479.17.3.225

Schraagen, J. M., Klein, G., & Hoffman, R. R. (2008). The macrocognition framework of naturalistic decision making. In J. M. Schraagen, L. G. Militello, T. Ormerod, & R. Lipshitz (Eds.), *Naturalistic decision making and macrocognition* (pp. 3–25). Aldershot, England: Ashgate.

Schraagen, J. M., Militello, L. G., Ormerod, T., & Lipshitz, R. R. (Eds.). (2008). *Naturalistic decision making and macrocognition*. Aldershot, England: Ashgate.

Shaban, R. Z. (2005). Theories of clinical judgment and decision-making: A review of the theoretical literature. *Journal of Emergency Primary Health Care, 3*, 1–12.

Shah, A. K., & Oppenheimer, D. M. (2008). Heuristics made easy: An effort-reduction framework. *Psychological Bulletin, 134*, 207–222. http://dx.doi.org/10.1037/0033-2909.134.2.207

Shilling, H. N. (2012). *How integrative and eclectic therapists make treatment selection decisions: A qualitative study* (Unpublished doctoral dissertation). University of Wisconsin–Madison.

Shoben, E. J., Jr. (1962). The counselor's theory as personal trait. *The Personnel & Guidance Journal, 40*, 617–621. http://dx.doi.org/10.1002/j.2164-4918.1962.tb02171.x

Sinclair, M., Sadler-Smith, E., & Hodgkinson, G. P. (2009). The role of intuition in strategic decision making. In L. A. Costanzo & R. B. MacKay (Eds.), *Handbook of research on strategy and foresight* (pp. 393–417). Northampton, MA: Edward Elgar. http://dx.doi.org/10.4337/9781848447271.00032

Singer, J. A. (2005). *Personality and psychotherapy: Treating the whole person*. New York, NY: Guilford Press.

Singer, J. A., & Conway, M. A. (2011). Reconsidering therapeutic action: Loewald, cognitive neuroscience and the integration of memory's duality. *The International Journal of Psychoanalysis, 92,* 1183–1207. http://dx.doi.org/10.1111/j.1745-8315.2011.00415.x

Slovic, P., Finucane, M. L., Peters, E., & MacGregor, D. G. (2004). Risk as analysis and risk as feelings: Some thoughts about affect, reason, risk, and rationality. *Risk Analysis, 24,* 311–322. http://dx.doi.org/10.1111/j.0272-4332.2004.00433.x

Smith, E. R., & DeCoster, J. (2000). Dual-process models in social and cognitive psychology: Conceptual integration and links to underlying memory systems. *Personality and Social Psychology Review, 4,* 108–131. http://dx.doi.org/10.1207/S15327957PSPR0402_01

Spence, D. P. (1982). *Narrative truth and historical truth: Meaning and interpretation in psychoanalysis.* New York, NY: Norton.

Spunt, R. P., & Lieberman, M. D. (2013). The busy social brain: Evidence for automaticity and control in the neural systems supporting social cognition and action understanding. *Psychological Science, 24,* 80–86. http://dx.doi.org/10.1177/0956797612450884

Stanovich, K. E. (2005). *The robot's rebellion.* Chicago, IL: University of Chicago Press.

Stanovich, K. E. (2009). Distinguishing the reflective, algorithmic, and autonomous minds: Is it time for a tri-process theory? In J. St. B. T. Evans & K. Frankish (Eds.), *In two minds: Dual processes and beyond* (pp. 55–88). New York, NY: Oxford University Press. http://dx.doi.org/10.1093/acprof:oso/9780199230167.003.0003

Stanovich, K. E. (2011). *Rationality and the reflective mind.* New York, NY: Oxford University Press.

Stanovich, K. E., & Toplak, M. E. (2012). Defining features versus incidental correlates of Type 1 and Type 2 processing. *Mind & Society, 11,* 3–13. http://dx.doi.org/10.1007/s11299-011-0093-6

Sullivan, H. S. (1953). *The collected works of Harry Stack Sullivan* (Vol. 1). New York, NY: Norton.

Thompson, V. A., Prowse Turner, J. A., & Pennycook, G. (2011). Intuition, reason, and metacognition. *Cognitive Psychology, 63,* 107–140. http://dx.doi.org/10.1016/j.cogpsych.2011.06.001

Todd, P. M., & Gigerenzer, G. (2007). Environments that make us smart: Ecological rationality. *Current Directions in Psychological Science, 16,* 167–171. http://dx.doi.org/10.1111/j.1467-8721.2007.00497.x

Tversky, A., & Kahneman, D. (1974). Judgment under uncertainty: Heuristics and biases. *Science, 185,* 1124–1131. http://dx.doi.org/10.1126/science.185.4157.1124

Wachtel, P. L. (1997). *Psychoanalysis, behavior therapy, and the relational world.* Washington, DC: American Psychological Association. http://dx.doi.org/10.1037/10383-000

Wiers, R. W., Gladwin, T. E., Hofmann, W., Salemink, E., & Ridderinkhof, K. R. (2013). Cognitive bias modification and cognitive control training in addiction and related psychopathology: Mechanisms, clinical perspectives, and ways forward. *Clinical Psychological Science, 1,* 192–212. http://dx.doi.org/10.1177/2167702612466547

Wiggins, J. S. (1979). A psychological taxonomy of trait-descriptive terms: The interpersonal domain. *Journal of Personality and Social Psychology, 37,* 395–412. http://dx.doi.org/10.1037/0022-3514.37.3.395

Zeelenberg, M., Nelissen, R. M. A., Breugelmans, S. M., & Pieters, R. (2008). On emotion specificity in decision making: Why feeling is for doing. *Judgment and Decision Making, 3,* 18–27.

4

CLINICAL PRACTICE GUIDELINE DEVELOPMENT AND DECISION MAKING

LYNN F. BUFKA AND ERIN F. SWEDISH

Clinical practice guidelines (CPGs) are increasingly becoming a vital component of clinical decision making. The complexity of decision making requires both empirical evidence, which can be found in evidence-based guidelines, and clinical expertise; neither alone is sufficient, as acknowledged in both Institute of Medicine (IOM; 2005) and American Psychological Association (APA; APA Presidential Task Force, 2006) policy. The development of CPGs is being fueled by a number of forces that are shaping how behavioral and mental health care will be delivered and reimbursed, not the least of which is the focus on improving care and patient satisfaction while containing costs. Most clinicians, when they understand the process of clinical guideline development and the checks and balances that are built into the system, will find that CPGs can be reliable resources to guide clinical decision making. Behavioral and mental health clinicians need to become acquainted with the process of developing CPGs. Familiarity with the processes of CPG

http://dx.doi.org/10.1037/14711-004
Clinical Decision Making in Mental Health Practice, J. J. Magnavita (Editor)
Copyright © 2016 by the American Psychological Association. All rights reserved.

development and the efforts undertaken to reduce potential forms of bias (see Chapter 2, this volume, for an in-depth presentation of these forms) is critical for their acceptance and uptake. In this chapter, we discuss how CPGs enhance clinical decision making. We also provide an overview of the development of CPGs and the efforts expended to reduce biases.

WHAT ARE CLINICAL PRACTICE GUIDELINES?

Over the past 2 decades there has been an increasing call for evidence-based practice in all of health care, including treatment for behavioral and mental health disorders. Both internal and external pressures, such as demands for accountability, marketplace changes, technological advances, and the explosion of research literature, have resulted in increased attention to the quality and content of psychotherapy (Goodheart, 2010). Currently, numerous empirically supported treatments (ESTs) for individuals with mental health problems have been shown to be efficacious. More specifically, sophisticated methodological designs have shown robust effects for various ESTs for anxiety, depression, posttraumatic stress disorder, and bipolar disorder, to name a few (Barlow, Levitt, & Bufka, 1999; Barrett & Ollendick, 2003). Large-scale efforts to disseminate ESTs have occurred as the state of science in psychology advances (Chorpita, 2002). However, other widely practiced psychotherapy approaches have not yet accumulated corresponding supportive bodies of research. Although lack of evidence does not indicate lack of efficacy (APA Presidential Task Force, 2006), the lack of evidence is problematic when payers and other third parties determine practices or otherwise demand certain clinical treatment approaches.

CPGs are one tool to help link research and practice. CPGs as defined by the IOM are "systematically developed statements to assist practitioner and patient decisions about appropriate health care for specific clinical circumstances" (Field & Lohr, 1990, p. 38). The development of quality CPGs for the treatment of behavioral and mental health disorders has the potential to help patients, mental health practitioners, policymakers, and administrators make better decisions about how to proceed with care.

Evidence-based CPGs are vital for effective clinical decision making and efficient patient care. The three-circle model for evidence-based clinical decisions (see Figure 4.1) was developed to promote a clear process for decision making to inform clinicians' treatment decisions (Haynes, Sackett, Gray, Cook, & Guyatt, 1996). Separately, the three circles illustrate that evidence-based clinical decisions use the best available research; clinical expertise; and patient values, characteristics, and circumstances. The

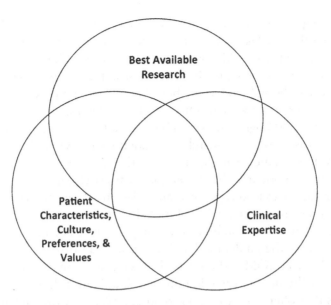

Figure 4.1. Three-circle model of evidence based practice in psychology. Data from Haynes, Sackett, Gray, Cook, and Guyatt (1996).

convergence of the circles highlights the importance of integrating all three sources of data in clinical decision making. By incorporating these three distinct yet overlapping circles, the model recognizes the need for the synthesis of available information and knowledge, both from research and clinical expertise, to provide the best treatment for each individual patient on a case-by-case basis.

The three-circle model of decision making emerged as a part of the evidence-based medicine (EBM) movement or the "conscientious, explicit, and judicious use of current best evidence in making decisions about the care of individual patients" (Sackett, Rosenberg, Gray, Haynes, & Richardson, 1996, p. 71). Sackett et al. (1996) also noted the importance of clinical expertise and that both research evidence and clinical expertise must be evaluated with an understanding of patients' values and preferences. A definition of EBM was later adapted for policy by both the IOM (2001) and the APA (APA Presidential Task Force, 2006). Evidence-based CPGs are critical tools for assisting clinicians with the inherent complexity of decision making in the clinical situation. The aim is to enhance the quality and efficiency of health care and to identify gaps in knowledge by providing the pros and cons of different interventions. Well-developed guidelines serve as an important protection against the inherent biases that are common in clinical decision making (see Chapter 5, this volume).

It is important to note that CPGs are explicit and actionable recommendations that are based on a critical appraisal of scientific evidence where attempts are made to avoid biasing the results so that they represent a valuable and reliable resource for clinicians. Research contains biases, and therefore CPGs can be vulnerable to those biases, but the process of guideline development provides some mechanisms for evaluating the literature for key sources of bias, although it does not eliminate all of it. For instance, the stringent standards by which research for guidelines is reviewed results in only very well-done studies being included in the analyses, and emerging areas of research or informative but lesser quality research might not be included in the final analyses leading to recommendations. Users of CPGs can generally feel confident in the quality of included evidence but should recognize that other sources of research evidence may not have been considered in the development of the guideline. CPGs are not a substitute for clinical judgment, and in fact, IOM and APA both recognize the importance of clinical expertise in the decision-making process. Guidelines should be viewed as resources that offer basic rules, but rigid compliance with guidelines is not in service of the patient; rather, the combination of high-quality evidence and clinical expertise is the basis for professional accountability. At times, depending on the clinical circumstances, such as patient preferences, cultural and ethnic factors, comorbidities, and so forth, there may be reasons for not complying with a guideline. Thus, guidelines offer one reliable source of information among many essential to effective clinical decision making.

Furthermore, CPGs are not established standards of care that have legal implications, although this may change as research advances and guidelines become more sophisticated. Informed clinical decision making combines the best available information with ethical standards. Practitioners may be concerned that CPGs reduce autonomy or create "cookbook" treatment (Arkowitz & Lilienfeld, 2008), but implementing the recommendations in CPGs requires training and clinical expertise (see Chapter 5, this volume). Additionally, CPGs do not determine what form of care ought to be covered by both public and private health benefit plans, but it is likely that as their credibility is established they will serve as resources that will be used as guideposts for policymakers, patients, and third-party payers. Guidelines are not synonymous with reimbursement policies, but those policies may certainly be informed by CPGs.

The National Guidelines Clearinghouse (http://www.guideline.gov) is sponsored by the Agency for Healthcare Research and Quality (AHRQ). The current criteria for guideline inclusion, effective June 2014, are that guidelines contain systematically developed recommendations; they are developed by an organization; they are based on a systematic review (SR) of evidence; they contain an assessment of the benefits and harms of recommended and alternative care options; and the full text of the document, including the most recent published version, is available. These criteria are consistent with emerging best practices in guideline development (IOM, 2011a, 2011b). Examples of CPGs that meet current quality criteria include screening for cognitive impairment in older adults (developed by the U.S. Preventive Services Task Force) and the use of fluoride to prevent cavities (developed by the American Dental Association). Furthermore, U.S. Department of Veterans Affairs (VA) and the Department of Defense generate joint CPGs relevant to health care providers in the Veterans Health Administration and Military Health systems. In the United Kingdom, high-quality guidelines have been developed by the National Institute for Health and Care Excellence. Currently, APA is generating CPGs for mental and behavior health problems in the United States to help guide mental health clinicians in the decision-making process. The APA process is consistent with the emerging best practices in guideline development (Hollon et al., 2014).

HISTORY OF GUIDELINE DEVELOPMENT

In the United States, unlike some other countries, the federal government has not assumed responsibility for creating CPGs. Typically, professional associations or health care organizations either singly or collaboratively create these guidelines in the United States. The U.S. Agency for Health Care Policy and Research was established in 1989 with responsibilities that included outcomes research and practice guideline development (Gray, Gusmano, & Collins, 2003). In the mid 1990s, the agency faced criticism over its work. Although the agency ultimately survived, it was renamed the Agency for Healthcare Research and Quality, and its focus shifted to comparative effectiveness research rather than guideline development. It is in this context that guideline development by organizations and professional associations increased, and standards for guideline development emerged in 2011.

Although the development of CPGs flourished in the 1990s and 2000s, guidelines had strong opponents (Abrahamson & Saakvitne, 2000; Reed, McLaughlin, & Newman, 2002). Criticism of existing guidelines included lack of generality or objectivity, suggesting potential bias in their content and therefore application or concerns regarding the presentation of the science (Craske & Zucker, 2001). For instance, guidelines from government entities, such as the VA, are focused on specific populations and therefore might not be applicable to other populations. Additionally, guidelines developed by professional societies were seen as potentially slanting toward the interests of specific guilds, and guidelines funded by industry were potentially biased toward industry interest, whether that funding and interest might be pharmaceutical, device, or managed care. The current evolution in the development of guidelines is heavily grounded in the advances in decision analytics presented in this volume.

For many years, APA weighed the relative merits of developing CPGs (also known in many settings as *treatment guidelines* or *practice parameters*). APA chose not to develop such guidelines in the 1990s but instead developed the "Criteria for Evaluating Treatment Guidelines," a document that was adopted as policy in 2002 (APA, 2002). This document offered criteria to evaluate CPGs promulgated by health care organizations, government agencies, professional associations, and other entities and proved useful for this purpose, especially in light of APA's decision not to develop CPGs at that time. This document also provided an APA definition of treatment guidelines (CPGs), as distinct from professional practice guidelines, which "consist of recommendations to professionals concerning their conduct and the issues to be considered in particular areas of clinical practice rather than on patient outcomes or recommendations for specific treatments or specific clinical procedures at the patient level" (APA, 2002, p. 1052).

However, since the 1990s, the environment for provision of psychological services has changed, and many health disciplines are utilizing guidelines for the purposes of synthesizing the research and conveying what is known about best practices in treating various conditions and disorders. In 2005, APA adopted a policy statement defining evidence-based practice in psychology as "the integration of the best available research with clinical expertise in the context of patient characteristics, culture, and preferences" (APA Presidential Task Force, 2006, p. 273). An accompanying report elaborating on these principles was subsequently published (APA Presidential Task Force, 2006). These documents were met with some controversy: Some critics thought research was undervalued, whereas others wanted greater emphasis on the value of clinical expertise. Nevertheless, these documents laid the foundation for future APA policy developments, underscoring the research foundation of psychological practice.

After this policy statement was adopted, leaders in psychology began to reexamine the role of CPGs in health care and asked if now was the time for APA to begin developing CPGs. Concerns about APA noninvolvement in CPG development included the possibility that topical guidelines that did not include psychosocial interventions would regulate treatment reimbursement and institutional quality controls and that existing guidelines overemphasize medications to the relative neglect of often more preferred and effective psychosocial interventions. Additionally, psychological science undergirds clinical practice, and CPGs would be an opportunity to highlight that connection and bring that evidence more broadly into health care decision making. Also, psychologists' research training provides the knowledge base and analytic skills necessary to understand, use, and oversee the development of evidence-based guidelines. For these reasons, APA's Council of Representatives approved the undertaking of a strategic initiative to develop CPGs and appointed an advisory steering committee in 2010. The committee has reviewed key issues in the arena of guideline development to create a process for APA that could best meet the needs of the organization and best utilize all potential resources (Hollon et al., 2014). These processes are consistent with the standards described in two recent IOM reports, *Clinical Practice Guidelines We Can Trust* and *Finding What Works in Health Care: Standards for Systematic Reviews* (IOM, 2011a, 2011b).

Evidence-based guideline generation typically involves (a) the conduct of a comprehensive SR of the empirical literature and (b) presentation of the findings from the SR to a *guideline development panel* (GDP). The GDP, consisting of practitioners, scientists, methodological experts, and patient representatives, is then asked to generate recommendations that are informed by the empirical literature but take clinical experience into account (Falck-Ytter & Schünemann, 2009). This results in CPG recommendations derived from the best available research evidence as filtered through expert clinical judgment and reflective of patient values and preferences.

The recently published IOM standards promise to lead to major changes in the way CPGs are developed (Kung, Miller, & Mackowiak, 2012). One standard addresses the formation and functioning of GDPs tasked with generating the treatment recommendations (IOM, 2011a). Standards for the basis of those recommendations, SRs of the literature, are addressed in the second IOM publication (IOM, 2011b). Prior CPGs have been quite diverse with respect to the methods followed and the way their recommendations were made. To create uniformity in guideline quality, the IOM created standards by which all CPGs should be developed. These standards are summarized in Exhibit 4.1 and discussed in the following section.

EXHIBIT 4.1
Institute of Medicine Standards for Developing
Trustworthy Clinical Practice Guidelines

- Transparency in development and funding
- Disclose, manage and resolve conflicts of interest
- Panels multidisciplinary, balanced and include patient/community involvement (adversarial collaboration)
- Systematic reviews of literature are basis for guideline recommendations
- Rate quality of evidence and recommendation strength
- Recommendations framed as actionable statements
- Submit draft guideline for public review and comments
- Update guideline periodically as necessary

Note. Data from Institute of Medicine (2011a).

INSTITUTE OF MEDICINE STANDARDS FOR CLINICAL PRACTICE GUIDELINES

Transparency

To ensure that guideline development is perceived to be as free of bias as possible, developers need to be transparent in reporting the processes of guideline development and sources of funding. Although reporting alone does not ensure lack of bias, the public is able to discern potential sources of influence and weigh those contributions in the development process. Additionally, transparency in the steps of guideline development ensures that all those not directly involved are at least familiar with the processes for how panel members were selected, how decisions were made, how recommendations were derived, and other key components of the development process.

Conflicts of Interest

Much attention has been focused on the potential impact of financial conflicts of interest (COI), such as industry support or grant funding, financial remuneration for training, and royalties from related publication, but increasingly the potential bias from nonfinancial, primarily intellectual, COI has also been addressed (Akl, Karl, & Guyatt, 2012; Guyatt et al., 2010). Guideline panel members with strong allegiance to particular clinical practices or orientations may not be able to review dispassionately the evidence regarding particular methods or practices. Or, in discussions about the evidence and potential recommendations, GDP members with a particular COI may attempt to exert their point of view when it coincides with their areas of expertise or areas of research funding. Hence it becomes important for all involved to first disclose any potential or actual COI so that the panel is informed. Then the panel can make determinations regarding how to manage any such conflicts. Management of such conflicts may range from basic acknowledgement of potential allegiance to abstention from voting to nonparticipation in deliberations to outright removal from the panel itself. And, of course, documentation of such disclosure and management of COI ensures transparency for those who will later read, evaluate and use the guidelines.

Guideline Development Panel Composition

Guideline panels composed of experts with a variety of perspectives promote the possibility for "adversarial collaboration," that is, for competing ideas to be evaluated and challenged in order to arrive at recommendations. Even when guidelines are developed by one professional organization, formally including other professionals such that panels are multidisciplinary can increase the likelihood that multiple perspectives are considered and addressed in the guideline. Guidelines developed by researchers, clinicians, and community members who represent a broad swath of potential contributors and users have a greater potential for reducing bias and incorporating key considerations from multiple perspectives in the final product. Additionally, strategies to incorporate public feedback during guideline development also provide an opportunity to ensure that key ideas are addressed in guidelines and content is framed in a manner applicable to a variety of users. The risk of one perspective possibly dominating or biasing the guideline is reduced by the adversarial collaboration, so such guidelines have the potential to serve as useful tools for decision making because users may feel confident in the final recommendations.

Interaction With the Systematic Review Team

CPGs based on high-quality SRs can serve as a foundation for clinical decision making. Many practitioners are not familiar with the methodology of SRs, but that process itself has several procedures to reduce the potential for bias. These procedures ensure that only research that meets specific standards are included in the review, and many, if not all, guideline developers are moving to adopt these procedures. One potential downside of the rigorous decision making regarding inclusion and exclusion of research studies is that some potentially informative research may not be included in the review. However, when guideline panels work with the SR team (usually these are distinct entities), panel members can provide input to the process and convey important information. Keeping the review team distinct from the panel supports the SR team's standard approach to reviewing the literature without undue influence from the panel, but some interaction between the two ensures that the end review will be of use to the GDP. Users of finished guidelines can be assured that those based on SRs represent the strongest findings in the professional literature.

Recommendation Evidence and Articulation

Recommendations are at the heart of any guideline document, and those formulated with a clear rationale and with reference to the strength of the research evidence will engender confidence in their use for decision making. Recommendations that convey the strength (and gaps) of the relevant evidence as well as discussion of the potential benefits and harms are likely to be most useful. Although there are many areas where abundant empirical findings can be culled, others may have a dearth of evidence and need further research. The quality ratings of recommendations indicate not only confidence in the effect of an intervention but also that the evidence supports a particular clinical decision by considering the benefit of the intervention, potential risks, problems of not intervening, and potential patient values (Balshem et al., 2011). Factors such as directness of evidence, precision, and publication bias are all important considerations in evaluating the body of evidence in writing recommendations. Guideline developers are also encouraged to explain how panel members' values, opinions, theory, or experiences may have informed the recommendations. This context, along with clear information regarding ratings in the confidence of the evidence underpinning the recommendations and the general strength of the recommendation, can make it easier for users to determine the value of particular recommendations to their specific decision making. Each of these elements reduces the potential for bias in the guidelines statements.

Also, clearly articulated recommendations make it easy to determine what the recommended action is and when it should be done, thus facilitating clinical decision making because the user can determine whether the specific recommendation applies to the case at hand. Recommendations that are actionable are preferred in CPGs. Although actionable recommendation statements have more to do with implementing the end product, such statements are also more readily measurable, and the impact of the CPG can be evaluated. Such evaluations reflect the quality and usefulness of the guidelines for end users.

External Review

Subjecting guidelines to a rigorous external review process enhances their usability for decision making. External review that encompasses feedback from relevant stakeholders, such as scientific and clinical experts, agencies and organizations, patients, and the public, provides an opportunity for a broad spectrum of perspectives to be considered. Potential biases may be identified through this process, and revisions can be made to correct for these. When guideline developers document comments received and responses to such comments, users have a clearer understanding of the process as well as the potential strengths and limitations of any such guideline when used in decision making.

Updating

Users need to know that guidelines are current. Literature on particular topics and interventions is continually in development, and guideline developers must stay attuned to the professional literature to be certain that emerging evidence is either incorporated into guideline updates or determined to not alter the validity of the existing document. Guidelines deemed to be too far afield from the extant research literature do not deserve significant consideration by users. Out-of-date guidelines will not reflect current knowledge, leading to possible errors in recommendations. Best practices suggest that CPGs need to be reviewed and updated, minimally, every 5 years.

To the extent possible, the APA guideline development process follows these standards. By so doing, APA's guidelines will be perceived as trustworthy and useful tools that are essential and relevant for effective clinical decision making.

SYSTEMATIC REVIEWS

Systematic reviews, which undergird the CPG development process, are rigorous, planned reviews of the literature that focus on specific questions. Those who conduct SRs are focused on the quality of the evidence for the effect of the intervention, while other factors of evidence quality are relevant in writing recommendations (Balshem et al., 2011). The IOM (2011b) has published standards for SRs in order to provide guidance to those who conduct such reviews and to improve the overall quality of SRs. AHRQ has provided guidance for managing COI as it relates to the development of SRs and recommends balancing expertise, independence, and transparency in the conduct of reviews (Viswanathan et al., 2013). These IOM and AHRQ guidelines include creating a team to conduct the review that has the appropriate expertise and experience, managing the bias and COI of team members and those providing input into the SR, soliciting user and stakeholder input as the review is designed and conducted, developing an analytic framework to define key clinical questions to be addressed and to link health interventions to outcomes, and developing an SR protocol and submitting that protocol for peer review. Developing the SR protocol is one of the more rigorous aspects of the process and includes specifying the screening and selection criteria of studies, describing precisely what will be addressed (outcomes, interventions, comparison groups, and so on), defining the search strategy to identify relevant evidence and the procedures for selecting studies, describing the data extraction strategy, and determining the process for identifying and resolving disagreement between researchers conducting the SR. In addition, the SR team must have specified practices for critically appraising identified studies and evaluating the body of evidence.

These components, including specified search strategies, identification of studies, and specified strategies for critically appraising and evaluating the evidence, serve to safeguard the review from bias. Although eliminating all bias is not likely, careful attempts to reduce sources of bias, such as lack of randomization, differences between comparison groups at baseline, and high rates of attrition, and highlighting points of bias lead to higher quality SRs and the potential to then have more confidence in final guideline products based on high-quality reviews. When efforts are not made to control for sources of bias, the potential for compounding these problems in the final product increases.

A variety of methodological sources of bias can influence the SR process and the quality of the recommendations derived from such reviews. GRADE (Grading of Recommendations Assessment, Development, and Evaluation) was developed to address many of these concerns (see http://www.gradeworkinggroup.org/index.htm). Some of the methodological sources of bias that are addressed include strategies for evaluating research studies on a variety of components, such as how participants were allocated to conditions, whether conditions were concealed, and how dropouts were managed. Additionally, as the evidence across a body of research is evaluated, inconsistencies and imprecision in findings as well as whether the evidence is direct or indirect are noted and evaluated before recommendations are made. Last, publication bias can also influence the results of SRs and the available evidence from which conclusions can be made. GRADE, and adaptations of GRADE, provide methods for addressing each of these areas during the recommendation development process. The more confidence users have that these sources of bias were addressed, the more confidence they can have in the final guideline product.

ROLE OF CLINICAL PRACTICE GUIDELINES IN REDUCING BIAS IN DECISION MAKING

Although CPGs have important external functions, such as providing guidance to policymakers regarding appropriate services for various disorders, CPGs are fundamental to practitioners' clinical decision making. CPGs that are built on high-quality SRs have the potential to reduce clinician bias and support optimal clinical decision making. Although many factors can influence decision making and introduce bias, such as the misuse of decision heuristics and cognitive errors, one source of bias is an individual's inability to stay current with the exploding research literature. APA alone publishes more than 80 journals in psychology, and many other relevant, peer-reviewed journals exist. More than 10 years ago, Bazian Limited (http://www.bazian.com/) estimated that 25,000 medical journals were in print and 8,000 articles were published daily. Even in the circumscribed field of mental and behavioral health, individual clinicians cannot keep up with the literature. Adding to that, the vast majority of studies are not sufficient, on their own, to reliably guide clinical decisions. An individual reader may not be familiar with the breadth of research on a given topic, but his or her decision making could be strongly influenced by the portion of literature with which he or she is familiar. If that portion covers only a segment of the relevant topic, the reader's capacity to derive appropriate conclusions is limited as well. Even the most dedicated scientist–practitioner can feel overwhelmed when attempting to keep up with the complete breadth of the scientific literature.

CPGs serve as a synthesis of the research with a systematic strategy for deriving recommendations. This reduces the tendency to base clinical decisions on the most recent literature but ensures that such decisions are based on a systematic, comprehensive, objective evaluation of the entire evidence base. CPGs are not themselves without bias, but the conduct of the SR serves to limit some of the bias in the research literature, and the transparent development process allows users to evaluate where and whether bias may have occurred in the panel's decision making. Of course, clinical decision making is not based simply on CPGs or even the empirical clinical research; other sources of evidence also contribute to the process, such as professional knowledge from related fields (e.g., developmental or cognitive psychology), clinical interview and observation, theory, and patient response to the interaction and intervention (Goodheart, 2006).

Increasingly, health care has focused on shared decision making, where clinician and patient collaboratively arrive at and refine treatment decisions. When treatment recommendations are relatively straightforward, decision making can be as well, but this is rarely the case. When multiple options exist, with differing balances of harms and benefits, understanding the individual patient's values and preferences becomes critical in making treatment decisions. Effective CPGs can facilitate shared decision making with clear recommendations and a clear explanation of the relative harms and benefits of each recommendation. CPGs that do not provide that information are less useful to the patient in decision making, but there may be times when that information simply does not exist in the literature. The CPG still affords some benefit, but the clinician must then interpret and utilize appropriately the content of the CPG.

Shared decision making can be accomplished with the use of a variety of decision support tools, generated for both clinicians and patients. Decision support tools can range from simple printed disease fact sheets containing symptom and treatment information to straightforward clinical algorithms to sophisticated electronic algorithms embedded in electronic health records. Even something as basic as a checklist has proven to be effective and lifesaving (Gawande, 2009). As CPGs are developed and refined, they are an important source of information for developers using decision analytics to provide support tools, although they have not always been developed with this in mind. Greater collaboration between developers of CPGs and decision support tools will likely result in products of greater use to patients and their providers (van der Weijden, Boivin, Burgers, Schünemann, & Elwyn, 2012). Tools developed from the same evidence base will be able to both highlight the same range of interventions and considerations and provide consistent information to all those involved in evaluating options.

RELEVANCE OF CLINICAL PRACTICE GUIDELINES FOR DECISION MAKING

Evidence-based CPGs can have numerous advantages in informing clinical decisions in mental and behavioral health settings. For example, it is nearly impossible for mental health clinicians to stay current on all of the available literature on prevention and treatment of behavioral and mental health problems; therefore, CPGs can provide clinicians with a clear and concise reference to navigate the scientific research. By using CPGs, mental health clinicians can ensure that their patients receive care that is informed by the best up-to-date evidence.

Additionally, research suggests that recommendations provided by CPGs can improve clinical decision making. For example, Grimshaw and colleagues found that CPGs can produce positive changes in clinical practice and patient outcome (Grimshaw et al., 1995). Furthermore, the VA has found a positive impact on clinical practice patterns and patient outcomes in several studies examining clinician use of CPGs in treating a variety of diseases (e.g., chronic obstructive pulmonary disease, asthma, sexually transmitted diseases). For instance, the use of CPGs in the treatment of pressure ulcers led to a 25% reduction in the development of additional pressure ulcers (Berlowitz & Halpern, 1997).

Furthermore, the development of rigorous evidence-based guidelines that consolidate results of numerous studies has the potential to improve consistency in clinical decision making by avoiding the inherent biases to which we are all subject. The consolidation of recent evidence from the literature about the relative effectiveness of various treatment options can also help simplify the inherent complexity of decision making. Evidence-based CPGs promote rational, informed clinical decision making that reflects the best available scientific evidence. Often in psychotherapy practice, decisions need to be made quickly (see Chapter 2, this volume), so guidelines can help clinicians to more rapidly recognize options and choice points. Ultimately, this helps to improve the quality of care and to reduce the inconsistency with which it is delivered. CPGs can also reduce variations in service delivery by informing public and scientific policy to ensure that interventions are appropriately covered and thus available to every patient.

An important benefit of CPGs is that they serve as decision-making and educational aids not only for providers but for patients, as well. CPGs allow for patient participation in clinical decision making, coordination of care, and use of best practices. To counter the inconsistent recommendations about best practices in health care settings promoted via the media, CPGs can provide credible and consistent information that increases patient understanding about the best treatments for health conditions. As such, guidelines can help inform patients' decisions and clarify patient preferences.

Concerns have been raised that CPGs will replace clinical judgment, although this should not be considered their purpose. Optimal treatment requires clinical expertise to synthesize the most relevant high-quality information to make clinical decisions. CPGs are recommendations based on the best available research evidence at the time of their development. They are not substitutes for clinical judgment, but they are used in conjunction with clinical judgment to provide the best possible care. The responsibility remains with the clinician to combine the evidence from CPGs with clinical expertise and patient values in managing individual patients and achieving the best possible outcomes. Evidence is used in practice to help reduce uncertainty in decision making, not to eliminate it. Used properly, guidelines can improve health care quality and be a support system in the decision-making process not only for the clinician but also for the patient.

IMPLEMENTATION OF CLINICAL PRACTICE GUIDELINES

The development of quality CPGs is challenging; however, implementation is an even greater challenge. It is crucial that implementation strategies take guidelines out of the developmental phase and into the professional health care settings of decision making. Efforts to implement guidelines have met with limited success (see Dopson & Fitzgerald, 2005). There are various barriers to successful implementation, and these can be related to the practitioner or the organization.

Guidelines need to be prepared and presented to practitioners so the value and the benefits are readily apparent. If this information is in an easily accessible format and is useful, it is likely that more practitioners will refer to guidelines and use them as an important foundation for practice. Guideline recommendations that are clear and concise are more readily utilized in decision making. Guidelines that are perceived as confusing or overgeneralized may have little impact on practice and may even be perceived as unreliable, so guideline developers need to consider the end user throughout the development process to facilitate the eventual use of the guidelines. Addressing potential barriers to use from the beginning may make it more likely that CPGs are implemented in daily practice.

Addressing organizational factors such as structural characteristics, management, philosophy, objectives, and operational capacities when introducing guidelines increases the likelihood of successful implementation. Additionally, factors that may affect potential users of guidelines include amount of insurance coverage and methods of institutional or practitioner payment. Financial incentives and disincentives may also contribute to the uptake and implementation of CPGs. Some systems are already piloting pay for performance measures (providing incentives for specific clinical behaviors or practice outcomes) that can be linked to CPGs, although additional data are necessary to determine whether such strategies increase guideline use or result in improved care.

Research has examined implementation strategies, and the results are mixed on their effectiveness. For example, Grimshaw et al. (2004) found that dissemination of educational materials, audit and feedback, and reminders of CPGs had modest effects in changing clinicians' behavior. Additionally, implementation is difficult to analyze, and studies often have methodological weaknesses (Grimshaw et al., 1995). It will be important to review the literature on dissemination and implementation of evidence-based psychological treatments (e.g., McHugh & Barlow, 2010, 2012) to identify strategies to adapt for use with CPGs. Therefore, it is essential for future research to examine behavior change in clinicians in order to develop effective implementation strategies.

SUMMARY

The implementation and use of high-quality CPGs has the potential to reduce some of the biases inherent in decision making. However, behavioral and mental health clinicians need to become acquainted with the process of developing those high-quality CPGs in order to determine which CPGs are worthwhile. The IOM has provided clear guidance on best practices in guideline development, and as more developers follow these practices, we will see increased quality in guidelines, reduced bias in the production of them and the underlying SRs, and uniformity in development procedures. Familiarity with the processes of CPG development and the efforts undertaken to reduce all forms of bias is critical for their acceptance and uptake. This should contribute to improved acceptance and uptake of guidelines, with the overall aim of improving clinical care and reducing the biases in clinical decision making.

The development of quality CPGs for the treatment of behavioral and mental health disorders has the potential to help patients, mental health practitioners, policymakers, and administrators make better decisions about how to proceed with care. High-quality CPGs can reduce bias in decision making and ensure that such decisions are based on a systematic, comprehensive, objective evaluation of the entire evidence base. CPGs can be trustworthy and useful tools that are essential in enhancing clinical decision making.

REFERENCES

Abrahamson, D. J., & Saakvitne, K. W. (2000). Quality management in practice: Re-visioning practice guidelines to improve treatment of anxiety and traumatic stress disorders. In G. Stricker, W. G. Troy, & S. A. Shueman (Eds.), *Handbook of quality management in behavioral health* (pp. 217–235). New York, NY: Springer. http://dx.doi.org/10.1007/978-1-4615-4195-0_12

Akl, E. A., Karl, R., & Guyatt, G. H. (2012). Methodologists and context experts disagree regarding managing conflicts of interest of clinical practice guidelines. *Journal of Clinical Epidemiology, 65,* 734–739. http://dx.doi.org/10.1016/j.jclinepi.2011.12.013

American Psychological Association. (2002). Criteria for evaluating treatment guidelines. *American Psychologist, 57,* 1052–1059. http://dx.doi.org/10.1037/0003-066X.57.12.1052

APA Presidential Task Force on Evidence-Based Practice. (2006). Evidence-based practice in psychology. *American Psychologist, 61,* 271–285. http://dx.doi.org/10.1037/0003-066X.61.4.271

Arkowitz, H., & Lilienfeld, S. (2008). Psychotherapy on trial. In S. Lilienfeld, J. Ruscio, & S. Lynn (Eds.), *Navigating the mindfield: A user's guide to distinguishing science from pseudoscience in mental health* (pp. 103–110). Amherst, NY: Prometheus.

Balshem, H., Helfand, M., Schünemann, H. J., Oxman, A. D., Kunz, R., Brozek, J., . . . Guyatt, G. H. (2011). GRADE guidelines: 3. Rating the quality of evidence. *Journal of Clinical Epidemiology, 64,* 401–406. http://dx.doi.org/10.1016/j.jclinepi.2010.07.015

Barlow, D. H., Levitt, J. T., & Bufka, L. F. (1999). The dissemination of empirically supported treatments: A view to the future. *Behaviour Research and Therapy, 37*(Suppl. 1), S147–S162. http://dx.doi.org/10.1016/S0005-7967(99)00054-6

Barrett, P. M., & Ollendick, T. H. (Eds.). (2003). *Handbook of interventions that work with children and adolescents: Prevention and treatment.* West Sussex, England: John Wiley & Sons.

Berlowitz, D. R., & Halpern, J. (1997). Evaluating and improving pressure ulcer care: The VA experience with administrative data. *The Joint Commission Journal on Quality Improvement, 23,* 424–433.

Chorpita, B. F. (2002). Treatment manuals for the real world: Where do we build them? *Clinical Psychology: Science and Practice, 9,* 431–433. http://dx.doi.org/10.1093/clipsy.9.4.431

Craske, M. G., & Zucker, B. G. (2001). Consideration of the APA practice guideline for the treatment of patients with panic disorder: Strengths and limitations for behavior therapy. *Behavior Therapy, 32,* 259–281. http://dx.doi.org/10.1016/S0005-7894(01)80005-8

Dopson, S., & Fitzgerald, L. (Eds.). (2005). *Knowledge to action? Evidence based health care in context.* Oxford, England: Oxford University Press. http://dx.doi.org/10.1093/acprof:oso/9780199259014.001.0001

Falck-Ytter, Y., & Schünemann, H. J. (2009, September). *Rating the evidence: Using GRADE to develop clinical practice guidelines.* Paper presented at the annual meeting of the Agency for Health Care Research and Quality, Bethesda, MD.

Field, M. J., & Lohr, K. N. (Eds.). (1990). *Clinical practice guidelines: Directions for a new program.* Washington, DC: National Academies Press.

Gawande, A. (2009). *The checklist manifesto: How to get things right.* New York, NY: Henry Holt.

Goodheart, C. D. (2006). Evidence, endeavor, and expertise in psychology practice. In C. D. Goodheart, A. E. Kazdin, & R. J. Sternberg (Eds.), *Evidence-based psychotherapy: Where practice and research meet* (pp. 37–61). Washington, DC: American Psychological Association. http://dx.doi.org/10.1037/11423-002

Goodheart, C. D. (2010). Economics and psychology practice: What we need to know and why. *Professional Psychology: Research and Practice, 41,* 189–195. http://dx.doi.org/10.1037/a0019498

Gray, B. H., Gusmano, M. K., & Collins, S. R. (2003). AHCPR and the changing politics of health services research. *Health Affairs.* http://content.healthaffairs.org/content/early/2003/06/25/hlthaff.w3.283.full.pdf

Grimshaw, J., Freemantle, N., Wallace, S., Russell, I., Hurwitz, B., Watt, I., . . . Sheldon, T. (1995). Developing and implementing clinical practice guidelines. *Quality in Health Care, 4,* 55–64. http://dx.doi.org/10.1136/qshc.4.1.55

Grimshaw, J. M., Thomas, R. E., MacLennan, G., Fraser, C., Ramsay, C. R., Vale, L., . . . Donaldson, C. (2004). Effectiveness and efficiency of guideline dissemination and implementation strategies. *Health Technology Assessment, 8*(6), iii–iv, 1–72. http://dx.doi.org/10.3310/hta8060

Guyatt, G., Akl, E. A., Hirsh, J., Kearon, C., Crowther, M., Gutterman, D., . . . Schünemann, H. (2010). The vexing problem of guidelines and conflict of interest: A potential solution. *Annals of Internal Medicine, 152,* 738–741. http://dx.doi.org/10.7326/0003-4819-152-11-201006010-00254

Haynes, R. B., Sackett, D. L., Gray, J. M. A., Cook, D. J., & Guyatt, G. H. (1996). Transferring evidence from research into practice: 1. The role of clinical care research evidence in clinical decisions. *ACP Journal Club, 125*(3), A14–A16.

Hollon, S. D., Areán, P. A., Craske, M. G., Crawford, K. A., Kivlahan, D. R., & Magnavita, J. J., . . . Kurtzman, H. (2014). Development of clinical practice guidelines. *Annual Review of Clinical Psychology.* Advance online publication.

Institute of Medicine. (2001). *Crossing the quality chasm: A new health system for the 21st century.* Washington, DC: National Academies Press.

Institute of Medicine. (2005). *Improving the quality of health care for mental and substance use conditions: Quality chasm series*. Washington, DC: National Academies Press.

Institute of Medicine. (2011a). *Clinical practice guidelines we can trust*. Washington, DC: National Academies Press.

Institute of Medicine. (2011b). *Finding what works in health care: Standards for systematic reviews*. Washington, DC: National Academies Press.

Kung, J., Miller, R. R., & Mackowiak, P. A. (2012). Failure of clinical practice guidelines to meet institute of medicine standards: Two more decades of little, if any, progress. *Archives of Internal Medicine, 172,* 1628–1633. http://dx.doi.org/10.1001/2013.jamainternmed.56

McHugh, R. K., & Barlow, D. H. (2010). The dissemination and implementation of evidence-based psychological treatments. A review of current efforts. *American Psychologist, 65,* 73–84. http://dx.doi.org/10.1037/a0018121

McHugh, R. K., & Barlow, D. H. (Eds.). (2012). *Dissemination and implementation of evidence-based psychological interventions*. New York, NY: Oxford University Press.

Reed, G. M., McLaughlin, C. J., & Newman, R. (2002). American Psychological Association policy in context: The development and evaluation of guidelines for professional practice. *American Psychologist, 57,* 1041–1047. http://dx.doi.org/10.1037/0003-066X.57.12.1041

Sackett, D. L., Rosenberg, W. M., Gray, J. A., Haynes, R. B., & Richardson, W. S. (1996). Evidence based medicine: What it is and what it isn't. *BMJ (Clinical Research Ed.), 312*(7023), 71–72. http://dx.doi.org/10.1136/bmj.312.7023.71

van der Weijden, T., Boivin, A., Burgers, J., Schünemann, H. J., & Elwyn, G. (2012). Clinical practice guidelines and patient decision aids. An inevitable relationship. *Journal of Clinical Epidemiology, 65,* 584–589. http://dx.doi.org/10.1016/j.jclinepi.2011.10.007

Viswanathan, M., Carey, T. S., Belinson, S. E., Berliner, E., Chang, S., & Graham, E., . . . White, C. M. (2013). *Identifying and managing nonfinancial conflicts of interest for systematic reviews* (Methods Research Report No. 13-EHC085-EF). Rockville, MD: Agency for Healthcare Research and Quality. Available at http://www.ncbi.nlm.nih.gov/books/NBK148586/

5

DEVELOPING CLINICAL PRACTICE GUIDELINES TO ENHANCE CLINICAL DECISION MAKING

STEVEN D. HOLLON

The clinical situation is complex, and no two clients are ever exactly alike. At times only limited empirical evidence exists to guide the decision-making process, and what evidence exists is often open to dispute. Clinical practice guidelines (CPGs) are intended to help guide the decision-making process. They are not a substitute for clinical judgment but when well crafted can provide a basis for the decisions to be made. Clinicians need to understand the basics underlying how these guidelines are developed in order to get maximum benefit from their use.

The American Psychological Association (APA) has decided in recent years to begin developing CPGs. That decision was not without some controversy and represents an evolution of the position that the APA has taken over the years (see Chapter 4, this volume, for a discussion of that evolution). It formed an advisory steering committee (ASC) to guide the process, and I was fortunate enough to be selected as its initial chair. The issues I describe in this

http://dx.doi.org/10.1037/14711-005
Clinical Decision Making in Mental Health Practice, J. J. Magnavita (Editor)
Copyright © 2016 by the American Psychological Association. All rights reserved.

chapter represent my own perspective on the questions that we confronted and do not necessarily represent the views of the ASC or the larger APA.

In this chapter I describe the evolving science that underlies the development of CPGs and its implications for the clinical decision-making process. Guideline development has moved from a process based largely on unsystematic clinical consensus to a more deliberative process in which a systematic review (SR) of the scientific data is conducted and the resultant evidence presented to a panel of individuals with diverse perspectives and expertise (including service utilizers to provide input concerning patient preferences). The goal is to ground the discussion in the best science currently available as filtered through the differing perspectives and expertise of the panelists in a manner that balances out whatever biases and blind spots each may possess.

INSTITUTE OF MEDICINE RECOMMENDATIONS FOR GENERATING CPGs

Not long after the APA steering committee was formed, the Institute of Medicine (IOM) published two sets of recommendations for generating CPGs. These reports had been in process of development for several years and did (in my opinion) a marvelous job of summarizing the current state of the knowledge regarding how to generate guidelines that the public could trust. The first report described the process of forming the guideline development panels (GDPs) charged with generating the treatment recommendations (IOM, 2011a), and the second dealt with the execution of the SRs on which those recommendations would be based (IOM, 2011b). The reports themselves are available to the public and summarized in recent articles (Hollon et al., 2014) and chapters (Chapter 4, this volume). Therefore, I highlight only certain aspects of the reports (and the larger process of guideline development) that I think are most relevant to their subsequent use.

It is important to note in that regard that both the IOM (2001) and the APA Presidential Task Force on Evidence-Based Practice (2006) explicitly adhere to a tripartite model of clinical decision making in which the best available evidence (represented by the CPG) is filtered through the expertise of the treating clinician to arrive at the best decisions consistent with the preferences and values of the individual patient. In essence, the goal of guideline development is to put the best available evidence before the patient and treating clinician, but the clinician trumps the guideline and the patient trumps the clinician.

What this means to me is that I have an obligation to provide my patients with the most complete and accurate information possible (drawing when possible on the CPG in the process) and to make my recommendations regarding those potential options (even when they are not wholly consistent with the guideline) but that the ultimate decision as to what is to be done rests with the patient I am treating (so long as he or she is competent). When I disagree with what the guideline recommends, I have an obligation to be clear about the basis for that disagreement, and if I am unwilling to go along with what the patient prefers, then I have an obligation to provide a referral to someone else who will. I have in the past worked with patients diagnosed with bipolar disorder who wanted to come off their lithium; both instances resulted in clinical disasters that I do not recommend repeating. Prospective patients also have asked me to treat them with an approach that I was not competent to provide and that had not impressed me with its success. When that happens I explain the reasons for my reticence and offer to make a referral. In other instances I have scrambled to add strategies to my basic cognitive approach that had been found to have specific benefit for the kinds of problems that my clients faced (although I tend to specialize in the treatment of depression, it is not unusual for clients to have comorbid problems with posttraumatic stress disorder or obsessive–compulsive disorder or panic attacks). The basic approach that I have taken throughout my career is to ground whatever I do in the best available scientific evidence as filtered through my own perceptions of what I think might work best for my particular client but always guided by his or her individual preference.

Forming the Guideline Development Panels

Several key aspects of the guideline development process are particularly relevant to the clinical decision-making process (and their inclusion influences whether I am likely to be willing to adhere to the guideline). The first is *transparency*. The IOM lays out a series of steps to ensure that the guideline user can understand how the recommendations were developed. Each step in the process is carefully documented, and a written record is made available to the public for review at multiple steps along the way. What this means is that the recommendations do not have to be taken on the basis of faith. Anyone who questions a specific recommendation can see just how it was generated and the evidential basis on which it rests. This allows the clinician (myself included) to gauge the extent to which he or she agrees with the recommendation.

Two recent guidelines on the treatment of depression highlight differences in how this issue was approached and the resultant impact that these differences had on the confidence that I have in each guideline. The National Institute for Health and Clinical Excellence (NICE) is charged by the National Health Service in the United Kingdom with generating CPGs to guide service provision within their single-payer system. The guidelines they develop are always based on an SR, and the organizations are meticulous in documenting what they do and why they do it. Their guideline on the treatment of depression was no exception (National Collaborating Centre for Mental Health, 2010).

By way of contrast, the American Psychiatric Association generated their guideline on the treatment of depression in the absence of any SR and with no clear documentation of how they arrived at their decisions (American Psychiatric Association, 2010). Neither course inspires much confidence in their recommendations. I was particularly struck by two "oversights" on their part that both worked to overstate the benefits of medications. Citing a study by Turner, Matthews, Linardatos, Tell, and Rosenthal (2008) that showed that withholding negative results in some instances and "spinning" results in others to make them more favorable to medications inflated the apparent efficacy of medications, the guideline's only comment was that "those factors do not appear specific to particular medications or medication classes" (American Psychiatric Association, 2010, p. 31). This comment was disingenuous because the factors were true for all antidepressant medications. An awareness of how *confirmation bias* can lead to favoring results that support one's thinking may have reduced the likelihood of these cognitive traps.

The second "oversight" involved a thrice-replicated finding that antidepressant medications only separate from pill-placebo (show a specific pharmacological effect) among patients with more severe depressions (Fournier et al., 2010; Khan, Leventhal, Khan, & Brown, 2002; Kirsch et al., 2008). The American Psychiatric Association guideline's comment with respect to those findings was that there was "some evidence suggesting greater efficacy relative to placebo in individuals with severe depressive symptoms as compared to those with mild to moderate symptoms" (American Psychiatric Association, 2010, p. 31). The guideline neglected to say that the lesser efficacy relative to placebo for those patients with mild to moderate depression dropped to zero and that although those patients get better on medications, they get better for psychological rather than pharmacological reasons. A less biased guideline would do better.

The second key aspect is management of *conflict of interest* (COI). Potential panelists often have secondary interests that might strongly bias their judgments. Financial conflicts represent one obvious source of bias, but intellectual passions can be a source of bias as well. Many of these have been reviewed in Chapter 4 of this volume. The IOM recommends requiring a full disclosure of potential COI at the time the GDP is formed (with periodic updates as needed). In our experience, it was necessary to work with potential panelists to educate them about just what might constitute a potential COI in the eyes of others.

We chose not to exclude panelists with strongly held perspectives or potential financial COI (as the IOM suggests) but elected instead to follow a strategy of balancing such conflicts rather than excluding them altogether. Our concern was that we not exclude participants with the necessary expertise but instead provide an internal check on any undue influence through a process that cognitive psychologists refer to as *adversarial collaboration* (Mellers, Hertwig, & Kahneman, 2001). This led us to include panelists with competing interests and expertise that spanned the major approaches to treatment. For example, our depression guideline panel includes members with recognized expertise in dynamic, behavioral, experiential, family, and pharmacological approaches. It also is diverse with respect to members who are primarily involved in clinical practice, treatment research, and health care administration. What this means to the practicing clinician is that each recommendation will have had to survive a fierce and lively debate among advocates for the major schools of treatment and professional career paths.

NICE handles potential COI in a similar fashion, and one of their directors (Stephen Pilling, professor from the University College of London) met with our steering committee early in our organizational process to discuss how they handled this and other issues. Many research psychiatrists (including most of the members of the guideline panel) receive money from the pharmaceutical industry in the form of speaker's fees and research grants (Angell, 2005). This was enough of a concern that the psychiatric association added an advisory committee of senior psychiatrists who no longer accepted industry funding to pass judgment on the final product. Once again, although I know many of the psychiatrists involved and have often published with them, I have more confidence in the way NICE handled the issue than the American Psychiatric Association guideline.

A third recommendation from the IOM was that the GDPs be *multidisciplinary* in nature. This was something that we wholeheartedly embraced. Most mental health disorders and problems in living can be treated with a variety of interventions (including psychotherapy and medications), and we wanted to be sure that we provided adequate coverage of all relevant treatments. Our guiding principle was that we wanted to produce guidelines that were in the public interest and not just in the interest of one profession or another. (Our sense was that if the guidelines were good for the public then they would be good for psychology as a discipline.) This principle extends to our desire to make common cause with other relevant professional organizations to generate joint guidelines in the future.

NICE guideline panels are invariably multidisciplinary in nature. Although a few psychologists were listed as commenting on the draft of the psychiatric guideline, all of the participants on the GDP itself and the oversight advisory board were psychiatrists. Once again I have greater confidence in the process followed by NICE than the one used by the American Psychiatric Association.

The IOM also recommends including current or former patients or patient care advocates in the process, although no clear consensus exists as to how this can best be done. My own sense is that inclusion of such members helps to keep the professionals on the panel honest and focused on the public welfare. After some deliberation and prodding from the first GDPs we constituted, that is what we finally decided to do. What this means is that users of the guidelines can expect that they will be broad in the interventions that they cover and focused on what the public needs. NICE always includes patients on their guideline panels; the American Psychiatric Association does not.

A fourth set of IOM recommendations specifies the nature of *interaction between the GDP and the SR team*. We opted to keep the two groups separate (to minimize bias in the conduct of the reviews) but to have them interact from the beginning in terms of formulating the questions to be asked and the nature of the evidence to be covered. In essence, the GDP determines what it wants to know (in consultation with the SR team regarding how best to formulate those questions), and the SR team conducts the actual review (with the ongoing feedback and subsequent requests for additional information from the GDP). The analogy that we like to use is that the GDP functions like a jury, determining what it wants to know, and the SR team functions like both the prosecution and the defense, reporting back on the evidence. What this means is that the guideline user can have some confidence that the questions addressed are clinically relevant and that the evidence examined is not constrained by preexistent bias.

I had the opportunity to sit in on a meeting of the NICE depression guideline panel several years ago and was struck by how the members were able to ask for clarifications in the data and have their queries answered within a matter of minutes (the requests were made to Pilling who communicated them to the SR team). The psychiatric guideline conducted no SR, so there was no one to whom to put a question regarding the data.

Once the SR has been conducted and the relevant evidence presented, the GDP is charged with generating and *rating the strength of the recommendations*. In some instances the evidence is quite clear, but in others, not so much. Strong recommendations indicate that the benefits of a given approach to treatment clearly outweigh its potential harms (or vice versa), but weak recommendations indicate a less clear balance. Moreover, the quality and amount of the evidence need to be taken into consideration. For example, although quantitative reviews often suggest that different types of psychotherapies are comparably efficacious for nonpsychotic patients, some types of treatments have been studied more extensively and stringently than others.

A relative *absence of evidence is not evidence of absence* (of effect), but it does limit certainty of recommendations. What this means is that clinicians using the guidelines can tell from the rated strength just how strong is the evidence base that underlies a given recommendation. NICE grades the strength of their recommendations, whereas the psychiatric guideline did not.

The IOM also suggests *articulating recommendations* in a manner that makes it clear what actions are being recommended. We plan to ask our GDPs to generate recommendations in the form of clear action statements that correspond to specific behaviors on the part of the clinician. That does not mean that the clinician will have to follow any given recommendation (clinical judgment still trumps any specific guideline), but it does mean that the clinician will know exactly what is being recommended and how best to follow that advice. NICE formulates its recommendations in terms of action statements; the psychiatric guideline did not.

The IOM also recommends subjecting the recommendations to *external review* and carefully documenting the changes that are made as a consequence. Drafts will be made available for public scrutiny at various points throughout the process. What this means is that there will be ample opportunity for individuals not directly involved in guideline generation to pass judgment on the wisdom of the recommendations and their relevance to clinical practice. NICE subjects its guidelines to intensive public scrutiny before publication; the psychiatric association only invites comments from selected individuals and does not publish their responses.

Finally, the IOM recommends *updating the recommendations* on a periodic basis. Precisely when and how will be determined by the growth of information in a given area, but the goal is to keep the guidelines current and up to date. What this means is that the guideline user can have reasonable assurance that the recommendations presented are current with the times. Both NICE and the psychiatric association update their guidelines on a periodic basis.

On the whole, I am much more impressed with the fairness and the balance provided by the procedures followed by NICE (most of which anticipated the IOM guidelines) than I am with those followed by the psychiatric guideline. As a consequence, I am much more likely to take the NICE recommendations seriously when it comes to areas that I do not know as well as depression. I particularly like that fact that I can track the basis for the recommendations to see if I concur with the conclusions that are drawn. It was clear to me that the IOM recommendations for guideline construction (most of them anticipated by NICE) are more likely to produce guidelines that I (or any other clinician) can trust than the procedures followed by the psychiatric association. I have every expectation that future psychiatric guidelines will follow those same IOM guidelines, and I hope our two associations will join forces to produce subsequent guidelines.

Conducting Systematic Reviews

The IOM also laid out a series of steps for conducting SRs. The details of these steps are rather technical in nature and will not be reviewed in any detail, but several aspects of the process deserve to be highlighted. First, *conducting an SR is broader and more inclusive than simply conducting a meta-analysis*, and in some instances (when studies are weak or few) conducting a meta-analysis might not even be indicated. Meta-analyses provide a quantitative summary of the empirical literature and can serve as a real guide to the recommendation development process, but like all summaries they often obscure relevant information. It is important for the GDPs to know just how many and how strong the studies are that contribute to a given body of the literature and whether systematic limitations exist that ought to be reflected in the nature and the strength of the resultant recommendations.

Second, *publication bias* is often a concern and tends to inflate the apparent efficacy of the given interventions. This is true not only for medication treatment (as previously noted) but also with respect to psychotherapy, although likely for noncommercial reasons (Cuijpers, Smit, Bohlmeijer, Hollon, & Andersson, 2010). There is a tendency for small studies with weak effects to not find their way into the literature, whereas small studies with large effects (often a consequence of chance) are much more likely to be published. Therefore, it can be important to search the "gray literature" for studies that were never published. The IOM recommends working with a reference librarian or other personnel experienced in the conduct of SRs to ensure adequate coverage. What this means is that the clinician and the public will not be misled by inflated estimates of efficacy; it is important to know not only what works but also how well it works. Paul Meehl (1987) once said that the basic attribute that ought to distinguish psychologists from the other helping professions is "the general scientific commitment not to be fooled or to fool anybody else" (p. 9). Whether we devote the bulk of our time to research or (more often) clinical practice, the one defining aspect of psychology as a profession is that we were all trained as scientists and in its application.

Most current reviews start with the *formulation of an analytic framework* that lays out the kinds of questions that the SR is intended to address. This might involve questions such as, "Do the interventions produce the desired changes in outcomes of interest (positive or negative)?" and if so, "Do they do so through the mechanisms specified?" We have opted to ask the GDPs to meet with the SR teams in the beginning of the process to generate the analytic framework that they want the review to address. The reason that this is important is because the GDP can focus the review on any aspect of clinical change that seems important. It is not necessary to limit attention to symptom change (although that will likely be one component), and most current reviews now address broader aspects of life satisfaction and adjustment. There will be times when the existing literature has little to say about these broader outcomes of interest, but one purpose of guideline development is to call attention to important aspects of human existence that have not received adequate empirical attention. The goal is not just to provide an aid to clinical decision making but also to suggest additional issues for the science to address.

The second key step involves *generating structured questions* based on the analytic framework to guide the actual review process. We plan to adopt the widely used PICOTS format in generating these questions. PICOTS is a mnemonic that stands for populations (P), interventions (I), comparisons (C), outcomes (O), time (T), and settings (S). Thus a specific PICOTS question might take the following form: For patients with major depressive disorder (P), does cognitive therapy (I) compared with medications (C) have an enduring effect that prevents subsequent relapse (O) following treatment termination (T) in outpatient settings (S)?

Using PICOTS to organize the SRs facilitates asking questions of clinical interest. The goal of personalized medicine is to find the best treatment for the given individual. Looking for variation in response as a function of differences in populations (P) can help to address that goal. For example, in an earlier study we found that cognitive therapy and the antidepressant medication paroxetine were comparably efficacious (on average) and both superior to pill-placebo in the acute treatment of patients with moderate to severe depression (DeRubeis et al., 2005). However, further exploration of the data indicated that patients with personality disorders did better in medication treatment than in cognitive therapy whereas patients without personality disorders did better in cognitive therapy than on medications (Fournier et al., 2008). One common critique of the treatment outcome literature is that it has tended to focus in the past on uncomplicated patients with single diagnoses (Westen, Novotny, & Thompson-Brenner, 2004). This is no longer as true as it once was, and to the extent that it remains a problem the CPG can highlight the issue.

The technical term for this phenomenon is *moderation*, and it typically is detected as an interaction between some patient characteristic and treatment condition. It is not just patient characteristics that are relevant in this regard; any aspect of the clinical situation that could influence treatment outcome can be examined as a potential moderator. Factors such as time (T), the length or frequency of treatment, and setting (S), exactly where and under what conditions treatment takes place, can be explored as moderators. Among recent examples, an intensive week of daily sessions of cognitive therapy for posttraumatic stress disorders was just as efficacious and much more rapidly so than the same number of weekly sessions spread out over a 2-month period

(Ehlers et al., 2014), and 20 weekly sessions of cognitive behavior therapy for bulimia was considerably more efficacious than 2 years of weekly dynamic psychotherapy (Poulsen et al., 2014). Adopting the PICOTS format practically guarantees that the SR will be broad in its focus with respect to the complexities involved in clinical practice and the inclusion of expert clinicians in the GDP guarantees that it will relevant to the clinical situation.

SELECTING THE BEST TREATMENT FOR A GIVEN PATIENT

One of the most important clinical decisions to be made is how to identify the best treatment for a given patient. There is a critical distinction between prognostic versus prescriptive information that has real implications for the clinical decision making process. *Prognostic indices* are individual difference variables that predict how someone will do over time (possibly during the course of treatment), whereas *prescriptive indices* are individual difference variables that predict differential response to one treatment versus another (Fournier et al., 2009). For example, in our work on depression, we have found that chronicity predicts poorer response regardless of treatment (cognitive therapy vs. medications). That means that it is worse to have a chronic depression (an episode that has lasted 2 years or longer) than a nonchronic depression; you will be less likely to get better no matter what treatment you receive than someone who does not have a chronic depression. On the other hand, employment status is prescriptive in that patients who are unemployed do worse in medication treatment than they do in cognitive therapy (patients who are employed do comparably well in either). What that means is that employment status can be used to make a decision regarding what kind of treatment a given patient should receive (if unemployed pick cognitive therapy), whereas chronicity cannot.

Where clinicians (and scientists) get in trouble is when they confuse the two kinds of information, and that is an especially easy thing to do. Prognostic information can be gleaned by holding treatment constant and allowing patient characteristics to vary. Prescriptive information, on the other hand, requires holding individual differences constant and systematically varying the nature of the treatment (as is done in randomized controlled trials). Because most clinicians do similar things with different patients (rather than different things with similar patients), what we are most likely to learn in the context of our clinical practice is what kind of patients best respond to the things we typically do (prognostic) rather than what kinds of things are best to do with a given patient (prescriptive). That means that typical clinical practice is best suited to teach us how to select the best patients for our preferred treatment rather than how to select the best treatment for a given patient. You do not have to try to fall prey to this logical fallacy when doing clinical work; you have to try hard not to be fooled in this fashion. When we ask ourselves who responds to what, we are most likely to recall prognostic information. We are particularly likely to recall patients who did particularly well or particularly poorly. That is what cognitive psychologists call the *availability heuristic* (Kahneman, Slovic, & Tversky, 1982). That is not an indictment of the practicing clinician (I do the same thing myself when asked in workshops who is most likely to respond to cognitive therapy); it is just a reflection of how we are wired to think.

Most clinical lore is based on the wrong kind of information to draw inferences about what treatment to select for a given patient. That is, most of what we see in the course of our daily practice is purely prognostic in nature. Prescriptive information can be ascertained, but it is a more difficult thing to do and requires forethought. The clinician would have to systematically vary the way he or she treated similar patients, and that is something that most of us do not do. The best way to do so is on the basis of a randomized controlled trial (RCT) in which similar patients are randomly assigned to different treatments. No matter how astute the clinician, recalling who did well in a given treatment compared with other patients is no basis for treatment selection; what is needed is what treatment did better than other treatments for similar patients.

One problem with addressing anything as complex as clinical change is that there are a lot of possible factors (patient or otherwise) that can influence treatment outcome, and it is not always easy to put them all together. That is where clinical experience can come into play. It is well understood that experience and expertise often confer special advantage in terms of pattern recognition. Master chess players can anticipate what their opponent is likely to do several moves in advance, and professional quarterbacks in football describe the game "slowing down" with experience in a manner that allows them to do a better job of anticipating the position of the pass defenders. It is likely that experienced clinicians become more skilled in integrating multiple patient and setting characteristics in a manner that allows them to select the optimal treatment for a given patient. On the other hand, there is ample evidence that statistical prediction is more accurate than clinical prediction (Meehl, 1954). We all have the very human tendency to rely too much on intuition; that is why casinos rarely go bankrupt.

DeRubeis and colleagues may be on the verge of developing a strategy that allows them to integrate multiple patient characteristics in a manner that facilitates identifying the optimal treatment for a given individual (DeRubeis et al., 2014). Working with data from the placebo-controlled comparison between cognitive therapy versus medication treatment previously described, the authors developed a system for generating equations that predict how each patient would have been expected to do in either cognitive therapy or medication treatment on the basis of presence of a personality disorder and other predictive indices. About a third of the patients would have been predicted to do better in cognitive therapy than on medications, whereas another third of the patients would have been predicted to show the opposite pattern (the remaining patients would have shown no advantage either way). Assigning patients to treatment on the basis of this selection algorithm would have improved outcomes by as much as the difference between either of the active treatments versus pill-placebo.

HIERARCHY OF EVIDENCE

Treatments are intended to produce change (or to prevent bad things from occurring in the case of preventive interventions). What this means is that they are intended to have a causal effect. Even humanistic interventions that presume that the locus of change is within the client specify certain necessary and sufficient conditions that must be provided by the therapist for the self-actualizing potential of the client to be realized (Rogers, 1957). There are two major sources of outcome whenever someone enters treatment: how they would have done in the absence of treatment (patients), and what gets done to them in treatment (procedures). CPGs are intended to identify the best treatment for the given patient, and that means that they are intended to identify that treatment that produces the best balance of benefits to harm. In essence, CPGs are all about personalizing causal inference and "guessing" what procedures work best for a given patient.

A hierarchy of evidence exists with respect to what kinds of research designs provide the best evidence with respect to the detection of causality (APA Presidential Task Force, 2006). Uncontrolled case studies rank lowest on this hierarchy. That is not because they are without value (most of the greatest breakthroughs in clinical practice have come about as a consequence of careful clinical observation) but because they do not provide a particularly good basis for distinguishing between patients and procedures as the source of that change. Philosophers of science distinguish between the context of discovery and the context of verification (Popper, 1934; Reichenbach, 1938); uncontrolled case studies are a rich source of the former but a poor basis for the latter. Open trials that follow multiple patients treated with the same procedures over time are somewhat more informative in that they provide prognostic information but again confound patient with procedure. Nonrandomized contrasts between two or more different treatments are more informative still in that they allow some sense as to how different patients respond to different treatments, but they still are susceptible to confounding patient prognostic with treatment effects. RCTs seek to control for patient characteristics by distributing them comparably across conditions. When patient characteristics are comparably distributed (on average), then any observed differences in outcomes can be attributed to differences in procedures and not to patients.

The controversy over hormone replacement therapy (HRT) illustrates the risk of not controlling assignment to treatment. For more than 2 decades, women going through menopause were encouraged to go on estrogen to minimize aversive symptoms like hot flashes and to reduce risk for osteoporosis and coronary heart disease. The common consensus (based on open trials and clinical experience) was that women who were treated with HRT did better than those who were not. However, these findings confounded patients with procedures; it was women who took better care of themselves and had access to better health care who typically sought out HRT. When the first RCTs were finally done it turned out that HRT increased risk for heart disease (Manson et al., 2003) and breast cancer (Chlebowski et al., 2003). In essence, differences in prognosis favoring women who received HRT (patients) masked problems inherent in the treatment (procedures).

What we have just described goes under the rubric of *internal validity* (Campbell & Stanley, 1963), which refers to the certainty with which we can attribute the differences we observe at the end of treatment to the procedures we manipulated experimentally. RCTs typically are privileged in SRs because they provide the strongest basis for drawing a causal inference. However, external validity also is relevant. *External validity* refers to the extent to which the causal inference drawn generalizes to the context of interest. Early analogue studies that treated less than fully clinical populations with poorly implemented approximations of more traditional interventions (often for unreasonably brief periods of time) lacked external validity and did not tell us all that much about what worked best for the kinds of patients typically seen in clinical practice. One of the reasons that we wanted to include practicing clinicians on the GDPs was to ensure that the recommendations formulated reflected a sophisticated understanding of the kinds of patients likely to be treated and the nature of the interventions likely to be used.

The C in PICOTS stands for the comparison condition, and it is here that studies differ most in the kinds of questions that they can address. *Construct validity* refers to the extent that we actually understand how our treatments work (Cook & Campbell, 1979). The first question that we want to address about a given treatment is whether it actually works (*efficacy*), and this can be addressed by simply comparing it with its absence. The second question that we typically want to address is whether that treatment works for the reasons specified by theory (*specificity*). That typically is best addressed by comparisons with nonspecific control conditions like pill-placebos (in the case of medications) or supportive treatments that provide all the typical accouterments of going into treatment without whatever is presumed to make the treatment unique. A third question is whether anything works better than its alternatives (*superiority*). That is typically tested by direct comparisons between different presumably active treatments.

Although there is ample evidence that most of the major existing types of treatments work (have efficacy), it is not so clear that they work for the reasons specified by theory (specificity). There exists a major debate in the psychotherapy literature as to whether different treatments work for different reasons (as is typically promulgated by their advocates) or whether they work for nonspecific reasons inherent in any helping relationship (Wampold, 2001). The answer to that question may differ as a function of disorder, and it clearly differs as a function of severity with respect to depression. Just as for medication treatment, psychotherapy for depression only separates from nonspecific attention controls among patients with more severe depressions (Driessen, Cuijpers, Hollon, Dekker, 2010). It may be the case that specific effects only will be found (if they are found at all) for patients with more severe (or chronic or comorbid) disorders. If so, then whether you provide an active treatment (something that goes beyond the nonspecific effects of simply going into treatment) may only matter for those latter patients.

DRAWING CONCLUSIONS REGARDING TREATMENT EFFICACY

There are at least two ways that the field has tried to determine what works with respect to treatment, and they tend to result in somewhat different answers. With respect to medications, the Food and Drug Administration requires at least two well-conducted trials conducted by different research groups that each produce positive findings (relative to pill-placebo) before it will let a new medication go to market. That is, we require evidence of specificity (which presumes efficacy) before we will allow a novel medication to be sold to the general public. (We also require evidence of safety as well but that is another story.) A similar approach (albeit one that only requires that a treatment is better than its absence to say that it is *efficacious* and that adds the modifier *specific* when it exceeds a nonspecific control condition) has been applied to the psychotherapy literature (Chambless & Hollon, 1998). Application of these criteria results in support for the efficacy of the cognitive and behavior therapies, along with interpersonal psychotherapy, and has earned them the appellation of "empirically supported treatments" (ESTs) with respect to depression (DeRubeis & Crits-Christoph, 1998). This approach tends to be favored by research scientists (who developed the ESTs) and viewed with suspicion by the majority of practicing clinicians (who tend to practice more traditional treatments).

The other approach is to conduct meta-analyses of the existing treatment literature, often without regard to quality of study or treatment implementation. The results of this approach are also quite clear; everything works better than nothing, and nothing works better than anything else (Smith, Glass, & Miller, 1980). Meta-regressions sometimes are used to tease out important moderating factors but can only be applied to information that can be coded (Cuijpers, van Straten, van Oppen, & Andersson, 2008). Researchers who conduct treatment trials (usually of their own preferred approach) tend to revile this approach because it lumps strong and weak studies together in an uncritical fashion.

It is likely that the truth lies somewhere between those two extremes. Several of the more traditional and widely practiced types of interventions that tend to be favored by practicing clinicians simply have not been adequately tested against nonspecific controls in the kinds of trials with more fully clinical patients that might allow specific treatment effects to emerge if they did in fact exist. That is not to say that these more traditional approaches would not produce such effects if given the opportunity (absence of evidence is not evidence of absence), just that they have had no such opportunity to succeed or fail. Studies of these interventions that do exist (and are available for meta-analysis) typically are older trials in smaller samples of patients who were not all that severely depressed. The typical finding is that something beats nothing (comparisons with no treatment typically produce effect sizes in the .6–.8 range) and that nothing beats anything else (effect sizes between the "active" treatments are negligible). It is hard to imagine that such trials could have produced any other outcome.

Those same studies also tend to produce modest advantages relative to supportive psychotherapy comparable in magnitude with typical drug–placebo differences (with effect sizes of about .3) but only when supportive psychotherapy is treated as a control condition for some other approach that the investigator prefers. When supportive psychotherapy is the featured intervention in the trial (i.e., when it is the intervention that the investigator is actually interested in and not just a nonspecific control condition), it tends to produce larger effects similar to those produced by "active" treatments (Cuijpers et al., 2012). Cuijpers et al. (2012) estimated the proportion of the variance in change in depression associated with the different components of treatment in the set of studies that included supportive psychotherapy as one condition; about a third of the change observed was associated with the simple passage of time (spontaneous remission), about half was associated with the nonspecific aspects of simply going into treatment, and only about a sixth was associated with the specific aspects of treatment. Given that most of the studies on which these estimates were based were conducted in less severely depressed samples (with whom it was ethical to conduct no-treatment controls), it is likely that the proportion of change associated with specific aspects of treatment (a pharmacologically active agent or a psychologically active causal mechanism) would account for a larger proportion of change in more severely depressed patients. Nonetheless, the proportion of change produced by nonspecific factors alone was striking and wholly consistent with the notion that for patients with less severe depressions "anything beats nothing and nothing beats anything else" (aka "all have won and all must have prizes"; Luborsky, Singer, & Luborsky, 1975).

Tie scores in the empirical literature may reflect any of several different possibilities: (a) limitations in the existing literature in terms of the quality of the studies that are available for review; (b) different treatments work through different mechanisms but just happen to produce comparable outcomes (possible but unlikely); (c) different treatments work through common mechanisms to produce comparable change in different clients (nonspecifics); or (d) different people respond to different treatments, but those differences get "washed out" when results are averaged across a number of individuals (moderation). I think that all of these potential explanations remain plausible, and I look to the guideline panels to do the best they can to work things out. The EST approach typically favors the cognitive and behavioral therapies, perhaps because they have been the most often tested against stringent control conditions and are the most likely approaches to have generated a sufficient number of studies with successful outcomes to pass muster. The meta-analytic approach typically suggests that everything works better than nothing and that nothing works better than anything else. If that is true then it does not matter what the therapist does so long as it is done with sufficient interpersonal skill.

How then is a guideline panel supposed to resolve these issues? My previous experience sitting in with the NICE depression guideline panel suggests a possible path to resolution. What impressed me most was the way that the diversity of professions and backgrounds represented in the group facilitated the decision-making process. Some were practicing clinicians and some were research scientists, some professionals with experience treating depression and others were former patients with experience being treated for depression. Some were pharmacotherapists and others were psychotherapists. All were interested in depression and its treatment, and each provided a perspective that enhanced the overall discussion. It was a classic example of adversarial collaboration in operation. The panelists came from different backgrounds and had different biases, but all were committed to generating the best possible recommendations given the existing information and all were committed to doing so in the public interest.

The discussions were informed by a review of the empirical data. Whenever the panel considered the evidence supporting a particular approach to treatment, they had in front of them (projected on a screen) a *forest plot* with findings from all the studies relevant to a particular PICOTS question. For example, when considering the question of whether cognitive therapy had an enduring effect that prevented the return of symptoms following successful treatment (relapse), they had a display in front of them that showed all the comparisons of prior cognitive therapy versus prior medication treatment. Prior cognitive therapy does appear to have an enduring effect (as is evident in six of the eight studies), but that effect is not evident in all trials (no differences were evident in a seventh, and the findings went in the opposite direction in the eighth). That means the finding is relatively robust (it holds up across most studies) but it is not universal. Had they simply presented a summary of the findings in a numerical fashion (an effect size or odds ratio) as typically is done in a meta-analysis, the GDP would have had no idea how little variance there was in this set of findings.

This process can be even more instructive when the findings are not robust. Cognitive therapy generally has done well in the acute treatment of clinical depression, but that has not always been the case. On the one hand, two of the four relevant trials have found it to be as efficacious as medications and each superior to pill-placebo in fully clinical populations (DeRubeis et al., 2005; Jarrett et al., 1999), whereas the other two relevant trials have found it less efficacious than medications and no better than pill-placebo among patients with more severe depressions (Dimidjian et al., 2006; Elkin et al., 1989, 1995). The reasons for that variability in outcomes are open to dispute, but it is important to know that such variability exists. For that you need to see the actual forest plots. A moderate-sized effect could be the consequence of a consistently mediocre intervention or an intervention with a big effect that requires competence in its execution. It also could be a consequence of heterogeneity in the treated populations. Either of the last two explanations represents an instance of moderation; the first on the basis of procedure and the second on the basis of patient characteristics.

Both represent instances of external validity. Studies can differ with respect to the representativeness of the patients studied and the fidelity with which the treatments are implemented. My sense is that you are unlikely to get more than one or two strong showings just by chance (the odds of doing that once might be one in 20, but the odds of doing that twice are one in 400). What is more likely is that an otherwise efficacious treatment is poorly implemented in a given trial. We did that in an early trial comparing cognitive therapy with medications (we set our dosages too low and withdrew the medications prematurely), and as a consequence found an advantage for cognitive therapy over medications that has been hard to replicate subsequently (Rush, Beck, Kovacs, & Hollon, 1977). Simply reporting the average effect size from a meta-analysis that includes this study underestimates the strength of medications relative to cognitive therapy (as does the Treatment of Depression Collaborative Research Program in the opposite direction). Graphing both studies in a forest plot allows the GDP to see just which studies are contributing to the variability in outcomes in a given literature and forces them to consider other factors that might account for this variation.

SUMMARY

I am a strong proponent of basing clinical decisions on the empirical evidence, but I am an even stronger proponent of bringing human judgment to bear on the way that evidence is evaluated. I recognize that we all have our biases (myself included), and I like the notion of balancing those different biases and perspectives in the context of reviewing the empirical evidence. I have confidence that the GDPs will do a better job on the basis of a full and fair evaluation of the empirical evidence than if I generated the recommendations myself.

Whether I agree with the recommendations in any given situation depends on my confidence in the quality of the evidence on which they are based and the process that was followed in their formulation. When I disagree I want to tell my clients why I disagree and make it clear to them what the consensus recommendation happens to be. I always want to be guided by the preferences and values of my clients. I will at times follow my clinical intuition, but I am reluctant to do that in the face of good evidence to the contrary. In most instances I rely on intuition to "fill in the blanks" only when no good evidence exists to guide the process of shaping the strategies I adopt to fit the needs of my particular patient.

REFERENCES

American Psychiatric Association. (2010). *Practice guideline for the treatment of patients with major depressive disorder* (3rd ed.). Washington DC: American Psychiatric Press. Retrieved from http://www.psychiatryonline.com/pracGuide/pracGuide Topic_7.aspx

Angell, M. (2005). *The truth about the drug companies: How they deceive us and what to do about it*. New York, NY: Random House.

APA Presidential Task Force on Evidence-Based Practice. (2006). Evidence-based practice in psychology. *American Psychologist, 61*, 271–285. http://dx.doi.org/10.1037/0003-066X.61.4.271

Campbell, D. T., & Stanley, J. C. (1963). *Experimental and quasi-experimental designs for research and teaching*. Chicago, IL: Rand McNally.

Chambless, D. L., & Hollon, S. D. (1998). Defining empirically supported therapies. *Journal of Consulting and Clinical Psychology, 66*, 7–18. http://dx.doi.org/10.1037/0022-006X.66.1.7

Chlebowski, R. T., Hendrix, S. L., Langer, R. D., Stefanick, M. L., Gass, M., Lane, D., . . . McTiernan, A. (2003). Influence of estrogen plus progestin on breast cancer and mammography in healthy postmenopausal women: The Women's Health Initiative randomized trial. *JAMA, 289*, 3243–3253. http://dx.doi.org/10.1001/jama.289.24.3243

Cook, T. D., & Campbell, D. T. (1979). *Quasi-experimentation: Design and analysis issues for field settings.* Chicago, IL: Rand McNally.

Cuijpers, P., Driessen, E., Hollon, S. D., van Oppen, P., Barth, J., & Andersson, G. (2012). The efficacy of non-directive supportive therapy for adult depression: A meta-analysis. *Clinical Psychology Review, 32*, 280–291. http://dx.doi.org/10.1016/j.cpr.2012.01.003

Cuijpers, P., Smit, F., Bohlmeijer, E., Hollon, S. D., & Andersson, G. (2010). Efficacy of cognitive–behavioural therapy and other psychological treatments for adult depression: Meta-analytic study of publication bias. *The British Journal of Psychiatry, 196*, 173–178. http://dx.doi.org/10.1192/bjp.bp.109.066001

Cuijpers, P., van Straten, A., van Oppen, P., & Andersson, G. (2008). Are psychological and pharmacologic interventions equally effective in the treatment of adult depressive disorders? A meta-analysis of comparative studies. *Journal of Clinical Psychiatry, 69*, 1675–1685. http://dx.doi.org/10.4088/JCP.v69n1102

DeRubeis, R. J., Cohen, Z. D., Forand, N. R., Fournier, J. C., Gelfand, L. A., & Lorenzo-Luaces, L. (2014). The Personalized Advantage Index: Translating research on prediction into individualized treatment recommendations. A demonstration. *PLoS ONE, 9*, e83875. http://dx.doi.org/10.1371/journal.pone.0083875

DeRubeis, R. J., & Crits-Christoph, P. (1998). Empirically supported individual and group psychological treatments for adult mental disorders. *Journal of Consulting and Clinical Psychology, 66*, 37–52. http://dx.doi.org/10.1037/0022-006X.66.1.37

DeRubeis, R. J., Hollon, S. D., Amsterdam, J. D., Shelton, R. C., Young, P. R., Salomon, R. M., . . . Gallop, R. (2005). Cognitive therapy vs medications in the treatment of moderate to severe depression. *Archives of General Psychiatry, 62*, 409–416. http://dx.doi.org/10.1001/archpsyc.62.4.409

Dimidjian, S., Hollon, S. D., Dobson, K. S., Schmaling, K. B., Kohlenberg, R. J., Addis, M. E., . . . Jacobson, N. S. (2006). Randomized trial of behavioral activation, cognitive therapy, and antidepressant medication in the acute treatment of adults with major depression. *Journal of Consulting and Clinical Psychology, 74*, 658–670. http://dx.doi.org/10.1037/0022-006X.74.4.658

Driessen, E., Cuijpers, P., Hollon, S. D., Dekker, J. J. M. (2010). Does pretreatment severity moderate the efficacy of psychological treatment of adult outpatient depression? A meta-analysis. *Journal of Consulting and Clinical Psychology, 78*, 668–680.

Ehlers, A., Hackmann, A., Grey, N., Wild, J., Liness, S., Albert, I., . . . Clark, D. M. (2014). A randomized controlled trial of 7-day intensive and standard weekly cognitive therapy for PTSD and emotion-focused supportive therapy. *The American Journal of Psychiatry, 171,* 294–304. http://dx.doi.org/10.1176/appi.ajp.2013.13040552

Elkin, I., Gibbons, R. D., Shea, M. T., Sotsky, S. M., Watkins, J. T., Pilkonis, P. A., & Hedeker, D. (1995). Initial severity and differential treatment outcome in the National Institute of Mental Health Treatment of Depression Collaborative Research Program. *Journal of Consulting and Clinical Psychology, 63,* 841–847. http://dx.doi.org/10.1037/0022-006X.63.5.841

Elkin, I., Shea, M. T., Watkins, J. T., Imber, S. D., Sotsky, S. M., Collins, J. F., . . . Parloff, M. B. (1989). National Institute of Mental Health Treatment of Depression Collaborative Research Program: General effectiveness of treatments. *Archives of General Psychiatry, 46,* 971–982. http://dx.doi.org/10.1001/archpsyc.1989.01810110013002

Fournier, J. C., DeRubeis, R. J., Hollon, S. D., Dimidjian, S., Amsterdam, J. D., Shelton, R. C., & Fawcett, J. (2010). Antidepressant drug effects and depression severity: A patient-level meta-analysis. *JAMA, 303,* 47–53.

Fournier, J. C., DeRubeis, R. J., Shelton, R. C., Gallop, R., Amsterdam, J. D., & Hollon, S. D. (2008). Antidepressant medications versus cognitive therapy in people with depression with or without personality disorder. *The British Journal of Psychiatry, 192,* 124–129. http://dx.doi.org/10.1192/bjp.bp.107.037234

Fournier, J. C., DeRubeis, R. J., Shelton, R. C., Hollon, S. D., Amsterdam, J. D., & Gallop, R. (2009). Prediction of response to medication and cognitive therapy in the treatment of moderate to severe depression. *Journal of Consulting and Clinical Psychology, 77,* 775–787. http://dx.doi.org/10.1037/a0015401

Hollon, S. D., Areán, P. A., Craske, M. G., Crawford, K. A., Kivlahan, D. R., Magnavita, J. J., . . . Kurtzman, H. (2014). Development of clinical practice guidelines. *Annual Review of Clinical Psychology, 10,* 213–241. http://dx.doi.org/10.1146/annurev-clinpsy-050212-185529

Institute of Medicine. (2001). *Crossing the quality chasm: A new health system for the 21st century.* Washington, DC: National Academies Press.

Institute of Medicine. (2011a). *Clinical practice guidelines we can trust.* Washington, DC: National Academies Press.

Institute of Medicine. (2011b). *Finding what works in health care: Standards for systematic reviews.* Washington, DC: National Academies Press.

Jarrett, R. B., Schaffer, M., McIntire, D., Witt-Browder, A., Kraft, D., & Risser, R. C. (1999). Treatment of atypical depression with cognitive therapy or phenelzine: A double-blind, placebo-controlled trial. *Archives of General Psychiatry, 56,* 431–437. http://dx.doi.org/10.1001/archpsyc.56.5.431

Kahneman, D., Slovic, P., & Tversky, A. (Eds.). (1982). *Judgment under uncertainty: Heuristics and biases.* New York, NY: Cambridge University Press. http://dx.doi.org/10.1017/CBO9780511809477

Khan, A., Leventhal, R. M., Khan, S. R., & Brown, W. A. (2002). Severity of depression and response to antidepressants and placebo: An analysis of the Food and Drug Administration database. *Journal of Clinical Psychopharmacology, 22,* 40–45. http://dx.doi.org/10.1097/00004714-200202000-00007

Kirsch, I., Deacon, B. J., Huedo-Medina, T. B., Scoboria, A., Moore, T. J., & Johnson, B. T. (2008). Initial severity and antidepressant benefits: A meta-analysis of data submitted to the Food and Drug Administration. *PLoS Medicine, 5*(2), e45. http://dx.doi.org/10.1371/journal.pmed.0050045

Luborsky, L., Singer, B., & Luborsky, L. (1975). Comparative studies of psychotherapies: Is it true that "everyone has won and all must have prizes"? *Archives of General Psychiatry, 32,* 995–1008. http://dx.doi.org/10.1001/archpsyc.1975.01760260059004

Manson, J. E., Hsia, J., Johnson, K. C., Rossouw, J. E., Assaf, A. R., Lasser, N. L., ... Cushman, M. (2003). Estrogen plus progestin and the risk of coronary heart disease. *The New England Journal of Medicine, 349,* 523–534. http://dx.doi.org/10.1056/NEJMoa030808

Meehl, P. E. (1954). *Clinical versus statistical prediction: A theoretical analysis and a review of the evidence*. Minneapolis: University of Minnesota Press. http://dx.doi.org/10.1037/11281-000

Meehl, P. E. (1987). Theory and practice: Reflections of an academic clinician. In E. F. Bourg, R. J. Bent, J. E. Callan, N. F. Jones, J. McHolland, & G. Stricker (Eds.), *Standards and evaluation in the education and training of professional psychologists: Knowledge, attitudes, and skills* (pp. 7–23). Norman, OK: Transcript Press.

Mellers, B., Hertwig, R., & Kahneman, D. (2001). Do frequency representations eliminate conjunction effects? An exercise in adversarial collaboration. *Psychological Science, 12*(4), 269–275. http://dx.doi.org/10.1111/1467-9280.00350

National Collaborating Centre for Mental Health. (2010). *Depression: The treatment and management of depression in adults (updated edition)* (NICE Clinical Guidelines, No. 90). Leicester, England: British Psychological Society. Retrieved from http://www.ncbi.nlm.nih.gov/pubmedhealth/PMH0016605/

Popper, K. (1934). *The logic of scientific discovery*. London, England: Routledge.

Poulsen, S., Lunn, S., Daniel, S. I. F., Folke, S., Mathiesen, B., Katznelson, H., & Fairburn, C. G. (2014). A randomized controlled trial of psychoanalytic psychotherapy versus cognitive behavior therapy for bulimia nervosa. *American Journal of Psychiatry, 171,* 109–116. doi:10.1176/appi.ajp.2013.12121511

Reichenbach, H. (1938). *Experience and prediction: An analysis of the foundations and the structure of knowledge*. Chicago, IL: University of Chicago Press. http://dx.doi.org/10.1037/11656-000

Rogers, C. R. (1957). The necessary and sufficient conditions of therapeutic personality change. *Journal of Consulting Psychology, 21,* 95–103. http://dx.doi.org/10.1037/h0045357

Rush, A. J., Beck, A. T., Kovacs, M., & Hollon, S. D. (1977). Comparative efficacy of cognitive therapy and pharmacotherapy in the treatment of depressed outpatients. *Cognitive Therapy and Research, 1*, 17–37. http://dx.doi.org/10.1007/BF01173502

Smith, M. L., Glass, G. V., & Miller, T. I. (1980). *The benefits of psychotherapy.* Baltimore, MD: Johns Hopkins University Press.

Turner, E. H., Matthews, A. M., Linardatos, E., Tell, R. A., & Rosenthal, R. (2008). Selective publication of antidepressant trials and its influence on apparent efficacy. *The New England Journal of Medicine, 358*, 252–260. http://dx.doi.org/10.1056/NEJMsa065779

Wampold, B. E. (2001). *The great psychotherapy debate: Models, methods, and findings.* Mahwah, NJ: Erlbaum.

Westen, D., Novotny, C. M., & Thompson-Brenner, H. (2004). The empirical status of empirically supported psychotherapies: Assumptions, findings, and reporting in controlled clinical trials. *Psychological Bulletin, 130*, 631–663.

6
USING TECHNOLOGY TO ENHANCE DECISION MAKING

FRANZ CASPAR, THOMAS BERGER, AND LUKAS FREI

Clinical decision making involves a number of issues we have dealt with on other occasions in previous publications, such as decision under time pressure, multiple constraint satisfaction, intuition, dealing with soft information, prescriptive models for information processing and decision making, research on expert performance, the use of technology in psychotherapy training and in clinical psychology in general, and more (Berger, 2004; Berger, Hohl, & Caspar, 2010; Caspar, 1997, 2004; Caspar, Benninghoven, & Berger, 2004; Caspar, Berger, & Hautle, 2004). Although there are relations between these topics and the use of technology for decision making, we concentrate on the latter, profiting from our larger background, yet making links only when necessary. Caspar (2004) stated,

> We are getting used to receiving all kinds of services in life without assistance by human beings: French fries are prepared by machines, autopilots fly us over the ocean, phone numbers and timetables are searched on the

http://dx.doi.org/10.1037/14711-006
Clinical Decision Making in Mental Health Practice, J. J. Magnavita (Editor)
Copyright © 2016 by the American Psychological Association. All rights reserved.

Internet, even English essays can be graded by computers without human English teachers. Just a few years or decades ago, who would have expected that all this could work, apart, maybe, from Jules Verne? The world has changed, and in a dramatically changing world clinical psychology/ psychotherapy does not have the choice of standing still. (p. 222)

Some of the applications are really new, and some are extensions and continuous developments of preexisting technological and nontechnological approaches. Ten years after Caspar's comment, as technology in general and computers in particular increasingly permeate all domains of life, it would be astonishing if they were not used for clinical decision making. The task of decision making includes many subtasks with which technology can help. In this chapter, we go through these tasks, depicting what technology can do and which technology is actually available and in use or in development, and we give a tentative evaluation of how each is utilized. As we all know, in the domain of technology, predictions about what will turn out to be useful in the long run can be terribly wrong, so the best we can do is provide perspectives and arguments.

In line with our view of *decisions* we have presented on earlier occasions, the term is not reserved for big, conscious, deliberate decisions. Decisions are often made in an implicit process of accumulating premises, which ultimately determine a decision, or rather, a course of action, even though a deliberate decision is never made (see Chapter 2, this volume). It is plausible that technology could be used in support of more deliberate decisions, but this should not make us forget the less deliberate processes that determine our actions as clinicians and psychotherapists. These less deliberate processes dominate all the more in *adaptive treatment* tuning processes (*adaptive Indikation* in German), in which small adaptations are made to details in the process of the actual procedure and in which *selective treatment* (*selektive Indikation*) is fine tuned and set into action.

We focus here on decision making in the everyday clinical situation and do not address decision making in politics and administration, although obviously it affects clinical practice and vice versa. For example, decisions against providing sufficient face-to-face psychotherapy is one factor that may increase the demand for Internet therapy, and vice versa—that is, the use of technology for therapy, as in Internet therapy, might influence to what extent face-to-face therapy needs to be provided. It is obvious that the aggregation of information for political and administrative decisions can take advantage of technology. If technology is used professionally, this should contribute to better informed decisions and less dependency on information provided by lobbyists who might not work in the interest of high-quality service for those who need it. An optimistic view is thus that technology works in favor of patients on this level as well.

In the interest of keeping the focus of this chapter manageable, we also do not address treatments fully delivered over the Internet or computers, as for the example described in Comer and Barlow (2014), although such treatments, as they unfold, of course also include decision making.

REASONS TO USE TECHNOLOGY FOR DECISION MAKING

To be attractive, technology needs to be superior in some way to humans doing the task traditionally. It is possible that sellers of technology could make a buyer or user believe in such superiority as well as the emphasizing new tasks that a human is not able to do. The superiority may refer to various dimensions, such as speed, efficiency, reliability, validity, information and concepts or data that can be included, and costs. These dimensions are not independent of each other. For example, speed may lower costs and enable the inclusion of large databases; the greater speed and efficiency of computer-based testing may lead to shorter testing, which in turn would be more valid because patients are less tired toward the end of shorter testing; and so on. The following sections provide an overview of tasks for which technology is potentially superior.

MAKING INFORMATION AVAILABLE

Theories and Findings

For how many disorders and problems do you currently have all available information that can have an impact on decisions made for an actual patient? It can be assumed that the honest answer from most clinicians (as well as clinical scholars!) is at best three or four. How would the gaps be filled when one of the other disorders or problems showed up? If the clinician has good professional connections she or he may ask a knowledgeable colleague, most probably by phone. The probability is high that information will be gathered through the Internet, or, if the clinician is more thorough, by books selected and/or ordered via Internet. Even a clinician who does not use technology-provided information him- or herself has to deal with the fact that patients access these sources. Maggio (2008) described how practitioners can expand their knowledge of evidence-based practice by gathering background information, searching filtered resources, and tracking down original studies through unfiltered databases. Some of the reported resources and affiliated advances are especially worth mentioning:

- *Online textbooks.* In contrast to traditional paper textbooks, so called e-texts, for instance *Goodman and Gilman's Pharmacological Basis of Therapeutics* (Brunton, Chabner, & Knollman,

2010), can be updated frequently, providing the most recent information available.
- *Knowledge databases*. Professional resources such as the *eMedicine Clinical Knowledge Database* (http://www.emedicine.com) provide instant access on constantly updated and reviewed articles. According to Maggio (2008), approximately 10,000 health care professionals contributed to this database, resulting in articles on more than 6,500 conditions. Other websites contain comprehensive information on specific topics, such as a collection of mental health and substance abuse interventions (http://www.nrepp.samhsa.gov/find.asp), lists of available practice guidelines (http://www.guideline.gov, http://www.nice.org.uk), and systematic reviews (e.g., the Cochrane Database). Often, direct links to considered studies or further resources are provided. Internet surveys with experts are a good means for extending and actualizing databases, thus contributing to decision making based on the best available knowledge (Gore & Leuwerke, 2008).

Together with large databases containing original research studies (e.g., MEDLINE, PsycINFO), these resources provide a powerful tool to assist the decision-making process.

Information on Mental Problems and Treatments on the Internet

Beyond the specific information mentioned in the previous paragraphs, therapists as well as patients and their relatives gather information of all kind on the Internet—for example, on locally available treatment alternatives, emergency services, legal information, self-help books providing psychoeducation and intervention programs complementing face-to-face therapy, patient reports on experiences with different forms of therapy, and so on, which may influence treatment decisions. In fact, seeking health information is one of the most popular reasons for going online (Fox, 2011).

The use of web-derived health information may have several advantages and disadvantages. For instance, web-based health information may make patients better informed, leading to better health outcomes and more appropriate use of health services. It may also improve the therapeutic alliance by sharing the burden of responsibility for knowledge and enhancing communication in general (Gerber & Eiser, 2001). The possibility of easily accessing all kinds of health information may also empower patients and increase their sense of control over their disease. Furthermore, because basic knowledge of a disease can easily be gained over the Internet, the scheduled time during treatment may be used more efficiently, for instance for more in-depth and higher level discussions about treatment options and clinical decision making. Moreover, the fact that patients are well informed fosters participatory and informed decision making, which may increase compliance with treatment (Gerber & Eiser, 2001). On the other hand, the quality of many health websites is questionable. Thus, web-based information may be misleading, compromising health behaviors and resulting in unnecessary anxiety or inappropriate requests for clinical interventions.

Making Individualized Psychoeducative and Therapeutic Information Available to a Patient

This is a special possibility, for which we have seen demonstrations (first with Carlos Mirapeix in Spain). A therapist selects one- to two-page psychoeducative documents with relevance for the patient during a session. At the end of the session, an individualized stack of information is printed out and given to the patient. This information, read between the sessions, can be a basis for shared decision making about the further course of therapy. More generally, one of the growing developments in the field of Internet- and computer-based treatments is their blending with traditional treatments. For instance, in a recent study, Månsson, Skagius Ruiz, Gervind, Dahlin, and Andersson (2013) evaluated an Internet-based support system for face-to-face cognitive behavior therapy (CBT). The web-based platform used within and between sessions included a library with both text and media resources used in psychoeducation and as homework assignments. The platform was built to give support to both therapists and patients in the delivery of face-to-face CBT. In this proof of concept study, therapists found several major benefits to delivering treatment in this format, such as the possibility of focusing more on the relational aspects of treatment during sessions because basic therapeutic tasks such as the delivery of psychoeducational information were supported by the platform. Moreover, most of the patients expressed largely positive opinions about sharing information and homework over the Internet.

Data Related to a Specific Patient

Computer-assisted questionnaires and tests (Coyle, Doherty, Matthews, & Sharry, 2007) can be administered in a clinical setting, sometimes with a clinician standing by (usually referred to as *computer-assisted testing*), or they can be run over the Internet, providing the client with the possibility for answering it from any place preferred (usually referred to by such terms as *web assessment*, *Internet-based testing*, and *online testing*). Although important, this distinction is not always very clear, because web assessment can be seen as a subcategory of computer-assisted testing, and even in a clinical setting, a test can be run over the Internet. However, web assessments raise several additional questions when it comes to psychometric properties and the validity of such tests. The validity of frequently used questionnaires has been examined in several studies (Butcher, Perry, & Hahn, 2004), and it is generally good and comparable to the validity of paper-and-pencil versions (Carlbring et al., 2007; Coles, Cook, & Blake, 2007; Herrero & Meneses, 2006; Holländare, Andersson, & Engström, 2010). On the other hand, Buchanan et al. (2005) reported several studies finding differences between web-based and paper-and-pencil assessments. Differences are found not only in score distribution, impairing the use of earlier norms, but also in the factor structure of the measured constructs, raising questions about the validity of web-based assessment. In a recent publication, Weigold, Weigold, and Russell (2013) identified several factors that may account for at least some of the differences, such as unequal recruitment procedures and self-selection on behalf of participants.

Generally, utilizing validated web-assessment instruments is recommended. Differences do not necessarily speak against the Internet version. A meta-analysis showed advantages of a web version over a paper version in precision (Butcher et al., 2004). Further advantages include less embarrassment, more control, time saved, possibility of repeating, no interpersonal interferences with the presence of other persons, possibility of giving immediate reports or recommendations; these, as well as disadvantages, were discussed by Coyle et al. (2007). Computerized tests can also be adaptive; that is, during the testing and depending on given answers, decisions are made on what further items are presented, so noninformative items can be left out (Butcher et al., 2004; Coyle et al., 2007). This saves time, makes the procedure less annoying, and contributes to patient motivation and validity.

The assessment of biological states is another goal typically requiring technical equipment. Biofeedback is mainly used as an intervention in which the effective factor is information a patient receives about physiological states that can otherwise not be validly monitored by the patient him- or herself. For this, technology is needed. On the basis of biofeedback information, patients can learn to influence body functions that are otherwise out of their control. Biofeedback is commonly used as an intervention method, not a tool in decision making, yet it can also be used to monitor change, compliance, and emotional processing (Clough & Casey, 2011).

More sophisticated and expensive tools would be needed to provide information on brain functioning as a basis of clinical decisions. For example, DeRubeis, Siegle, and Hollon (2008) proposed that the decision about psychotherapy versus antidepressants should depend on whether depression seems mainly related to amygdala hyperfunction or prefrontal cortex hypofunction. The determination of these conditions for each patient individually, for example via functional magnetic resonance imaging, is currently very expensive and cannot be considered a standard procedure. On the basis of the assumption that equipment for the assessment of brain states will become cheaper and more mobile, Grawe (2007), in his visionary work *Neuropsychotherapy*, proposed assessing temporary brain states of a patient to give a therapist information as a basis for deciding whether the conditions for a particular intervention are favorable or not. A recent development in this direction is *neurofeedback*, which is a type of biofeedback that uses real-time displays of electroencephalography to illustrate brain activity and to teach self-regulation.

Feedback Systems

Computers can be used not only for single assessments but also to keep track of the process and progress of an ongoing therapy, providing feedback to clinicians. Bickman, Kelley, and Athay (2012) designated such applications *measurement feedback systems* (MFSs), and according to them, "the primary purpose of an MFS is to provide feedback that is used to inform clinical practice" (p. 277), which, of course, means a use for decision making (See Chapter 9, this volume). What are the benefits of MFSs? One argument mentioned by Duncan (2012) is their potential to reduce the high dropout rates usually found in routine practice through the identification of at-risk patients. They are also being discussed as tools for quality assurance and for optimizing cost effectiveness of therapies (Strauss et al., 2015). Additionally, MFSs may enhance patients' active participation in an ongoing therapy (Sexton, Patterson, & Datchi, 2012).

Feedback systems can be used to predict the course of an individual treatment by using data from patients who are similar to the current patient to make assumptions about how this patient can be expected to develop (Lambert, 2007; Lutz, Tholen, Kosfelder, Grawe, & Schulte, 2005; Percevic, Lambert, & Kordy, 2004). Some trials have demonstrated several benefits, including a reduction in the duration of treatments, reduced failure rates for at-risk patients, greater success rates of clinically significant improvement, and reduced operating costs (Coyle et al., 2007); other studies did not find superiority (Strauss et al., 2015).

In sum, feedback systems show a considerable capacity to improve outcome, especially for problematic therapies, if the therapist is supported in interpreting and utilizing the feedback (see the section Support of a Decision-Making Process in Therapy later in this chapter) and if the patient is also informed (De Jong et al., 2014). It is important to note that technology does not do the job of improving the procedure but that it helps provide *extrinsic feedback* (feedback that is not naturally and without particular efforts provided by the therapeutic procedure), which can be an essential input for a therapist trying to understand a patient and an ongoing procedure.

Ambulatory Monitoring

Ambulatory monitoring or *ecological momentary assessment* (EMA; Axelson et al., 2003; Coyle et al., 2007; Marks, Cavanagh, & Gega, 2007; Matthews, Doherty, Coyle, & Sharry, 2008) is a special form of data collection that leads to more valid assessment than retrospective recall. EMA is a "noninvasive method of gathering real-time data from subjects" (Axelson et al., 2003, p. 255). Mobile phones and personal digital assistants can help a patient collect data in everyday life—for example, about mood, behavior, motivation, or social activities (Clough & Casey, 2011).

A recent development is to include sensors such as GPS, motion detectors, and sound recordings. These measures may enrich and enhance the validity of traditional EMA self-report measures. The monitoring of the activity or self-report data in real life and time offers the opportunity to obtain a wealth of information for decision making, to follow the treatment progress over time, and to adapt the intervention.

Video Recordings, Data From a Patient, and Their Use in Supervision and Peer Consulting

It has long been shown that therapist written records of therapy sessions are highly unreliable (Levenson & Strupp, 1999). Although there are still big differences between private practice and training or research settings, it has become common to video-record single psychotherapy sessions or even entire therapies. Not only research protocols but also some training programs require recording on a regular basis, and more and more therapists are finding that video is a useful source of information for regular practice as well. Video records can be used to complete the information a therapist has about a session in which his or her capacity for watching, listening, and interpreting was limited, or they can be used to give others insight into a therapy (for supervision or peer consulting; see the section Online Supervision later in this chapter). For patients, it has become common to be video-recorded, and hardly any of them ask anymore whether this will be on the TV news.

Manring, Greenberg, Gregory, and Gallinger (2011) described how to set up a video-recording system and which issues should be considered. In principle, only a computer with a webcam and a microphone (usually built in on a laptop) are needed for reasonably good records. Video-recording has become so inexpensive that the cost of a reasonably good picture and sound recording system is no longer an argument against installing and using video-recording systems. In advanced video systems using a server, as we have installed in our training clinic, video recordings are stored on a secured server and can be accessed during supervision sessions with external supervisors from their offices. The system has passed rigorous security checks, and risks of unauthorized access are smaller than losing video recordings through, for example, burglary of a supervisee's car. In any case, security and protecting video files at least with a password are important issues.

Support of a Decision-Making Process in Therapy

As Comer and Barlow (2014) argued, for problems that do not occur frequently it would be inefficient to train a large number of clinicians so that they would have all necessary information available at all times. Technology can help to quickly provide the information needed to make a clinical decision, and it also enables well-informed decisions for rare disorders. Providing conceptual and empirical information has been an issue, as described earlier. Here we discuss more direct support of decision making.

A branch of decision-making research has proposed basing clinical decisions on explicit probability calculations, even by a general practitioner on a home visit. An "actuarial" or "statistical" way of making decisions is claimed to be superior to "clinical" decision making, which includes soft information, qualitative decisions, and intuitive information processing. There is no doubt that statistical decision making would be a field for the use of technology. We are convinced, though, that although the inclusion of probability information in clinical decision making is highly recommended, primary reliance on it in mental health and psychotherapy-related clinical decision making is not a viable approach. We therefore do not detail here how technology and computers could be used in such an approach.

Beutler and Harwood (2004; Beutler, Williams, & Norcross, 2011; Harwood et al., 2011) described a web-based systematic treatment selection system approach that is based on an Aptitude × Treatment Interaction design, providing information about adequate interventions or therapeutic styles. Before intake, certain patient characteristics (e.g., the patient's therapist preferences, most dominant symptoms, demographic data) are assessed via a web-delivered self-report measure, resulting in a tailored self-help tool for the patient and a more detailed report for the clinician. During the treatment process, a patient's symptoms are continuously being assessed, and the resulting change trajectory is compared with a projected change trajectory, showing the expected development according to initial information. This corresponds largely to the feedback systems described earlier. Harwood et al. (2011) further described how certain patient characteristics, such as functional impairment, coping style, subjective distress, social support, reactance–resistance level, problem complexity–chronicity, and stages of change–readiness are being used by systematic treatment selection to assist treatment planning.

Although the concepts on which the system is based are empirically derived, so far no empirical evaluation of the program itself exists.

Beyond descriptive feedbacks, some MFSs provide further assistance by providing decision trees and suggesting interventions. Clinical support tools (CSTs), for instance, attempt to assess therapeutic alliance, patient motivation, social support, and errors in diagnostic and treatment planning. If one of those variables is identified as problematic, suggestions for possible interventions are made. In a summary of two studies (Lambert, 2010), the percentage of at-risk patients deteriorating during the continuing therapy process dropped from 20% in the control group to 8% in the "feedback + CST" group. At the same time, the percentage of at-risk patients showing significant improvement doubled from 22% in the control group to 45% in the "feedback + CST" group. However, these promising results should be considered with caution: One of the included studies used data from prior feedback studies as a control group (Harmon et al., 2007), and in the second study, therapists could decide whether to use CSTs for a particular at-risk patient or not (Whipple et al., 2003), resulting in selective comparison groups. Although this particular MFS used nonelectronic tools, it gives an idea of how electronic feedback systems might be further enhanced for decision making.

This nonexhaustive list of more recent MFSs shows a wide application spectrum: Computerized and sometimes web-based feedback systems can be used for initial treatment planning, for session planning during an ongoing therapy, for tracking therapy progress, and for identifying at-risk patients. Assessments can occur between, directly before, or directly after sessions, providing information on outcomes, alliance, and motivation. Feedback is not limited to mere descriptions but may also provide more or less specific suggestions. Aside from these promising possibilities, the number of sometimes very similar systems and their general lack of evaluation raise the assumption that the search for a more widely applicable MFS is not over yet.

A special topic is decision making in a stepped-care approach involving the use of Internet-based self-help. Although stepped care as such does not require technology-based decision making, Internet therapy—if involved—may render relevant data. In a study by Berger et al. (2011), the number of mouse clicks during the first week of Internet-based treatment turned out to be an extremely simple and predictive criterion, readily delivered by technology. Activity and time spent in the self-help program during the first week of treatment was significantly associated with treatment outcome. Such early process predictors can be used to step up clients to more intensive interventions such as face-to-face psychotherapy early in the treatment process.

CONTACT AND COMMUNICATION

Videoconferencing

Some uses of technology in the process of clinical decision making are very obvious: Regular phone and Skype contacts among clinicians need no further mention, and just like we can use videoconferencing for all kinds of other shared decision making, we can, of course, also use it for clinical decision making. Although meetings in person may be favorable to initially build a personal relationship and trust, once those are established, videoconferencing is a very efficient way of bringing clinicians together among each other or with experts. When distances forbid a personal contact, videoconferencing is an excellent alternative.

Webinars

Similarly, *webinars* (web-based seminars) have become a common tool to make the wisdom of international experts available for trainees and colleagues who cannot easily travel to conferences, or to complement these. For example, the Society for Psychotherapy Research offers webinars on a regular basis.

Blended Treatment

As we mentioned before, we are not covering in this chapter the extensive literature on Internet-based treatments that are fully delivered online. With regard to decision making in traditional psychotherapy, it may be relevant that therapists are becoming more accustomed to offering some elements of the treatment online (e.g., psychoeducational information; Månsson et al., 2013; see earlier discussion) and to communicating online in between sessions. There are several indications from the literature that blending of traditional with Internet-based treatment may be a promising venue. In a recent review, it was concluded that patients' treatment adherence may be improved through new technologies (Clough & Casey, 2011). For instance, e-mails between sessions may be useful in prompting patients to do homework reports, providing more frequent feedback on homework, adapting the homework according to patients' feedback, and encouraging reflection (Murdoch & Connor-Greene, 2000). As with ambulatory assessments (see earlier discussion), therapists also receive more real-time and real-life data as a basis for their decisions when they communicate with their clients between sessions. In addition, it has been shown that aftercare also may be improved by the use of technological adjuncts such as online chat or SMS interventions (e.g., Bauer, Percevic, Okon, Meermann, & Kordy, 2003).

Collaborative Problem Solving

Complementary profiles in knowledge and skills may make it desirable that professionals with, for example, psychological and medical backgrounds cooperate. Although the telephone may be good enough when the information on which the collaboration is based is sufficiently simple, the situation changes when the needed information is more complex. Then more sophisticated technical support may lead to better outcomes. Because the competent handling of such collaboration is not trivial, several forms of training have been developed and evaluated.

TRAINING

Applications Concentrating on Video Recordings

Some information has already been provided in the previous section on video and its use for supervision. However, there are many more uses of video recordings.

Video is prominent in several applications serving the training of therapists. Beyond the use of raw video recordings for supervision, several applications provide rating systems, further structuring the supervision process. One of them is the Internet-based training system (ITS) developed to observe, rate, and comment on videotaped mock sessions through the use of structured feedback items (Worrall & Fruzzetti, 2009). These ratings and comments can then be compared with those from other therapists.

One very similar tool is e-SOFTA (which stands for System for Observing Family Therapy Alliances, an electronic system for observing family therapy alliances; Escudero, Friedlander, & Heatherington, 2011). Although e-SOFTA is useful only for specific therapy settings and only for certain aspects related to the alliance, it is an example of a well-documented, frequently used, and freely available instrument. Both the documentation and the program can be accessed through the SOFTA website (http://www.softa-soatif.com). A therapist can use the software to rate videos of therapy sessions on engagement in the therapeutic process, emotional connection with the therapist, safety within the therapeutic system, shared sense of purpose within the family, and the therapist's contribution to the alliance. Ratings are linked to the respective time during a therapy session and can be supplemented with a comment. The same video can be rated by several persons (e.g., a therapist and a supervisor), and ratings as well as comments can be compared easily. The rating scales of e-SOFTA have been validated (Friedlander et al., 2006), and the tool has been successfully used in a training intervention for students

(Carpenter, Escudero, & Rivett, 2008), significantly improving their knowledge related to the therapeutic alliance (from 43% to 74%, $p < .001$) as well as their observation skills (from 43% to 65%, although without reaching statistical significance; $p = .08$). A related tool is Counselor Assisted Supervision, a program that trainees can use to watch and critique tapes of their counseling sessions (Gore & Leuwerke, 2008). All this is not directly related to decision making in a narrow sense, but abilities are trained that are plausibly relevant for decision making.

Computer-Based and Web-Based Training

The number of studies investigating the use of computer- and web-based training in schools of medicine, nursing, and allied sciences has increased substantially in the past few years. Obvious and documented advantages of computer- or web-based training in comparison with traditional classroom teaching are (a) self-paced learning—students can progress at their own pace and repeat as they please; (b) increased accessibility—as technical devices become more easily accessible, courses can be accessed when and where they create minimal intrusion into students' lives and when they are in the best possible learning state; (c) decreased costs—costs decrease in proportion to the number of learners using a specific program; and (d) constant quality—many students can use the same qualified training module (Berger, 2004). An example of such a web-based training program in the field of psychotherapy is Psychotherapy Training e-Resources (PTeR; Weerasekera, 2013). PTeR consists of 11 web-based modules with content information being presented in multiple forms, including clinical vignettes to demonstrate expert modeling of clinical skills. The program houses more than 70 video clips demonstrating several types of psychotherapy. The program also includes pre–post tests in each module so that performance can be monitored throughout training.

Another example is an interactive multimedia online training (OLT) in dialectical behavior therapy skills. In a controlled study, Dimeff et al. (2009) compared the OLT with a written treatment manual and a 2-day instructor-led training workshop (ILT). Participants in the OLT group outperformed participants in both other conditions in terms of knowledge. OLT and ILT further resulted in larger gains in self-efficacy than the manual-only condition. However, comparing the use of the training content in their clinical practice, self-reports of participants did not differ across conditions, nor did the observer-rated adherence or competence in a simulated clinical interaction.

In medicine and allied sciences, hundreds of studies comparing computer- and web-based trainings with conventional modes have found computer-based trainings to be either equivalent or superior to conventional instruction with regard to students' learning (Kulik, 1994). However, critics of these findings who cited various biases in the studies, such as different degrees of effort used in designing computer-based trainings and control conditions, should be taken seriously (Clark, 1994). In well-controlled studies in which the same material was used and the same teacher provided the instructions for the experimental and control groups, equivalent results were reported (Fletcher-Flinn & Gravatt, 1995). It seems plausible that learning outcomes are a function not of the delivery medium but of the instruction itself (Clark, 1994).

Computer-Based Training of Skills Related to Case Conceptualization

Our own group has developed computer-assisted trainings based on the concept that only limited skills can be taught in computer-supported training modules. In line with the deliberate practice model for the development of professional expertise in general (Ericsson, Krampe, & Tesch-Römer, 1993), it is assumed that the goals of learning need to be concrete, that success should be achievable within a reasonably short time to provide success experiences motivating further efforts, that the provision of feedback is crucial and that it needs to be fast and informative, and that trainees should have the possibility to improve their behavior in further rounds and get feedback again. It is further assumed that computer support should be used because there are not enough human masters from whom to learn, and if they were available, they would be too expensive. Because there are plenty of more complex tasks that can hardly be squeezed into computer-supported limited modules, there is no threat to the demand for human experts–trainers. There is also no concurrence between the training of relatively simple, limited skills and the training of more complex skills; instead, by using computer-supported learning for the structured, efficient training of basic skills, resources are freed for training in more complex skills in psychotherapy. In supervision, for example, supervisors would be confronted as little as possible with a lack of basic skills in their supervisees and therefore would not need to address such a lack in their supervision.

More concretely, as a first step, a training has been developed in *optimizing coherence*. This is based on the idea that coherence is a crucial criterion for the strength and plausibility of models in general (Thagard, 1989). In a computer-supported training, trainees were instructed to use a graphical tool to express their view of important aspects of the structure of their patient's functioning. The general goal is the development of abilities to see and explicitly express the structure with multiple links between its elements. Conflicts and contradictions residing within the patient can also be fed into the program and, if appropriately expressed, do not hamper the coherence fed back to the user. The user can get feedback on the achieved level of coherence any time while working on the network. Therapists can use their own patients because the program does not need to "understand" content.

Thirty-four users participated in a study on the effects of such a training module, 19 in the training, 15 in a control condition with a training of different content. Acceptance was good, and the networks representing the view these therapists had of their individual patients became richer and more complete, more complex in a positive sense, and more coherent, although the latter criterion did not reach significance. It is concluded that computer-supported training can be used to acquire specific skills that are relevant for case conceptualization and decision making (Caspar, Benninghoven, & Berger, 2004).

A second approach includes content as opposed to formal aspects of the structure in the coherence training. One would think that computer-supported training including content would require more standardization in the sense of using multiple choice answers and/or expert systems in which it is clearly defined which view of a patient is wrong or right. In our view, though, in clinical–psychotherapeutic reality the view of experts may differ, and out of different perspectives several may be of value. To pretend that the clinical world is simple would convey an incorrect view, and a program based on such a view would get little acceptance by those who know. Although we felt that content should be included, we renounced doing this in a simplistic way. The situation changed when we became acquainted with latent semantic analysis (LSA) through Kintsch and Landauer (Landauer, Foltz, & Laham, 1998). The second author of this chapter adapted this concept and the underlying programs so that the program could project users' typed-in formulations into a semantic space in which their views of videotaped cases could be compared with the views of a number of experts. How this works is based on mathematics, and an explanation is beyond the scope of this chapter (Landauer et al., 1998), although Figure 6.1 illustrates the principle.

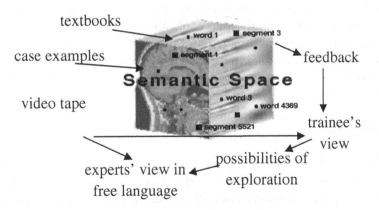

Figure 6.1. Feedback based on latent semantic analysis; see explanation in the text.

A semantic space is built up by feeding thousands of clinical texts (e.g., articles, case reports) into a computer program. This program analyzes how close together words are used and builds up a semantic space based on this information. This is very different from a classical expert system, which has to be constructed by experts deciding what is right or wrong. In a second step, experts watch a videotape of an intake interview and type in their view of the case. This information is then projected into the semantic space. Now the system is ready to be used by trainees. They also watch the videotape and type in their view of the case just like the experts did. They then get several forms of feedback. The first simply tells them which aspects of the observed case that were covered by the experts have also been addressed by the user and what percentage of what the experts have stated they have succeeded in covering as well. The goal is not to bring the histograms in the graphical feedback up to 100% because not all experts would agree with all that has been said by other experts. But if the percentage covered by the user is very low, this is a challenge to think about what could have been overlooked and to amend the originally typed-in view to drive up the percentage. Other forms of feedback follow, and ultimately the program, in exploring the views of the experts, supports the user. He or she also gets a realistic impression of potential variations in the experts' view.

The procedure and positive results of a first study were described in Caspar, Berger, and Hautle (2004). The breadth of those users who had a chance to practice repeatedly with the program was significantly superior to trainees who received another form of training. Acceptance was very good. In a second study, LSA-based feedback was compared with traditional written feedback received 2 weeks after sending in a text on the patient. In a third study, users typed in their verbal answer to a video scene and were then confronted with the answer of the patient, which was chosen by the program out of several alternatives depending on the quality of the user's written intervention. Then, the user typed in his or her next intervention and got feedback on this. Subsequently, users could also read what the experts would have said. This form of learning requires the user to act (albeit only in the form of typing), and the task is more dynamic because the dialogue develops over a short time. The acceptance for this program is also good; the effects are still in evaluation.

Online Supervision

Great possibilities lie in online supervision. About 10 years ago, Miller, Miller, and Evans (2002) stated that the counseling literature was full of studies examining the effectiveness of live supervision, and they provided a short overview of the different forms being used. Early live supervision was provided in person, through the "knock-on-the-door" method, where the supervisor interrupted a session to consult with the supervisee or to give additional input. Similarly, using the "telephone call-in" approach, a supervisor disrupted the session by calling in via telephone. Technological advances allowed less intrusive feedback, through the use of a microphone and an earpiece unit ("bug-in-the-ear"), or by providing visual feedback ("bug-in-the-eye"). The latter has the advantage of being less intrusive than a bug in the ear: Whereas a therapist unavoidably hears what a supervisor says, he or she has the freedom to look or not to look at a screen behind the patient displaying hints from a supervisor. There is limited empirical evidence for the effectiveness of the bug-in-the-eye method (Miller et al., 2002). Surprisingly, the past decade yielded little additional research on live supervision methods, and what there was has had mixed findings (Bartle-Haring, Silverthorn, Meyer, & Toviessi, 2009), which should not surprise us given that the balance between disturbing–intruding versus helping is not equal for all therapists, patients, supervisors, and situations. Nevertheless, live supervision seems to be quite common (Denton, Nakonezny, & Burwell, 2011), and both bug-in-the-ear and bug-in-the-eye have been further developed to be used in remote supervision (Jakob, Weck, & Bohus, 2013; Rousmaniere & Frederickson, 2013; Smith et al., 2007, 2012). Through videoconference software, the therapy session is streamed onto the supervisor's computer, and the supervisor, in turn, can give instructions to the supervisee, either via microphone and earpiece (bug-in-the-ear) or through text messages, which are then displayed on a laptop computer sitting next to the patient (bug-in-the-eye). Aside from some anecdotal evidence from the parties involved on "more intense" and "closer" experiences, no evaluation of this approach seems to exist so far.

Another branch of research is related to the use of videoconferencing for supervision. Abbass et al. (2011) provided a short survey on the respective literature and concluded that there has been limited research in this area. Existing studies mainly focused on the experiences of supervisors and trainees, whereas the impact on efficacy and client-based outcomes has been neglected (Reese et al., 2009; Sørlie, Gammon, Bergvik, & Sexton, 1999; Xavier, Shepherd, & Goldstein, 2007). Although videoconferencing offers promising possibilities for supervision, most researchers point out legal and ethical issues that need to be addressed (Worrall & Fruzzetti, 2009). According to Rousmaniere and Frederickson (2013), most guidelines concerning technology-assisted supervision and training are rather vague and do not provide specific instructions. As more specific guidelines, they cite *Best Practices in Clinical Supervision* by the Association for Counselor Education and Supervision (ACES Task Force, 2011), which mentions that "in using technology for distance supervision, the supervisor clearly approximates face-to-face synchronous contact" (p. 6); that the adopted technology has to be "in compliance with ethical guidelines and regulations promulgated by accreditation, certification, and licensure bodies" (p. 7); and that the supervisor "is competent in the use of the technology employed in supervision" (p. 7). As a fourth premise, password protection and encryption must be compliant with the Health Insurance Portability and Accountability Act to ensure confidentiality. Several videoconference tools seem to exist, where such compliance is given (e.g., https://liveconferencepro.com; http://www.talktoanexpertinc.com).

Collaborative Problem Solving

Collaborative problem solving with videoconferencing is not a trivial task. Extensive research has shown that the success of collaborative efforts does not occur on its own. Therefore, trainings for such collaboration have been developed and evaluated (Rummel & Spada, 2005). Rummel and Spada (2005) developed a program to train users for a collaboration between professionals with medical versus psychological backgrounds whose joint task is to formulate a report that includes a detailed diagnosis for the patient and a proposal of a suitable therapy. In this scenario, the two experts work at distant locations and cannot afford the time to meet in person. Instead, they decide to take advantage of a desktop videoconferencing system that has recently been implemented at both of their institutions. There are three constituent elements to such a collaboration: There is *symmetry* between the two; nobody is superior, but they have complementary competencies. Each of the partners is a "novice" in the other's domain and an "expert" in his own. They have *common goals*, namely, to solve the problem, and there is a *division of labor*. The presented task is both realistic and of high practical relevance. The findings show that observational learning from worked-out collaboration examples is a successful way to promote collaborative skills. If such an example is well conceived, it functions as a model for the people observing the collaboration, especially if they have the possibility to reflect on what they see and hear. Partners who work jointly on a problem-solving task following a cooperation script acquire collaborative skills that also improve collaboration in subsequent tasks.

Virtual Reality

Virtual reality has been used for the assessment of medication management skills (Kurtz, Baker, Pearlson, & Astur, 2007). Beutler and Harwood (2004) proposed a virtual reality–based training in their empirically supported and multifaceted systematic treatment selection model (see also the section Support for Decision Making earlier in this chapter). As far as we know, only a pilot model has been developed.

ACCEPTANCE AND SKILLFUL USE

Comer and Barlow (2014; Rogers, 2003) pointed out the importance of four factors for the acceptance of new approaches: (a) limited complexity; (b) trialability, which means the possibility of trying out something new before a decision for or against its permanent use is made; (c) compatibility with existing approaches; and (d) the testability of results. Acceptance will also depend on financial compensation; for example in telemedicine, face-to-face contact is replaced by virtual contact, but where technology complements human activity, the tools and procedures must also be financed.

Beyond acceptance, the skillful use of technology is an issue. Depending on how close the use of the technology is to the everyday use, it may be very demanding in terms of resources and motivation to introduce and effectively use technology. Dedication as well as communicative and didactic skills of personnel may become crucial, along with employee retention in the interest of not losing knowledge and experience with turnover on the job (Comer & Barlow, 2014). As a basis for appropriate training, requirements for competent use must be defined by the developers of applications (Comer & Barlow, 2014).

RISKS

There are some risks related to the use of technology:

- Fascination with technology could lead to an application in which costs and disadvantages outweigh the advantages, or technical aspects could blind users as well as developers to clinical aspects.
- The use of traditional expert systems as an aid in decision making may mislead users to believe that there are simple truths and solutions in this field.
- Responsibility for the quality of decisions and for errors could be diffuse or delegated to technology; this is a hot debate also in medicine, for example, in robotic surgery.
- Reduced practice in the own processing of information, such as recognizing patterns, may lead to a loss of abilities and to dependency on technology, just like abilities to read maps efficiently may deteriorate when people use a GPS on a regular basis (see also Chapters 4 and 11, this volume).
- Letting technology do jobs without really knowing what is done and how may lead to bad solutions, which translates into deterioration or failed improvement and its consequences for the patient's quality of life and, in the worst case, even loss of life.

- Technology supporting the dissemination of relevant information to practitioners not fully trained for their task may lead to superficial use of information. To have information available does not imply its competent use, so the availability of technology may contribute to an overestimation of the quality of service and may thus mask a need for better training.
- Risks from not seeing a patient in person exist, although Internet therapy applications show that even without a personal contact, individual emergency plans can be developed.
- Privacy–confidentiality is always an issue in applications involving exchanges over the Internet.

Overall, there are undeniably a number of risks, but if they are recognized and dealt with, the risks do not forbid a use of technology.

SUMMARY AND FUTURE DEVELOPMENTS

There are many aspects or parts of clinical decision making where technology contributes to or is even essential for the quality and efficiency of decisions. Applications utilizing technology for decision making in a narrow sense are rare, but technology contributes to gathering and passing on information and communication with patients, colleagues, supervisors, and experts. Some applications, like the use of telephones, have become so obvious that we are mostly not even aware of using technology. When we use highly sophisticated computer programs, we are aware of this, even if it is part of the quality of such programs that the user recognizes only the tip of the iceberg of the underlying technology. And then there are applications that are highly technological on the user side as well as on the provider side—such as Internet search—but that are becoming so much a part of everyday life that we soon may experience it as a use of technology on par with the telephone.

If seen as a complex process of accumulating premises—as opposed to making big decisions between clear alternatives at limited points of time—a large part of clinical decision making already is determined by technology. A big question is, of course, what further developments we have to expect or to strive for. When looking into models of the development of human professional expertise, there is a progression from the conscious, relatively crude, rule-based information processing of the novice to the more complex information of the expert. This takes into account more complex and subtle factors and circumstances to come up with a professional behavior that is much more flexible and adapted to the patient's individual, momentary situation. In principle, technology, and in particular computers with access to the Internet, can provide much of the information needed. Schäfer (Schäfer & Niederer, 2014), a German "Dr. House" in his Marburg clinic for unrecognized diseases, has said that even extremely rare cases can be diagnosed by doing a simple Google search with the right combination of symptoms. To what extent this applies also to the field of mental disorders, and what it takes to assess the symptoms correctly, is another question. Clinical decisions, at least in the field of psychotherapy, are not only a question of the right diagnosis. A good qualitative understanding of the functioning of a patient, as it is typically elaborated in case conceptualizations, is essential. Such a conceptualization is probably more than medical diagnosis based on subtle, soft information, on inferences requiring information processing such as pattern recognition, and the like. No clinician would survive a day without implicit and intuitive information processing. The question is whether this should and could be replaced by technology-supported rational decision making. Dreyfus and Dreyfus (1986) formulated concerns that the quest for rational, justifiable decisions might suppress the development of true expertise so that professionals would get stuck at a suboptimal, subexpert stage of development. We believe that this danger exists, but whether technology contributes to such a suboptimal development depends on ingenuity and the smart use of technology. For example, the speed and efficiency with which knowledge relevant for a case can be gathered today could set free resources that we can use to lean back and let our imagination and intuition do some work on our view of the patient's problems before we switch back to a more rational mode of thinking about the patient. Effective telecommunication or webinars enable us to tap into intuitive decision making of experts. The technology behind our LSA-based training program (Caspar, Berger, & Hautle, 2004) is so smart that we do not have to pretend that there is one correct view of a case or problem and that one arrives at it with answers to multiple choice questions. Rather, as described earlier, users can formulate their views freely, the program compares it with the views of several experts, and the user can see that there is not only one correct view and is supported in exploring the views of several experts.

If we use technology in such a way, without forcing our minds into a procrustean bed of one-sidedly rational thinking, we see a great potential in the future. Which concrete development we can expect is hard to predict.

> The task for clinical researchers and practitioners will be to make intelligent use of technology; "empty" technology is of little use.... One thing is clear: Many products developed will appear as "dinosaurs" in just a few years, but they are necessary stepping stones for further development. (Caspar, 2004, pp. 348–349)

REFERENCES

Abbass, A., Arthey, S., Elliott, J., Fedak, T., Nowoweiski, D., Markovski, J., & Nowoweiski, S. (2011). Web-conference supervision for advanced psychotherapy training: A practical guide. *Psychotherapy, 48,* 109–118. http://dx.doi.org/10.1037/a0022427

ACES Task Force. (2011, January 18). *Best practices in clinical supervision: ACES Task Force report.* Retrieved from http://www.saces.org/resources/documents/aces_best_practices.doc

Axelson, D. A., Bertocci, M. A., Lewin, D. S., Trubnick, L. S., Birmaher, B., Williamson, D. E., . . . Dahl, R. E. (2003). Measuring mood and complex behavior in natural environments: Use of ecological momentary assessment in pediatric affective disorders. *Journal of Child and Adolescent Psychopharmacology, 13,* 253–266. http://dx.doi.org/10.1089/104454603322572589

Bartle-Haring, S., Silverthorn, B. C., Meyer, K., & Toviessi, P. (2009). Does live supervision make a difference? A multilevel analysis. *Journal of Marital and Family Therapy, 35,* 406–414. http://dx.doi.org/10.1111/j.1752-0606.2009.00124.x

Bauer, S., Percevic, R., Okon, E., Meermann, R., & Kordy, H. (2003). Use of text messaging in the aftercare of patients with bulimia nervosa. *European Eating Disorders Review, 11,* 279–290. http://dx.doi.org/10.1002/erv.521

Berger, T. (2004). Computer-based technological applications in psychotherapy training. *Journal of Clinical Psychology, 60,* 301–315. http://dx.doi.org/10.1002/jclp.10265

Berger, T., Caspar, F., Richardson, R., Kneubühler, B., Sutter, D., & Andersson, G. (2011). Internet-based treatment of social phobia: A randomized controlled trial comparing unguided with two types of guided self-help. *Behaviour Research and Therapy, 49,* 158–169. http://dx.doi.org/10.1016/j.brat.2010.12.007

Berger, T., Hohl, E., & Caspar, F. (2010). Internetbasierte Therapie der sozialen Phobie: Ergebnisse einer 6-Monate-Katamnese [Internet-based therapy of social phobia: Findings in a 6-month follow-up]. *Zeitschrift für Klinische Psychologie und Psychotherapie, 39,* 217–221. http://dx.doi.org/10.1026/1616-3443/a000050

Beutler, L. E., & Harwood, T. M. (2004). Virtual reality in psychotherapy training. *Journal of Clinical Psychology, 60,* 317–330. http://dx.doi.org/10.1002/jclp.10266

Beutler, L. E., Williams, R. R., & Norcross, J. N. (2011). *Science and research.* Retrieved from http://innerlife.com

Bickman, L., Kelley, S. D., & Athay, M. (2012). The technology of measurement feedback systems. *Couple and Family Psychology, 1,* 274–284. http://dx.doi.org/10.1037/a0031022

Brunton, L., Chabner, B., & Knollman, B. (2010). *Goodman and Gilman's the pharmacological basis of therapeutics* (12th ed.). New York, NY: McGraw Hill Professional.

Buchanan, T., Ali, T., Heffernan, T. M., Ling, J., Parrott, A. C., Rodgers, J., & Scholey, A. B. (2005). Nonequivalence of on-line and paper-and-pencil psychological tests: The case of the prospective memory questionnaire. *Behavior Research Methods, 37,* 148–154. http://dx.doi.org/10.3758/BF03206409

Butcher, J. N., Perry, J., & Hahn, J. (2004). Computers in clinical assessment: Historical developments, present status, and future challenges. *Journal of Clinical Psychology, 60,* 331–345. http://dx.doi.org/10.1002/jclp.10267

Carlbring, P., Brunt, S., Bohman, S., Austin, D., Richards, J., Öst, L.-G., & Andersson, G. (2007). Internet vs. paper and pencil administration of questionnaires commonly used in panic/agoraphobia research. *Computers in Human Behavior, 23,* 1421–1434. http://dx.doi.org/10.1016/j.chb.2005.05.002

Carpenter, J., Escudero, V., & Rivett, M. (2008). Training family therapy students in conceptual and observation skills relating to the therapeutic alliance: An evaluation. *Journal of Family Therapy, 30,* 411–424. http://dx.doi.org/10.1111/j.1467-6427.2008.00442.x

Caspar, F. (1997). What goes on in a psychotherapist's mind? *Psychotherapy Research, 7,* 105–125. http://dx.doi.org/10.1080/10503309712331331913

Caspar, F. (2004). Technological developments and applications in clinical psychology and psychotherapy: Summary and outlook. *Journal of Clinical Psychology, 60,* 347–349. http://dx.doi.org/10.1002/jclp.10268

Caspar, F., Benninghoven, D., & Berger, T. (2004). Kohärenz in psychotherapeutischen Fallkonzeptionen—Grundlagen und Evaluation eines computergestützten Trainingsprogrammes [Coherence in psychotherapeutic case conceptualizations—Fundamentals and evaluation of a computer-based training program]. *Zeitschrift für Psychiatrie. Psychotherapie und Medizinische Psychologie, 54,* 320–329. http://dx.doi.org/10.1055/s-2003-815001

Caspar, F., Berger, T., & Hautle, I. (2004). The right view of your patient: A computer assisted, individualized module for psychotherapy training. *Psychotherapy: Theory, Research, Practice, Training, 41,* 125–135. http://dx.doi.org/10.1037/0033-3204.41.2.125

Clark, R. E. (1994). Media will never influence learning. *Educational Technology Research and Development, 42,* 21–29. http://dx.doi.org/10.1007/BF02299088

Clough, B. A., & Casey, L. M. (2011). Technological adjuncts to enhance current psychotherapy practices: A review. *Clinical Psychology Review, 31,* 279–292. http://dx.doi.org/10.1016/j.cpr.2010.12.008

Coles, M. E., Cook, L. M., & Blake, T. R. (2007). Assessing obsessive compulsive symptoms and cognitions on the internet: Evidence for the comparability of paper and Internet administration. *Behaviour Research and Therapy, 45,* 2232–2240. http://dx.doi.org/10.1016/j.brat.2006.12.009

Comer, J. S., & Barlow, D. H. (2014). The occasional case against broad dissemination and implementation: Retaining a role for specialty care in the delivery of psychological treatments. *American Psychologist, 69,* 1–18. http://dx.doi.org/10.1037/a0033582

Coyle, D., Doherty, G., Matthews, M., & Sharry, J. (2007). Computers in talk-based mental health interventions. *Interacting with Computers, 19,* 545–562. http://dx.doi.org/10.1016/j.intcom.2007.02.001

De Jong, K., Timman, R., Hakkaart-Van Roijen, L., Vermeulen, P., Kooiman, K., Passchier, J., & Van Busschbach, J. (2014). The effect of outcome monitoring feedback to clinicians and patients in short and long-term psychotherapy: A randomized controlled trial. [Advance online publication]. *Psychotherapy Research, 24,* 629–639. http://dx.doi.org/10.1080/10503307.2013.871079

Denton, W. H., Nakonezny, P. A., & Burwell, S. R. (2011). The effects of meeting a family therapy supervision team on client satisfaction in an initial session. *Journal of Family Therapy, 33,* 85–97. http://dx.doi.org/10.1111/j.1467-6427.2010.00518.x

DeRubeis, R. J., Siegle, G. J., & Hollon, S. D. (2008). Cognitive therapy versus medication for depression: Treatment outcomes and neural mechanisms. *Nature Reviews Neuroscience, 9,* 788–796. http://dx.doi.org/10.1038/nrn2345

Dimeff, L. A., Koerner, K., Woodcock, E. A., Beadnell, B., Brown, M. Z., Skutch, J. M., . . . Harned, M. S. (2009). Which training method works best? A randomized controlled trial comparing three methods of training clinicians in dialectical behavior therapy skills. *Behaviour Research and Therapy, 47,* 921–930. http://dx.doi.org/10.1016/j.brat.2009.07.011

Dreyfus, H. L., & Dreyfus, S. E. (1986). *Mind over machine: The power of human intuition and expertise in the era of the computer.* New York, NY: Free Press.

Duncan, B. L. (2012). The Partners for Change Outcome Management System (PCOMS): The Heart and Soul of Change Project. *Canadian Psychology/Psychologie canadienne, 53,* 93–104. http://dx.doi.org/10.1037/a0027762

Ericsson, K. A., Krampe, R. T., & Tesch-Römer, C. (1993). The role of deliberate practice in the acquisition of expert performance. *Psychological Review, 100,* 363–406. http://dx.doi.org/10.1037/0033-295X.100.3.363

Escudero, V., Friedlander, M. L., & Heatherington, L. (2011). Using the e-SOFTA for video training and research on alliance-related behavior. *Psychotherapy, 48,* 138–147. http://dx.doi.org/10.1037/a0022188

Fletcher-Flinn, C. M., & Gravatt, B. (1995). The efficacy of computer assisted instruction (CAI): A meta-analysis. *Journal of Educational Computing Research, 12,* 219–241. http://dx.doi.org/10.2190/51D4-F6L3-JQHU-9M31

Fox, S. (2011). *Health topics.* Pew Research Center website. Retrieved from http://pewinternet.org/Reports/2011/HealthTopics.aspx

Friedlander, M. L., Escudero, V., Horvath, A. O., Heatherington, L., Cabero, A., & Martens, M. P. (2006). System for observing family therapy alliances: A tool for research and practice. *Journal of Counseling Psychology, 53,* 214–225. http://dx.doi.org/10.1037/0022-0167.53.2.214

Gerber, B. S., & Eiser, A. R. (2001). The patient physician relationship in the Internet age: Future prospects and the research agenda. *Journal of Medical Internet Research, 3*(2), e15. http://dx.doi.org/10.2196/jmir.3.2.e15

Gore, P. A., Jr., & Leuwerke, W. C. (2008). Technological advances: Implications for counseling psychology research, training, and practice. In S. D. Brown & R. W. Lent (Eds.), *Handbook of counseling psychology* (4th ed., pp. 38–53). New York, NY: Wiley.

Grawe, K. (2007). *Neuropsychotherapy*. Mahwah, NJ: Erlbaum.

Harmon, S. C., Lambert, M. J., Smart, D. M., Hawkins, E., Nielsen, S. L., Slade, K., & Lutz, W. (2007). Enhancing outcome for potential treatment failures: Therapist–client feedback and clinical support tools. *Psychotherapy Research, 17*, 379–392. http://dx.doi.org/10.1080/10503300600702331

Harwood, T. M., Pratt, D., Beutler, L. E., Bongar, B. M., Lenore, S., & Forrester, B. T. (2011). Technology, telehealth, treatment enhancement, and selection. *Professional Psychology: Research and Practice, 42*, 448–454. http://dx.doi.org/10.1037/a0026214

Herrero, J., & Meneses, J. (2006). Short web-based versions of the Perceived Stress (PSS) and Center for Epidemiological Studies-Depression (CESD) Scales: A comparison to pencil and paper responses among Internet users. *Computers in Human Behavior, 22*, 830–846. http://dx.doi.org/10.1016/j.chb.2004.03.007

Holländare, F., Andersson, G., & Engström, I. (2010). A comparison of psychometric properties between internet and paper versions of two depression instruments (BDI-II and MADRS-S) administered to clinic patients. *Journal of Medical Internet Research, 12*(5), e49. http://dx.doi.org/10.2196/jmir.1392

Jakob, M., Weck, F., & Bohus, M. (2013). Live-Supervision: Vom Einwegspiegel zur videobasierten [Live supervision: From the one-way mirror to video-based online supervision]. *Verhaltenstherapie, 23*, 170–180. http://dx.doi.org/10.1159/000354234

Kulik, J. A. (1994). Meta-analytic studies of findings on computer-based instruction. In E. L. Baker & H. F. O'Neil Jr. (Eds.), *Technology assessment in education and training* (pp. 9–33). Hillsdale, NJ: Erlbaum.

Kurtz, M. M., Baker, E., Pearlson, G. D., & Astur, R. S. (2007). A virtual reality apartment as a measure of medication management skills in patients with schizophrenia: A pilot study. *Schizophrenia Bulletin, 33*, 1162–1170. http://dx.doi.org/10.1093/schbul/sbl039

Lambert, M. (2007). What we have learned from a decade of research aimed at improving psychotherapy outcome in routine care. *Psychotherapy Research, 17*, 1–14. http://dx.doi.org/10.1080/10503300601032506

Lambert, M. M. (2010). "Yes, it is time for clinicians to routinely monitor treatment outcome." In B. L. Duncan, S. D. Miller, B. E. Wampold, & M. A. Hubble (Eds.), *The heart and soul of change: Delivering what works in therapy* (2nd ed., pp. 239–266). Washington, DC: American Psychological Association. http://dx.doi.org/10.1037/12075-008

Landauer, T. K., Foltz, P. W., & Laham, D. (1998). Introduction to latent semantic analysis. *Discourse Processes, 25*, 259–284. http://dx.doi.org/10.1080/01638539809545028

Levenson, H., & Strupp, H. H. (1999). Recommendations for the future of training in brief dynamic psychotherapy. *Journal of Clinical Psychology, 55*, 385–391. http://dx.doi.org/10.1002/(SICI)1097-4679(199904)55:4<385::AID-JCLP2>3.0.CO;2-B

Lutz, W., Tholen, S., Kosfelder, J., Grawe, K., & Schulte, D. (2005). Zur Entwicklung von Entscheidungsregeln in der Psychotherapie: Die Validierung von Vorhersagemodellen mit einer sequenzanalytischen Methode [For the development of decision rules in psychotherapy: The validation of predictive models with a sequence analytical method]. *Zeitschrift für Klinische Psychologie und Psychotherapie, 34*, 165–175. http://dx.doi.org/10.1026/1616-3443.34.3.165

Maggio, L. A. (2008). Locating the best available research. In J. C. Norcross, T. P. Hogan, & G. P. Koocher (Eds.), *Clinician's guide to evidence based practices: Mental health and the addictions* (pp. 29–77). Oxford, England: Oxford University Press.

Manring, J., Greenberg, R. P., Gregory, R., & Gallinger, L. (2011). Learning psychotherapy in the digital age. *Psychotherapy, 48*, 119–126. http://dx.doi.org/10.1037/a0022185

Månsson, K. N. T., Skagius Ruiz, E., Gervind, E., Dahlin, M., & Andersson, G. (2013). Development and initial evaluation of an Internet-based support system for face-to-face cognitive behavior therapy: A proof of concept study. *Journal of Medical Internet Research, 15*, e280. http://dx.doi.org/10.2196/jmir.3031

Marks, I. M., Cavanagh, K., & Gega, L. (2007). Computer-aided psychotherapy: Revolution or bubble? *The British Journal of Psychiatry, 191*, 471–473. http://dx.doi.org/10.1192/bjp.bp.107.041152

Matthews, M., Doherty, G., Coyle, D., & Sharry, J. (2008). Designing mobile applications to support mental health interventions. In J. Lumsden (Ed.), *Handbook of research on user interface design and evaluation for mobile technology* (pp. 635–656). Hershey, PA: Information Science Reference. doi:10.4018/978-1-59904-871-0.ch038

Miller, K. L., Miller, S. M., & Evans, W. J. (2002). Computer-assisted live supervision in college counseling centers. *Journal of College Counseling, 5*, 187–192. http://dx.doi.org/10.1002/j.2161-1882.2002.tb00221.x

Murdoch, J. W., & Connor-Greene, P. A. (2000). Enhancing therapeutic impact and therapeutic alliance through electronic mail homework assignments. *The Journal of Psychotherapy Practice & Research, 9*, 232–237.

Percevic, R., Lambert, M. J., & Kordy, H. (2004). Computer-supported monitoring of patient treatment response. *Journal of Clinical Psychology, 60*, 285–299. http://dx.doi.org/10.1002/jclp.10264

Reese, R. J., Aldarondo, F., Anderson, C. R., Lee, S.-J., Miller, T. W., & Burton, D. (2009). Telehealth in clinical supervision: A comparison of supervision formats. *Journal of Telemedicine and Telecare, 15*, 356–361. http://dx.doi.org/10.1258/jtt.2009.090401

Rogers, E. M. (2003). *Diffusion of innovations* (5th ed.). New York, NY: Free Press.

Rousmaniere, T., & Frederickson, J. (2013). Internet-based one-way-mirror supervision for advanced psychotherapy training. *The Clinical Supervisor, 32*, 40–55. http://dx.doi.org/10.1080/07325223.2013.778683

Rummel, N., & Spada, H. (2005). Learning to collaborate: An instructional approach to promoting collaborative problem-solving in computer-mediated settings. *Journal of the Learning Sciences, 14*, 201–241. http://dx.doi.org/10.1207/s15327809jls1402_2

Schäfer, J., & Niederer, A. (2014, May 7). Mit Dr. House zu einer besseren Medizin [With Dr. House to a better medicine]. *Neue Zürcher Zeitung*, p. 56.

Sexton, T. L., Patterson, T., & Datchi, C. C. (2012). Technological innovations of systematic measurement and clinical feedback: A virtual leap into the future of couple and family psychology. *Couple and Family Psychology: Research and Practice, 1*, 285–293. http://dx.doi.org/10.1037/cfp0000001

Smith, J. L., Amrhein, P. C., Brooks, A. C., Carpenter, K. M., Levin, D., Schreiber, E. A., . . . Nunes, E. V. (2007). Providing live supervision via teleconferencing improves acquisition of motivational interviewing skills after workshop attendance. *The American Journal of Drug and Alcohol Abuse, 33*, 163–168. http://dx.doi.org/10.1080/00952990601091150

Smith, J. L., Carpenter, K. M., Amrhein, P. C., Brooks, A. C., Levin, D., Schreiber, E. A., . . . Nunes, E. V. (2012). Training substance abuse clinicians in motivational interviewing using live supervision via teleconferencing. *Journal of Consulting and Clinical Psychology, 80*, 450–464. http://dx.doi.org/10.1037/a0028176

Sørlie, T., Gammon, D., Bergvik, S., & Sexton, H. (1999). Psychotherapy supervision face-to-face and by videoconferencing: A comparative study. *British Journal of Psychotherapy, 15*, 452–462. http://dx.doi.org/10.1111/j.1752-0118.1999.tb00475.x

Strauss, B. M., Lutz, W., Steffanowski, A., Wittmann, W. W., Boehnke, J. R., Rubel, J., . . . Kirchmann, H. (2015). Benefits and challenges in practice-oriented psychotherapy research in Germany: The TK and the QS-PSY-BAY projects of quality assurance in outpatient psychotherapy. *Psychotherapy Research, 25*, 32–51. doi:10.1080/10503307.2013.856046

Thagard, P. (1989). Explanatory coherence. *Behavioral and Brain Sciences, 12*, 435–502. http://dx.doi.org/10.1017/S0140525X00057046

Weerasekera, P. (2013). Psychotherapy Training e-Resources (PTeR): On-line psychotherapy education. *Academic Psychiatry, 37*, 51–54. http://dx.doi.org/10.1176/appi.ap.11120215

Weigold, A., Weigold, I. K., & Russell, E. J. (2013). Examination of the equivalence of self-report survey-based paper-and-pencil and internet data collection methods. *Psychological Methods, 18*, 53–70. http://dx.doi.org/10.1037/a0031607

Whipple, J. L., Lambert, M. J., Vermeersch, D. A., Smart, D. W., Nielsen, S. L., & Hawkins, E. J. (2003). Improving the effects of psychotherapy: The use of early identification of treatment and problem-solving strategies in routine practice.

Journal of Counseling Psychology, 50, 59–68. http://dx.doi.org/10.1037/0022-0167.50.1.59

Worrall, J. M., & Fruzzetti, A. E. (2009). Improving peer supervisor ratings of therapist performance in dialectical behavior therapy: An Internet-based training system. *Psychotherapy: Theory, Research, Practice, Training, 46,* 476–479. http://dx.doi.org/10.1037/a0017948

Xavier, K., Shepherd, L., & Goldstein, D. (2007). Clinical supervision and education via videoconference: A feasibility project. *Journal of Telemedicine and Telecare, 13,* 206–209. http://dx.doi.org/10.1258/135763307780907996

7
CLINICAL DECISION MAKING WHEN THE STAKES ARE HIGH

JEFFREY J. MAGNAVITA

Many decisions made in clinical practice are relatively routine and automatic, whereas others are much more complex and more prone to the influence of biases. There are a number of disorders with high base rates associated with abundant information, along with a continuum of evidence-based treatment approaches, to guide clinical decision making (National Institute of Mental Health, 1999). Patients with uncomplicated clinical presentations generally do not demand multiple resources; clinical decision making is relatively straightforward in these cases. Internet searches can supplement knowledge and experience by supplying abundant information concerning uncomplicated presentations (see Chapter 6 in this volume).

However, clinical practice is often not routine. There are situations where the stakes are high because the clinical decision making involves complex and potentially risky outcomes, such as medical and legal risks. High-risk

---

This model of collaborative treatment for high stakes cases was developed and practiced with John Santopietro, MD.

http://dx.doi.org/10.1037/14711-007
Clinical Decision Making in Mental Health Practice, J. J. Magnavita (Editor)
Copyright © 2016 by the American Psychological Association. All rights reserved.

situations may be life threatening and the outcome possibly catastrophic in terms of harm to self or violence toward others. There are far too many examples of these high-stakes situations; for example, in recent years our nation has struggled to understand and prevent school shootings and other cases of mass murderers who have slipped through the treatment net. Most clinicians who have been in practice for some time have run into similar cases.

In this chapter, some of the important issues that are inimical to making decisions when the stakes are high are presented. A model is presented of collaborative–shared decision making, developed in collaboration with a psychiatrist colleague, that has been found to be effective. This model is different from most decision-making models in that it expands the traditional dyadic configuration (i.e., between patient and clinician) by utilizing a triadic configuration (i.e., among patient; two clinicians; treatment team; and other significant parties such as families, community representatives, etc.). This model is anchored in system theory, which we used as a framework for unifying and orienting our clinical work (Magnavita, 2012; Magnavita & Anchin, 2014). Human behavior and mental and relational processes can be understood by incorporating complexity or chaos theory, which are recent iterations of system theory. Using chaos and complexity theory allows one to see patterns in systems as they emerge and/or are repeated. These patterns represent attractor states, which are essentially convergent processes such as we might see in a severely eating-disordered family member who organizes the family system around the management of his or her illness (Magnavita, 2005a). Recurrent processes have been explained as follows:

> The strength of an attractor is measured by the depth of its basin. A deep attractor is well-developed and behavioral repertoires are frequently drawn to this attractor. As behavioral patterns are repeated, the attractor is strengthened. In any given interaction, there are likely to be several available attractors in the state space, with some presenting a stronger pull than others. (Stanton & Welsh, 2012, p. 21)

Complex systems operate in a nonlinear holistic fashion, viewed through the lenses of the various levels and domains of the biopsychosocial model (Magnavita & Anchin, 2014). The use of theory in decision analytics is covered in Chapter 3 in this volume.

HIGH-RISK CASES—WHEN THE STAKES ARE HIGH

Some cases give rise to fear in behavioral and mental health clinicians; most often these are cases where the stakes are high and the outcome uncertain. Most clinicians can easily recall those experiences in which decision making was risky and the potential for disaster loomed large. Such cases are generally emotionally laden not only for patients, families, and communities but also for the clinician. Examples of high-risk cases may include patients referred for follow-up care after a near lethal suicide attempt, severe psychotic decompensation, or patients with comorbid disorders such as traumatic brain injury and posttraumatic stress disorder that severely compromise executive functioning and make standard treatments difficult to administer.

We begin with a discussion of the central features of high-risk cases. High-risk cases tend to challenge our decision making because they generally do not follow the algorithms that we rely on for less complex cases. Often these cases are characterized by multiple pathologies, family dysfunction, trauma, and/or generational transmission processes that are quite powerful and are often carried forth by subsequent generations. There are often limited data available with which to make predictive decisions, so clinical decision-making processes must be employed along with clinical expertise to bring about a positive outcome. An overview of some of the common high-risk categories that are seen in clinical practice includes the following:

- severe eating disorders,
- severe personality disorders,
- complex trauma,
- severe treatment refractory affective disorders,
- nontreatment-compliant severe mental illness,
- severe treatment refractory addictive disorders,
- fibromyalgia and chronic fatigue syndrome, and
- chronic and some acute medical disorders.

This list is not meant to be comprehensive but represents a heuristic sampling to bear in mind when treating patients with these presentations. Other complicating factors for decision making include a high degree of co-occurring or comorbid disorders that may be interacting in complicated ways that make first-line treatments ineffective.

A HIGH INCIDENCE OF COMORBID DISORDERS

Generally speaking, patients with multiple comorbidities and a history of multiple treatment failures are likely to be categorized as high-stakes patients. Many high-risk patients suffer from a personality disorder as one of their primary conditions (Magnavita, 2004, 2010a). They also tend to have other comorbid presentations such as addictions; eating disorders; mood disorders; traumatic brain injury; chronic or acute medical disorders; complex trauma; and a spectrum of somatic conditions such as fibromyalgia, chronic fatigue syndrome, and severe sleep disorders.

When the stakes are high in clinical situations and the outcome is not certain, our decision-making capacity is tested. For some patients it may be that they have a behavioral or mental health condition, as previously discussed, which if not treated appropriately will likely result in an unfavorable outcome. For example, in one case a 50-year-old male who suffered from a severe alcohol addiction, which for a period of time was in remission, resumed drinking with a vengeance and was highly refractory to treatment. In this particular case, it was apparent to the clinician that this patient would eventually destroy himself as a result of his drinking. There had been many treatment interventions, hospitalizations, and rehabilitation efforts. It was clear that this was a high-stakes case. Unfortunately, the patient did end up drinking himself to death. Sometimes, a high-stakes patient is one who has had multiple treatments without any improvement, so they will not commit to a treatment even though we predict a positive outcome. In many similar cases, the complex disorders can have many negative consequences that impact employment and children's mental health and well-being and also tax community resources. There are common features present in high-risk cases. Patients with the disorders described in the previous section often share a high degree of self-destructive potential. This is another useful heuristic: When a pattern of chronic self-defeating or self-destructive behavior is apparent, one might consider this to be a high-stakes case. Occasionally, cases with a history of violence can become high-stakes cases. Another common indicator of a high-risk case is found with patients who engender intense countertransference reactions in their health care professionals.

A COLLABORATIVE SHARED DECISION-MAKING MODEL

Shared decision making is considered an important element of enhancing quality of care (Institute of Medicine, 2001). Typically, shared decision making is considered to be primarily dyadic—between patient and provider. The basic framework presented in this chapter is systemic—the patient as part of a larger system of nested, interactive structures. The original purpose of this model was to expand the dyadic framework to include as many appropriate stakeholders as reasonable and ethical in the patient's treatment, assuming the multiple benefits of enhanced "wisdom" in the participating group. In this model, the group is defined by the parameters of each case on an individual basis. Sometimes there are a number of other professionals who manage or treat a particular aspect of the patient's care, such as the family physician or community social worker. Often patients with complex issues become frustrated with their therapist, which is not an uncommon transference reaction. The advantage to this collaborative model is that it affords us the opportunity to "hold" the negative affect in the triad, enabling metabolization of these destructive impulses and negative emotions, which often would have resulted in a premature termination, acting out, or sabotaging treatment. Another central aspect of this model is the emphasis on active decision making based on shared data and open communication. This open feedback loop is essential for monitoring the system and was used as a barometer to track the cases, allowing interventions before the situation reached a dangerous tipping point. "The decision-making process refers to how information and values are combined to form preferences and to arrive at decisions" (Wills & Holmes-Rovner, 2006, p. 13). There is a range of treatments and modalities to offer patients, but in each case an attempt should be made to calculate the benefits and harms and to encourage a buy-in from the patient and system. Patients are key partners in shared decision making with health care providers, an assumption that is central to this model (Wills & Holmes-Rovner, 2006). Furthermore, patients are reinforced and welcomed when they seek out services independently.

The model presented in this chapter emerged from a 3-year collaboration between the author and a psychiatric collaborator. We sought to develop and pilot a model of collaborative and shared decision making that would allow us to offer patients whom we considered to be high risk an intensive treatment experience that would maximize their adaptive capacity and prevent overutilization of costly and often retraumatizing higher levels of care. "Patients' decisions impact behavior, such as treatment initiation and continuance, which in turn can influence individual and aggregate clinical health status and health systems outcomes" (Wills & Holmes-Rovner, 2006, p. 9). We strove to keep patient preferences at the center of our collaborative relationship. It is important for the clinician to maintain the dialectic between "expert with specialized knowledge" and "not knowing" by remaining curious and open to new perspectives.

> True experts, it is said, know when they don't know. However, nonexperts (whether or not they think they are) certainly do not know when they don't know. Subjective confidence is therefore an unreliable indication of the validity of intuitive judgments and decisions. (Kahneman & Klein, 2009, p. 524)

One of the findings that has emerged from converging sources is that we clinicians are prone to overestimating our expertise (see Chapter 2, this volume). We believe that working in a team with open and honest feedback is an important way to guard against this and the other biases we are prone to, which are presented in Chapter 2 and elsewhere in this volume. It is important to recognize that clinicians should present themselves as experts and try to be confident about their work, yet it is also important to critically analyze the quality of information that we use to make decisions. Falling back on unexamined beliefs about our expertise is potential source of bias for experienced and novice clinicians.

EXPECTED UTILITY THEORY

The "best" decisions maximize utility that we expect for an outcome. Expected utility (EU) theory, developed in the 1980s, provides a formula for considering and weighing competing and multiple goals, which may be in contradiction with one another, to achieve the optimal outcome (Schoemaker, 1982). EU can be represented as the following equation: multiplying the probability (p) of an outcome by its value/utility (u) and then summing the products of each outcome. EU offers a systematic approach for determining the optimal tradeoffs that should be made to attain the desired goal. Often the probabilities used in calculating outcome are unknown, but there is still utility in using the best evidence to make probabilistic statements. For example, a patient suffering from an anxiety disorder might consider a psychoanalytic treatment versus a cognitive behavior therapy (CBT) approach. We can compare treatments and ascertain various factors that assist us in making an appropriate determination as to what course to take. The analytic approach is likely to be of longer duration and costlier, and the evidence is weaker for a reduction of anxiety symptoms; on the basis of these factors it appears that CBT would optimize outcome. Other factors, however, may complicate the picture and must be considered. The prospective patient might be interested in developing a deeper appreciation of the inner workings of his or her mind or they might be contemplating pursuing psychoanalytic training and want to experience this form of treatment. These and other factors may overshadow the need for the quickest path to reduction of anxiety symptoms.

A SIMPLIFIED DECISION-MAKING MODEL

Rothert et al. (1997) developed a simplified decision model, which has been applied by Wills and Holmes-Rovner (2003) to depressed patients seen in primary care practice. The main elements are briefly summarized in the following paragraphs.

Information

The data relevant to decision making is the information used in determining a course of action. This includes the probability of risks and benefits and the evidence of effectiveness of a particular treatment approach. It is essential to stay informed about current treatment approaches and refer to trusted sources of information when making decisions. It is important to be able to share the most accurate and current information with patients and also to provide resources for patients that inform their choices.

Values

Values refers to the importance that a person places on aspects of his or her experience and other factors in the spectrum of decision making. Values are inherent to any decision-making process, and it is imperative that clinicians spend time determining the values that are important to each patient. For example, some patients hold the core value that medications are bad; others believe in their benefits. Extreme values and their underlying beliefs have important implications for treatment. For example, many patients hold the belief that therapeutic healing occurs and may be influenced by powerful placebo effects, whereas others may be described as being influenced by negative beliefs that nothing will help and they won't get better, a "nocebo" response. Clarifying and honoring each patient's value system is a fundamental part of the decision-making process.

Preferences

Preferences refers to the likelihood of preferring one alternative or treatment to another. We have found that although there are a number of effective treatments that we can offer, some patients have strong preferences for or against a certain course of action. For example, in the collaborative relationship developed when using this model, one of us provided psychotherapy and the other primarily pharmacotherapy. There tended to be a self-selection process whereby patients with preference for psychotherapy would often find their way to me, and those with preferences for pharmacotherapy found their way to my colleague. One of the benefits of a collaborative process was that we could introduce the potential benefits of each approach, providing relevant information valuable in decision making. We found that offering the alternatives for discussion was a very powerful educative and decision-making experience.

QUADRATIC DECISION-MAKING

To maximize our decision analytics, we have often used a quadratic decision-making model (see Table 7.1). This model is easy to use and helps to systematically weigh benefits and risk based on two ways of asking a question.

TABLE 7.1
Quadratic Decision Making

Benefit	Risk
Benefit associated with continuing Treatment A (e.g., patient on mood stabilizer with uncertain diagnosis) *Continued stable mood*	Risk associated with continuing Treatment A *Unnecessary burden of continued treatment; effects on fetus when pregnant; long-term effects of medication*
Benefit associated with discontinuing Treatment A *Reduce side effects and potential long-term damage; diagnostic confirmation; less risk for fetus*	Risk associated with discontinuing Treatment A *Potential relapse; possible loss of time from work; disruption in personal life; possible need for higher level of care*

As has been discussed earlier in this volume, the way a question is framed influences the answer. Quadratic modeling can guard against some of these framing risks.

An example is a case of a married woman in her early 30s who, prior to being seen by one of us, was hospitalized and diagnosed with bipolar disorder for which she was placed on a mood stabilizer. She was referred for pharmacological treatment and medication management. My colleague wondered if the diagnosis was accurate. The patient wanted to come off her medication because she was considering having a child. Quadratic decision making helped to assess the risks involved in weaning her off medication. The first question we sought to assess was the veracity of the diagnosis, and the question was, "Is the patient suffering from bipolar disorder?" Second, we wanted to decide if she should continue to be treated for bipolar disorder. The question we posed was, "Should she be supported in coming off her medication when she is trying to conceive a child?"

We addressed our questions in as systematic a fashion as possible. We wanted to know what evidence showed that the patient suffered from a bipolar disorder. The evidence we had on intake was that she was diagnosed with bipolar during a brief hospitalization. More information was gathered through a history and clinical interview and then a recommendation that she be further evaluated with psychometric testing for more data. A Millon Multiaxial Clinical Inventory–III (Millon, Millon, Davis, & Grossman, 2009) was administered and did not endorse bipolar disorder. Instead, from history and interview, it appeared that the patient suffered, at least in part, from an undiagnosed posttraumatic stress disorder (Magnavita, 2005b).

The quadratic questioning was then formulated as follows:

What is the risk of weaning the patient off her mood stabilizer? And conversely, *What is the benefit of weaning the patient off her mood stabilizer?* These questions represent two sections of the quadrant.

The subsequent question was formulated as follows:

What is the risk of maintaining the patient on a mood stabilizer if she does not have a bipolar disorder? And conversely, *What is the benefit of maintaining the patient on a mood stabilizer if she does not have a bipolar disorder?*

After jointly collaborating with the patient, it was agreed that she would be weaned off her medication and during this time undertake a more intensive course of trauma-focused psychotherapy. She was monitored closely by us both, and although she had some difficult times was able to successfully come off the mood stabilizer.

DECISION-MAKING AIDS

We sought to incorporate as many decision-making aids (DAs) as we thought useful to educate patients and inform their decisions. "DAs are interventions to help people make deliberative, effective choices about health treatment options (including maintaining a status quo position) for complex decisions" (O'Connor et al., 1999, p. 731).

> The current criteria for key DA elements include information about options, presentation of probabilities of outcomes, values clarification, use of patient stories/testimonials, guidance/coaching, disclosure of conflicts of interest, balanced information, use of plain language, use of current scientific information, and assessment of decision quality and effectiveness (IPDAS, 2005). (Wills & Holmes-Rovner, 2006, p. 14)

Where possible, we reviewed and offered information from the most current practice guidelines (see Chapters 4 and 5, this volume).

ELEMENTS OF A COLLABORATIVE JOINT DECISION-MAKING CARE TEAM

Establishing a collaborative joint decision-making care team is a necessary component for treating high-risk patients. In developing this collaborative model we were able to work in close physical proximity, with offices next to one another. While working with a patient, and if the timing seemed appropriate, we would often introduce the value of considering psychotherapy or pharmacology in addition to what we were each offering. By expanding the frame we opened up the possibility of exploring another treatment venue. If the timing seemed right we might ask if the patient was willing to meet our associate. At this point, if they were open to the possibility, we would often check to see if the other's consulting room door was open or closed. If open we would ask if the other could stop in and we would introduce, join, summarize, and model a collaborative relationship. Often the patient would agree to schedule an appointment, and at other times they would ask us questions and take our contact information. This physical proximity also afforded us tremendous opportunity to have a continuous feedback system where we could chat between sessions and meet patients when appropriate. There are some important elements that we think are crucial to this approach.

Team Approach

A team approach can sound like an overused cliché. Respect and trust are essential to a functional team. Part of the benefit of a multispecialty team approach is that the perspectives offered by various members can be a strong corrective to the bias of one's model and the underlying beliefs that inform one's clinical work. Our goal was to establish open and regular lines of communication with other health care providers who were involved in the cases we were treating.

Utilization of Experts to Enhance a Team's Breadth

One of the important aspects of this model is the inclusion of as many health care providers as necessary to manage the multifaceted physical and psychological needs of patients who are deemed to be high risk. This requires careful attention to competitive feelings that are often common between health care and related professionals. Often there are understandable turf issues about who controls the patients' care. Financial and ego issues often drive these dynamics and must be sensitively handled to assure that splitting does not occur among team members. *Splitting* refers to some patients' tendencies to divide therapists into dichotomous categories such as "bad" or "good," "rigid" or "flexible," "compassionate" or "uncaring," and so forth, which unsuspecting clinicians can fall prey to believing. These patient "projections" can intensify rivalrous feelings about compensation, status, and other dynamics among team members, which may result in them working at cross-purposes. When there is splitting, which is inevitable, there is a process for handling these feelings. We strove to be quick to acknowledge when we didn't have the required expertise and often referred to different prescribers or other therapists when there seemed to be a better fit. For example, we sought out consultation and management with addiction specialists when we were dealing with patients with opioid dependence or who required very complex pharmacological treatment. We attempted to keep all the treatment options open. We frequently referred to the literature to see what the empirical evidence suggested and when there were new approaches that we could incorporate such as heart rate variability biofeedback, neurofeedback, transcranial magnetic stimulation, and electrical cranial stimulation. We also made use of alternative approaches such as yoga and physical exercise training with practitioners we knew and trusted. One problem that we faced was determining which treatment element was beneficial while administering a comprehensive treatment package with multiple components. Some options such as exercise and structured activities such as yoga seem to have benefit. However, there are times when even these might be detrimental, and their use should be considered with decision-making processes. For example, patients with chronic fatigue and fibromyalgia often report that exercise makes them worse and forces them to spend days in bed.

Establishing a Supportive Core Care Team

Our core team included a board-certified psychiatrist who specialized in case consultation and pharmacological treatment and a board-certified clinical psychologist who specialized in the psychosocial treatment of high-risk and refractory cases. We also developed strong working relationships with an array of health care providers including nutritionists, family practitioners, neuropsychologists, physical trainers, educational specialists, vocational rehabilitation specialists, social workers, and other disciplines whom we trusted and felt would add a valuable component of care to the treatment team.

"Handing Off" Patient Systems

One important feature of our shared collaborative care model is what we describe as the patient "hand-off." We believe that this is a critical to expanding the scope of treatment. As we have observed in our practice and in those of our peers, there is often a tendency for patients who are seeking or referred for behavioral and mental health treatment to have preferences about the kind of treatment they expect will be efficacious. Some seek psychopharmacological treatment. This trend seems to be increasing and in our view is related to the increased advertising of medications in the media. Other patients have strong beliefs about medication and may believe they are toxic and or mind-controlling agents that should be avoided. There is some illuminating research on this issue. When clinicians believe that a behavioral or mental disorder is biologically based we are likely to refer them for pharmacological treatment, and when we believe that there is a psychological basis the referral tends to be for psychosocial treatment. It is also interesting that for those who are viewed as having a primarily biological basis to their disorder less stigma is attributed to the person compared with when one believes there is a psychological basis (Ahn, Proctor, & Flanagan, 2009).

Important components in the way this model of collaborative treatment evolved were friendship, mutual respect, and shared values. We attempted where possible to make our work flexible and consumer oriented in that we tried to offer the kind of treatment that we would expect for families, friends, and ourselves. Patients with complex presentations may often miss sessions or disappear from treatment. We always strove to nonjudgmentally accept patients when they returned after an absence. Patients were reinforced for appropriately contacting team members when they felt a need and were not made to feel that access to clinical care or our attention were misused. We strove to make patients feel they were most welcome to contact us. Much of what we did was psychoeducational. We both spent a great deal of time educating our patients about other modalities of treatment and the benefit of a pharmacological or psychotherapeutic approach if we thought that might be beneficial. We would often be a consultant to the patient about the other's role and work. For example, if a patient was opposed to medication, time might be spent educating the patient about the possible benefits as well as some of the risks and side effects.

The Consultation Model—Joint Collaborative Care Meetings

One of the most helpful experiences for many families was the opportunity to have both of us present at collaborative care meetings. These were often necessary in situations where there was deterioration in a patient, couple, or family's condition. These downward spirals are the situations that in the past would have resulted in a hospitalization. Instead, with a review of treatment and modification of the treatment plan we were often successful in averting hospitalizations or in keeping them limited except in cases of extreme necessity where stabilization required a longer episode of care.

COLLABORATIVE CARE MODEL GOALS

A collaborative care model for treating high-risk patients, although complex, includes a number of clear goals. Overall, the goals of collaborative care are to maximize communication, enhance access to vital information, and be aware of biases that might interfere with decision making. The goals include the following:

1. Manage risk in the least restrictive and most cost efficient manner.
2. Provide ongoing treatment planning and case formulation.

3. Encourage a feedback system among patient, families, team members, and other providers and institutions.
4. Create an optimal care environment that encourages use of our services.
5. Encourage use of appropriate decision aids.
6. Provide ongoing consultation for complex cases to team, agencies, and families.
7. Empower patient systems that utilize all available resources for maintaining high quality of life.

RISK MANAGEMENT

The management and tolerance for risk is a necessary function of treating high-risk patients. Clinicians who work with high-risk, treatment-refractory, or complex cases should have the necessary training and experience. A level of expertise can be attained through advanced training (Magnavita, Levy, Critchfield, & Lebow, 2010). An understanding of the challenges that other clinicians have faced is useful (see Chapter 10 in this volume).

TOLERANCE FOR UNCERTAINTY

Treating high-risk patients can cause high levels of anxiety for clinicians because of the chaos and uncertainty involved. Continual monitoring of the therapeutic alliance is critical for risk management. Shared collaborative decision making is one way to tolerate the uncertainty and risk. Anxiety in the care team can at times run rather high, and on occasion vicarious traumatization of the team or a team member is not uncommon. Many high-risk patients have suffered from a variety of traumatic experiences and developmental traumata. The clinicians who treat high-risk cases should be trained extensively in trauma and be alert to the possibility of suffering from compassion fatigue and vicarious traumatization.

CASE MANAGEMENT VERSUS PROVIDING A VEHICLE FOR UNDERSTANDING

Often the approach utilized for treating high-risk cases is based on a case management model. Our model sought to expand the case management aspect by providing a shared decision-making model offered in a containing framework of the team collaborative care context. One goal for this framework was to provide understanding and to tolerate the messiness of decision making when sufficient data were not available to fully inform the family and our efforts.

USING PATTERN RECOGNITION IN HIGH-RISK CASES

The use of pattern recognition heuristics in high-risk cases can be central to reducing the uncertainty and finding the leverage necessary to positively influence a patient system.

Essential Theoretical Constructs

The most fundamental pattern recognition tool in our minds is the biopsychosocial model used in a unifying framework (Magnavita & Anchin, 2014). This is a multiperspective and multipragamatic framework that emphasizes interdisciplinarity (Magnavita, 2005a). Important pattern recognition tools are essential to clinical decision making in high-risk cases. We rely on the four domain levels that included in a unifying framework. All theoretical frameworks are in part pattern recognition tools. The unifying framework that has been elaborated in a number of previous publications has been extremely helpful especially in complex cases.

Personality Systematics

Personality systematics is the study of the interrelationships among the domains of the personality system from the micro- to the macro-level (Magnavita, 2005a). The personality system can be conceptualized as four embedded subsystems that, at the microscopic level, involve biological–intrapsychic structure and processes integrally intertwined at increasingly macroscopic levels with dyadic, triadic, and sociocultural structures and processes.

MANAGING COUNTERTRANSFERENCE–TRANSFERENCE REACTIONS

Countertransference–transference phenomena are commonly activated in the treatment of high-risk cases (Magnavita, 2010b, 2013). "Countertransference–transference may be conceptualized using a systemic model that views the entire personality system embedded in various matrices" (Magnavita, 2013, p. 228). Countertransference reactions are evident in response to individuals (Muran & Hungr, 2013), couples dyads (Gottman

& Gottman, 2013), and family systems (Heatherington, Friedlander, & Escudero, 2013). We often noted that strong countertransference responses from referring clinicians were suggestive of high-risk and refractory cases. We also noted among our treatment team that when countertransference or transference reactions were high this was a sign of high-risk cases. Betan, Heim, Zittel Conklin, and Westen (2005) summarized, "Although every clinician and every therapeutic dyad is distinct, the significant correlations between countertransference factors and personality disorder symptoms suggest that countertransference responses occur in coherent and predictable patterns" (p. 234). Accordingly, it is not only clinicians who react in predictable ways; it is also likely that significant others respond in this manner as well.

SAFEGUARDS AGAINST COGNITIVE BIASES

It is of the utmost importance when treating high-risk cases to examine your personal biases (see Chapter 2, this volume) and to be continually mindful of the ways in which your biases can influence decision making. High-risk patients often have had multiple previous treatment episodes of various levels of intensity and may have had experiences with a number of health care professionals. These trajectories can be convergence points for a variety of biases discussed in Chapter 2. For example, a patient may have been diagnosed early in their mental health history, and this diagnosis then becomes an anchor, risky for later providers to challenge. For example, a patient who was diagnosed with an eating disorder and was refractory to treatment on further consideration showed signs of borderline personality disorder. The eating disorder, which was the focus of treatment for many years by many clinicians, took on a different set of considerations when the patient was viewed through the lens of a personality disorder.

SUMMARY

In this chapter we described a pilot model of collaborative treatment for high-risk cases and discussed various components. The stakes are high for clinicians and families when there are potentially negative outcomes, which are particularly common in certain clinical conditions. This model emerged during a collaboration that lasted over a period of 3 years between a board-certified psychiatrist and board-certified clinical psychologist offering a holistic model of treatment that integrated pharmacotherapy and psychotherapy. Also, this model incorporated many other behavioral and mental health specialists as well as medical practitioners to form a flexible team of behavioral and health care providers, so that a comprehensive treatment approach could be offered. A shared decision-making model with close collaboration allowed risk to be analyzed and options explored and agreed on by all the relevant members of the patient system and clinical team.

REFERENCES

Ahn, W. K., Proctor, C. C., & Flanagan, E. H. (2009). Mental health clinicians' beliefs about the biological, psychological, and environmental bases of mental disorders. *Cognitive Science, 33,* 147–182. http://dx.doi.org/10.1111/j.1551-6709.2009.01008.x

Betan, E., Heim, A. K., Zittel Conklin, C., & Westen, D. (2005). Countertransference phenomena and personality pathology in clinical practice: An empirical investigation. *American Journal of Psychiatry, 162,* 890–898.

Gottman, J. M., & Gottman, J. S. (2013). Difficulties with clients in Gottman method couples therapy. In A. W. Wolf, M. R. Goldfried, & J. C. Muran (Eds.), *Transforming negative reactions to clients* (pp. 91–112). Washington, DC: American Psychological Association. http://dx.doi.org/10.1037/13940-004

Heatherington, L., Friedlander, M. L., & Escudero, V. (2013). Managing negative reactions to clients in conjoint therapy: It's not all in the family. In A. W. Wolf, M. R. Goldfried, & J. C. Muran (Eds.), *Transforming negative reactions to clients* (pp. 113–137). Washington, DC: American Psychological Association.

Institute of Medicine. (2001). *Crossing the quality chasm: A new health system for the 21st century.* Washington, DC: Author.

Kahneman, D., & Klein, G. (2009). Conditions for intuitive expertise: A failure to disagree. *American Psychologist, 64,* 515–526. http://dx.doi.org/10.1037/a0016755

Magnavita, J. J. (Ed.). (2004). *Handbook of personality disorders: Theory and practice.* Hoboken, NJ: Wiley.

Magnavita, J. J. (2005a). Systems theory foundation of personality, psychopathology, and psychotherapy. In S. Strack (Ed.), *Handbook of personology and psychopathology* (pp. 140–163). Hoboken, NJ: Wiley.

Magnavita, J. J. (2005b). Using the MCMI–III for treatment planning and to enhance clinical efficacy. In R. J. Craig (Ed.), *New directions in interpreting the Millon Clinical Multiaxial Inventory—III (MCMI–III)* (pp. 165–184). Hoboken, NJ: Wiley.

Magnavita, J. J. (Ed.). (2010a). *Evidence-based treatment of personality dysfunction: Principles, methods, and processes.* Washington, DC: American Psychological Association. http://dx.doi.org/10.1037/12130-000

Magnavita, J. J. (2010b). When the evidence base is scant: Some considerations in the ethical treatment of personality dysfunction. In J. J. Magnavita, K. N. Levy, K. L. Critchfield, & J. L. Lebow, Ethical considerations in treatment of personality dysfunction: Using evidence, principles, and clinical judgment. *Profes-*

sional Psychology: Research and Practice, 41, 64–68. http://dx.doi.org/10.1037/a0017733

Magnavita, J. J. (2012). Advancing clinical science using system theory as a framework for expanding family psychology with unified psychotherapy. *Couple and Family Psychology: Research and Practice, 1*, 3–13. http://dx.doi.org/10.1037/a0027492

Magnavita, J. J. (2013). Pattern recognition in the treatment of narcissistic disorders: Countertransference from a unified perspective. In A. W. Wolf, M. R. Goldfried, & J. C. Muran (Eds.), *Transforming negative reactions to clients* (pp. 221–244). Washington, DC: American Psychological Association. http://dx.doi.org/10.1037/13940-010

Magnavita, J. J., & Anchin, J. C. (2014). *Unifying psychotherapy: Principles, methods, and evidence from clinical science*. New York, NY: Springer.

Magnavita, J. J., Levy, K. N., Critchfield, K. L., & Lebow, J. L. (2010). Ethical considerations in treatment of personality dysfunction: Using evidence, principles, and clinical judgment. *Professional Psychology: Research and Practice, 41*, 64–74. http://dx.doi.org/10.1037/a0017733

Millon, T., Millon, C., Davis, R., & Grossman, S. (2009). *MCMI–III manual* (4th ed.). Minneapolis, MN: Pearson.

Muran, J. C., & Hungr, C. (2013). Power plays, negotiation, and mutual recognition in the therapeutic alliance: "I never met a client I didn't like . . . eventually." In A. W. Wolf, M. R. Goldfried, & J. C. Muran (Eds.), *Transforming negative reactions to clients* (pp. 23–44). Washington, DC: American Psychological Association. http://dx.doi.org/10.1037/13940-001

National Institute of Mental Health. (1999). *Bridging science and service: A report by the National Advisory Mental Health Council Clinical Treatment and Services Research Workgroup*. Washington, DC: Author.

O'Connor, A. M., Rostom, A., Fiset, V., Tetroe, J., Entwistle, V., Llewellyn-Thomas, H., . . . Jones, J. (1999). Decision aids for patients facing health treatment or screening decisions: Systematic review. *British Medical Journal, 319*, 731–734. http://dx.doi.org/10.1136/bmj.319.7212.731

Rothert, M. L., Holmes-Rovner, M., Rovner, D., Knoll, J., Breer, L., Talarczyk, G., . . . Wills, C. (1997). An educational intervention as decision support for menopausal women. Research. *Nursing & Health, 20*, 377–387.

Schoemaker, P. J. (1982). The expected utility model: Its variants, purposes, evidence and limitations. *Journal of Economic Literature, 20*, 529–563.

Stanton, M., & Welsh, R. (2012). Systemic thinking in couple and family psychology research and practice. *Couple and Family Psychology: Research and Practice, 1*, 14–30. http://dx.doi.org/10.1037/a0027461

Wills, C. E., & Holmes-Rovner, M. (2003). Preliminary validation of the Satisfaction With Decision scale with depressed primary care patients. *Health Expectations, 6*, 149–159. http://dx.doi.org/10.1046/j.1369-6513.2003.00220.x

Wills, C. E., & Holmes-Rovner, M. (2006). Integrated decision making and mental health interventions research: Research directions. *Clinical Psychologist, 13*, 9–25.

8

USE OF EMPIRICALLY GROUNDED RELATIONAL PRINCIPLES TO ENHANCE CLINICAL DECISION MAKING

KEN L. CRITCHFIELD AND JULIA E. MACKARONIS

Recent clinical science has demonstrated the importance of taking into account underlying principles of change when implementing interventions in clinical practice (e.g., Castonguay & Beutler, 2006). Our focus here is the contextual use of relationally based treatment principles to enhance treatment efficacy for specific individuals. In addition to being evidence based, relational principles apply across the spectrum of clinical work, from collaborative setting of treatment goals to moment-by-moment word choice. Our conceptualization of interventions emphasizes the use of underlying principles and mechanisms of change, in contrast to emphasizing specific techniques or treatment packages for specific symptoms or disorders. From our principles-based viewpoint, the same underlying change mechanisms may be activated by techniques and procedures used across schools. An advantage to the use of principles is that treatment response can be measured, articulated, and applied in ways that are responsive to context. Magnavita (Magnavita,

http://dx.doi.org/10.1037/14711-008
Clinical Decision Making in Mental Health Practice, J. J. Magnavita (Editor)
Copyright © 2016 by the American Psychological Association. All rights reserved.

Levy, Critchfield, & Lebow, 2010) has emphasized that use of principles is essential for ethical intervention in areas where there is little empirical evidence, such as decision making for patients with comorbid disorders; patients with understudied disorders; patients with unusually severe or chronic disorders or unusual cultural experience; or patients who have shown little benefit from previous treatment trials.

A focus on principles represents a return to the conceptual origins of most manualized approaches, which are premised on guiding principles about the etiology, maintenance, and change processes governing psychopathology. For example, the psychodynamic "blank screen" of neutrality—a technique—is intended to make transference patterns more available for interpretation, insight, and change. Similarly, in cognitive behavior therapy (CBT) for anxiety disorders, graduated exposure protocols are intended to inhibit avoidance responses and stimulate new learning. In each approach, specific techniques serve as tools for engaging a deeper change principle. Presumably, if a given principle is validly linked to problems and change processes, any technique that activates it in a specific context will be effective.

Psychotherapy research has shown that many therapy approaches have efficacy for a wide variety of disorders. Generally equivalent results, however, have been found across protocols for the same disorders (Wampold, 2001). One possible explanation for equivalent results is that these protocols may use techniques that activate the same or similar underlying mechanisms. For example, cognitive restructuring, eye movement desensitization and reprocessing, and psychodynamic–interpersonal approaches all impact trauma symptoms to some degree (Chard, Schuster, & Resick, 2012; Gallagher & Resick, 2012; Nayak, Powers, & Foa, 2012; Schottenbauer, Glass, Arnkoff, & Gray, 2008). This may be because they all require some degree of "being with" traumatic material in the context of a safe, therapeutic "secure base" (Cloitre, Stovall-McClough, Miranda, & Chemtob, 2004; Keller, Zoellner, & Feeny, 2010; Kinsler, 2014).

Research to establish treatment efficacy has primarily emphasized the randomized controlled trial (RCT). RCTs frame the primary research question as, "Do a set of specific techniques applied in a systematic way produce an average benefit for a specified population?" Internal controls are strong, largely owing to random assignment to groups and clear operationalization of techniques. Evidence produced from RCTs is powerful for answering whether average effects can be attributed directly to the impact of the treatment package. However, RCTs tell us relatively little about how individuals might respond to the treatment, especially those differing significantly from RCT samples, such as those with comorbid diagnoses or any number of cultural differences (Holt et al., 2013). RCTs also do not aid clinicians in selecting or tailoring treatments to best match individual strengths, weaknesses, or preferences. The same standardization procedures that are essential for establishing scientific certainty about a given effect also produce treatment approaches that are not easily adapted to new contexts.

Since the advent of RCTs, the idea that a treatment is based on underlying principles seems to have been supplanted with the idea that treatment consists only of techniques. If this notion is pursued too strictly, we become unable to address the question usually faced in the clinical encounter: "What does my particular patient need in order to feel and function better in life?" Here, the American Psychological Association has provided important perspective in the form of evidence-based practice of psychology (EBPP; APA Presidential Task Force, 2006):

> It is important to clarify the relation between EBPP and empirically supported treatments (ESTs). EBPP is the more comprehensive concept. ESTs start with a treatment and ask whether it works for a certain disorder or problem under specified circumstances. EBPP starts with the patient and asks what research evidence (including relevant results from RCTs) will assist the psychologist in achieving the best outcome. (p. 273)

In keeping with EBPP, a focus on principles allows clinicians to keep the primary focus on individual clients in their particular contexts. Some work has been done already to identify principles supported by the existing evidence base.

EMPIRICALLY DERIVED PRINCIPLES SPANNING TREATMENT APPROACHES

In 2006, Castonguay and Beutler convened a task force of APA Division 12 (Society of Clinical Psychology) and the North American Society for Psychotherapy Research (hereafter referred to as the Task Force) to distill principles from the empirical literature on psychosocial treatments for mood, anxiety, personality, and substance use disorders. Principles were identified on the basis of the presence of empirical data and/or their inclusion in treatments with empirical support and were organized as relating to participant characteristics, aspects of the therapeutic relationship, or elements of treatment technique associated with improved outcomes. As Castonguay and Beutler noted, there is an inherent connection between therapeutic relationships and techniques:

> One of the most salient controversies in the field of psychotherapy is whether client change is primarily due to the therapist's techniques or the quality of the therapeutic relationship. . . . this controversy reflects, more or less implicitly, an "either/or" assumption that is conceptually flawed and empirically untenable. (p. 353)

Connections between relational processes and techniques have been observed for many forms of treatment. For example, Critchfield, Henry, Castonguay, and Borkovec (2007) demonstrated the strong relational impact made by including a reflective–listening component in a treatment study of generalized anxiety disorder. Others have established connections in treatments such as psychodynamic (e.g., Ulberg, Amlo, Critchfield, Marble, & Høglend, 2014), process–experiential (Wong & Pos, 2014), CBT (Ahmed, Westra, & Constantino, 2012), and group work (Tasca et al., 2011).

The relevance of an interface between relationship and technique elements is most striking for those whose personality patterns are rigid, problematic, or qualify for a personality disorder (PD) diagnosis. The Task Force concluded that comorbid PD predicted poorer treatment response and longer treatments for other disorders. This is significant given that roughly half of community outpatients meet criteria for PD (Keown, Holloway, & Kuipers, 2002).

An integrative summary of factors associated with outcome for treatment of PD was distilled by Critchfield and Benjamin (2006). To be included, each principle had to be (a) linked to outcomes, (b) included as an element in empirically supported treatments, or (c) widely assumed to be relevant to this understudied area. Critchfield (2012) reorganized key relationship and treatment principles to aid mindful treatment with patients who show unique patterns of comorbidity (summary shown in Exhibit 8.1). A number of these principles were found to be shared across disorders and are relevant to this chapter. These include presence of a strong positive alliance, a clear case formulation that is transparent and addresses current concerns, and interventions that focus on increasing adaptive and decreasing maladaptive patterns (behaviors, affects, cognitions).

PRINCIPLES OF INTERPERSONAL RELATING RELEVANT TO CLINICAL DECISION MAKING

Relational elements clearly have powerful links to outcomes across disorders and treatments (Castonguay & Beutler, 2006; Norcross, 2002). The standard recommendation from the literature is thus that therapists should establish a strong alliance. This good advice is not accompanied by much detail as to how this blessed state should be achieved and maintained, however, and many disorders involve disruptions of interpersonal relationships (Kiesler, 1996). A hallmark of PDs in particular is difficulty in maintaining collaborative relationships.

One of the themes of Linehan's (1993) dialectical behavior therapy, initially developed for borderline PD, is that balance must be struck between validation and support for change. The particular balance may need to be different between patients or at various points in therapy. For example, provision

EXHIBIT 8.1
Questions to Aid Mindful Practice of PD Treatment Based on
Principles Summarized in Castonguay and Beutler (2006)
Principles of Therapeutic Change That Work

Features of the Therapeutic Relationship
- Is there evidence of a good therapeutic relationship: (a) a strong bond? (b) collaboration to reach shared goals?
- Am I able to be supportive?
- Do I communicate empathy and positive regard?
- Am I able to be open-minded, flexible, and creative?
- Am I able to have patience, tolerance, and remain congruent despite personal reactions to the patient and/or session content?
- Can I discuss the therapy relationship (including my own limits) in ways that will be helpful to the patient if needed?

Intervention Focus
- Are the goals of therapy clear, grounded in a clear rationale, and pursued in well-structured and sensible ways? Does my patient agree?
- Are interventions consistent with the case formulation and goals for treatment?
- Do interventions address current problems and concerns? Does my patient agree?
- Is there a shared understanding of what to do in crisis?
- Am I available and flexible enough to implement my part of the crisis plan if needed?

Intervention Quality
- Am I relatively active in sessions?
- Is treatment intensity (frequency, depth) appropriate for the level of patient impairment?
- Is there a focus on change, balanced with support and validation for the present?

Intervention Impacts
- Is motivation for change enhanced?
- Is there increased understanding of problems relative to environmental inputs, affect, cognition, and behavior?
- Are maladaptive ways of thinking and behaving decreased?
- Are adaptive ways of thinking and behaving increased?

Therapist Supports
- Do I have adequate access to support and consultation?
- Would specialized training enhance aspects of the treatment?

Note. From "Tailoring Common Treatment Principles to Fit Individual Personalities," by K. L. Critchfield, 2012, *Journal of Personality Disorders, 26*, p. 122. Copyright 2012 by Guilford Press. Reprinted with permission.

of warmly consistent structure may be an effective antidote to abandonment fears, affective dysregulation, and internal chaos for a particular patient with borderline PD. The same approach may discourage initiative in a dependent patient or lead to reactivity (to perceived control) from individuals with more antisocial, paranoid, or passive–aggressive personalities. Similarly, an open-ended, validating stance may do little to promote change among those with antisocial, narcissistic, or other PDs who tend to see "the problem" as external to them. Evidence addressing how alliance is best optimized and maintained in the face of such diverse patterns is still needed. A literature on alliance rupture and repair has explored part of the necessary territory, noting that markers of alliance rupture include patients "tuning out" or showing signs of hostility, distress, or resistance. They also include therapist and patient appearing not to understand each other (Eubanks-Carter, Muran, Safran, & Hayes, 2011; Safran, Muran, & Eubanks-Carter, 2011). This literature also suggests that alliance repairs may offset ruptures and sometimes strengthen subsequent outcomes.

Research supports the proposition that the interpersonal contributions of both therapist and patient impact outcomes (Benjamin & Critchfield, 2010) and demonstrate links with outcome not just for global views of the alliance but also for patterns of moment-by-moment interpersonal processes (Ahmed, Westra, & Constantino, 2012; Coady, 1991; Henry, Schacht, & Strupp, 1986, 1990; Karpiak & Benjamin, 2004; Tasca et al., 2011; Ulberg et al., 2014; Wong & Pos, 2014). The relational qualities of the therapist come into play especially in difficult therapeutic encounters and for patients with complex presentations. For example, treatments for PD and complex trauma are often long and can involve a quite difficult process. Intense feelings about the therapist or therapy may occur in the form of anger, fear, love, contempt, envy, or dependency. A therapist may easily become anxious, frustrated, critical, or overwhelmed. To prevent adverse outcomes, therapists need to be empathic, engaged, and willing to talk about the therapeutic relationship while still retaining a sense of boundedness and separation from the patient's patterns. The opposite also holds true. Henry et al. (1986, 1990) found that even small amounts of hostility expressed in therapeutic interactions can predict poorer outcomes. A therapist's use of interpersonal control can also produce poor outcome expectations when following patient resistance (Ahmed, Westra, & Constantino, 2012). Task Force principles emphasizing therapist empathy, tolerance, patience, and ability to acknowledge limits all relate to these challenges.

With these observations in mind, we turn next to a model for describing interpersonal behavior to anchor our discussion of how relational principles can be translated directly to moment-by-moment intervention and even word choices. We apply the model to specific case examples to illustrate use of relational principles designed to enhance adaptive responses.

STRUCTURAL ANALYSIS OF SOCIAL BEHAVIOR: A MODEL FOR PRACTICAL ANALYSIS OF RELATIONAL PROCESSES

According to Benjamin (1979, 1996), any interpersonal behavior (e.g., a sentence, a gesture) may be described using three dimensions: focus of the behavior (transitive focus on other vs. intransitive focus on self), degree of affiliation (friendliness to hostility), and degree of interdependence (enmeshment to differentiation). These dimensions are organized in the structural analysis of social behavior (SASB) model shown in Figure 8.1. Behaviors focused on others are boldface, and behaviors focused on the self are underlined. SASB's structure and internal and predictive validity have been well established (Benjamin, Rothweiler, & Critchfield, 2006). The version shown here is the simplified cluster model, which defines eight positions for each focus. The model can represent behavior that is loving, aggressive, controlling, and freeing (when focused on others) or delighted, submissive, recoiling, and separate (when focused on the self). There is "space" for forms of enmeshment (bottom of the model) as well as forms of differentiation and autonomy (top of the model). The model also accommodates "complex" behavior such as simultaneous hostility and friendliness or simultaneous focus on the self and another person. It can thus characterize double-bind and mixed-message behaviors as well as commonly encountered clinical dynamics such as demanding dependency ("You have to help . . . I can't do this without you," **Control** plus Trust), blaming interpretations ("It sounds to me like you went back to your old ways again by saying . . ."; **Protect** plus **Blame**), and defensive disclosure ("So I lost my cool again . . . what else do you expect from me?" Disclose plus Sulk).

In addition to characterizing one person's behavior in a moment, the model can be used to track or even predict interactive patterns. Perhaps the most important of these predictive principles is complementarity. According to complementarity theory (Benjamin et al, 2006; Carson, 1969; Kiesler, 1996), any interpersonal behavior "pulls for" a limited set of responses while constraining the likelihood of others. In the SASB model, complementary behaviors occupy the same position, differing only in their focus. For example, **Control** and Submit form behavioral complements (bottom center of Figure 8.1), as do **Ignore** and Wall-Off (top left of Figure 8.1). Certain pairings are common in therapeutic practice; for example, therapists often focus on patients with moderately friendly and autonomy-granting behaviors (Critchfield et al., 2007). Expressions by a therapist of affirmation, empathic reflection, or desire to understand a patient are all examples of these behaviors, seen in the upper right quadrant of Figure 8.1. Patients often adopt the complementary position of comfortable, open disclosure that is focused on the self. Another common pairing occurs in the lower right quadrant of the SASB model: A therapist provides friendly structure, advice, instruction, or didactic input while a patient adopts a stance of trusting or following the input. Complementary interactions are often stable over time.

Other configurations are also important. Similarity is defined as two individuals showing the same behavior (e.g., **Blame** is met with counter-**Blame**), whereas positions that are 180 degrees apart on the same surface

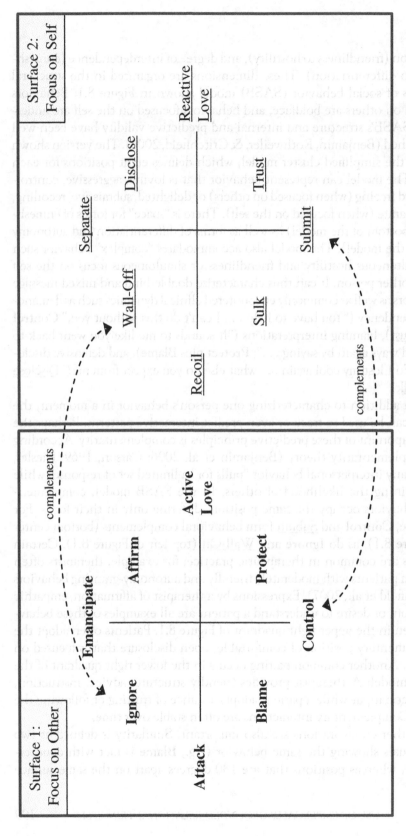

Figure 8.1. Structural analysis of social behavior simplified cluster model illustrating complementary behaviors. Behaviors focused on others are boldface, and behaviors focused on the self are underlined. In this adapted version, the focus on Other and Self are shown in separate "surfaces," and lines and arrow are added to illustrate complementary conceptual pairings. From *Interpersonal Diagnosis and Treatment of Personality Disorders* (2nd ed., p. 55), by L. S. Benjamin, 1996/2003, New York, NY: Guilford Press. Copyright 1996/2003 by Guilford Press. Adapted with permission.

are opposites (e.g., **Blame** and **Affirm**; **Protect** and **Ignore**). Similarity and opposition are predicted to be unstable. The *antithesis* or *antidote* refers to a position that is maximally different from another behavior on all three SASB dimensions.

DEFINING "NORMAL" THERAPY RELATING

The optimal therapy relationship can be thought of as a kind of attachment relationship in which the therapist provides a secure base characterized by friendliness, moderate enmeshment, and moderate differentiation (Benjamin et al., 2006; Florsheim, Henry, & Benjamin, 1996). The relationship is asymmetric in focus (both stay focused on the patient), and expressions of love occur only in limited, contextualized ways. Interventions are usually characterized by **Affirm** and **Protect**. Patients are in complementary positions of Disclose and Trust. Across studies, these positions characterize about 88% of all therapist and patient statements (Critchfield et al., 2007).

SASB-based studies of therapeutic process have repeatedly found that deviations from the optimal baseline are associated with poorer outcomes. Henry et al. (1986, 1990) found that even small amounts of therapist **Blame** and **Ignore**, or complementary patient behaviors of Sulk and Wall-Off, predict poorer symptomatic outcomes and more hostile self-treatment. These findings have been replicated in additional studies (Samstag et al., 2008; Schut et al., 2005; Von der Lippe, Monsen, Rønnestad, & Eilertsen, 2008). Poorer outcomes are also associated with extremes along the vertical dimension of SASB, especially therapist **Control**, and patient Separate (Ahmed, Westra, & Constantino, 2012; Macdonald, Cartwright, & Brown, 2007).

USING INTERPERSONAL PRINCIPLES TO INTERVENE WITH THE MOMENT-BY-MOMENT THERAPY PROCESS

The following example demonstrates use of the therapy relationship conforming to the optimal interpersonal patterning just described, with emphasis on the upper right of the SASB model (friendly differentiation). The interaction occurred at the beginning of a second session during an inpatient hospitalization for a patient with multiple diagnoses, including PD:

Therapist: I'd really like to just follow up on our meeting yesterday, sort of what thoughts and feelings you've had about that discussion, and maybe figure out where to go from here, or whether to go from here.

Patient: OK, I know it brought out a lot of emotions and a lot of feelings, some good, some bad, especially when we talked about how I needed to learn to cope on my own because I'm so dependent on people. That kinda freaked me out.

Therapist: Really, in what way?

Patient: Because I just, I don't think I can do it. I'm terrible at talking with people, so I don't know.

Therapist: So you feel freaked out by the idea.

Patient: Yeah, that I could help do it on my own and learn how to not depend on people and I just don't know how I—I've always had someone to help me.

Therapist: What would that look like? I mean, what would it be like to try and cope with things and build a life? Do you have any . . . ?

Patient: Well eventually I felt more suicidal. I hate to say that. But the thought of just doing it made me even more unsure. Because right now I'm dealing with the pain and trying to manage on my own, and trying to manage without pain pills, and it's just like . . . I lost my train of thought.

Therapist: That's all right, um, you were telling me about how thinking about this sounds like it's just overwhelming to add on top of . . .

The conversation returns to the patient's sense of hopelessness about being helped several times and develops as a theme for the session. She discusses how her mother had always been there in the past to "advocate" for her with doctors and others and that she now feels she doesn't have the strength to fill this role for herself. Later, she remembers her mother:

Patient: We all just laughed and that made her even madder. [*laugh*] We lived with her drama queen scene so much that it was just like every time she did something we ended up laughing, so . . . [*pause*]

Therapist: Do you miss her?

Patient: A lot.

Therapist: I imagine. I imagine it would be hard not to.

Patient: Mm-hmm.

Therapist: You said that even if she couldn't figure out a way to advocate or take the pain away, she'd be up here helping in whatever way she could think of.

Patient: Mm-hmm. She was really knowledgeable and she didn't believe in medicine and drugs. But she advocated for me because she saw I couldn't function and when it became that I was in too much pain she said, "OK, this needs to be done." But other than that like with her cancer just got into all these different things and so she'd probably get, if she couldn't find a doctor to prescribe or help with my pain she would try to find a way to bring me out of it, instead of feeling like giving up. . . .

Therapist: So it sounds like it just makes everything that much more intense that she isn't here, not just as your advocate, but as your mother.

Patient: Mm-hmm.

Therapist: And the idea of trying to take over some of that role for yourself.

Patient: I've lost all hope. I just don't care. There is a tiny piece in there that cares because I would have left here already and ended it. But, the majority of me has said, "I'm sick of this. I hate the way doctors treat me. I hate going in and out. I have to live like this the rest of my life." It makes it hard to have a relationship or friends or anything so I feel like, there is that little bit that would like to try, but the majority of it is still thinking to end it.

Therapist: Well, I hear you. And there's no one who could stop you if you make that choice in the long run, and you know that as well as anyone does. I do appreciate your honesty in just saying it how it is. And I hope you feel like I'm hearing you.

Patient: I do.

Therapist: And I also hear the tension in you between that part of you and the little part that has made it this far.

Patient: Mm-hmm.

Overall, the session sustains a clear process of collaboration around the central topic of developing a healthy capacity for self-care. The therapist carefully listens and tracks, softly but persistently returning to a key part of the patient's struggle (dependence vs. autonomy and self-care), exploring how the struggle developed and why it remains important given her history with her mother. The therapist makes optimal use of **Affirm** to understand and track the patient accurately. In this case, a dramatic positive shift occurred over the next few sessions of daily inpatient work that drew surprised comments from staff. Her focus between sessions appeared to parallel in-session conversations, shifting from hopelessness, suicidality, and craving for a return of her mother's advocacy and protection to the process of building a new, self-chosen life.

There are many ways to deviate from the optimal interpersonal baseline. Some deviations, such as hostility, distancing, or walling-off, can be cues that the alliance is troubled. Often, if caught quickly, these problems can corrected and discussed. Other deviations are more subtle. For example, in the following excerpt, a therapist briefly reverses focus from the patient to herself. The choice does not express hostility or obvious neglect of what the patient is saying, but the session does not deepen as opportunities are missed to focus on the patient's central theme (sense of being exploited and treated unfairly by those on whom he depends):

Therapist: How are things going?

Patient: OK. Looking forward to moving out. I have gone out and looked at some apartments.

Therapist: How did that go? How did you feel doing that?

Patient: Just a little overwhelming kind of, kind of reminds me of looking for a job. A lot of them are already filled, or you know, fill out this application and leave it with us and we will call you if, you know, we're interested. So I have an appointment to go look at a couple more tonight.

Therapist: OK. That sounds good. So as you were doing it you were feeling like it was kind of overwhelming?

Patient: I just, it just reminds me of looking for a job, and I hate that. I really hate that.

Therapist: Mhm. What's the worst part about it?

Patient: [pause] I guess it's just hard. To think that you know the money I'll be spending, I guess it's not my money, that it's my father's money, is just going in somebody's pocket.

Therapist: Mmm.

Patient: . . . and it doesn't bother me to buy a home, because the money is going to buy my home. But it just kinda bothers me that my money's just going into somebody else's pocket.

Therapist: Mmm. You like thinking of it as investing in something.

Patient: Yeah, I thought even if I got you know a lump sum, depending on how far back on my disability they go . . . I've got you know, heck I'd rather buy a fourplex or a duplex and rent out the other three units, or two units, and you know. I'd probably make enough to make the payment and you know just live there for free.

Therapist: Yeah, I mean I have an apartment too, and it's something to think about is buying duplexes. I've had people tell me it's a great investment especially if you are willing to live in half of it and have the other half almost pay for your mortgage usually.

Patient: Yeah.

Therapist: Well, it sounds like some good plans. I mean, I like the way you are thinking because even though you're feeling like it might not be the best and wisest use of the money that you're kind of still looking down the road to maybe what you might do differently in the future, which is good.

This session touches on several domains and relationships. In each one, the patient complains about unfair treatment by those on whom he is dependent. However, thoughts about how to understand and change this pattern, which is linked to his suicidality and depression, are never brought into clear focus. Even though there are some occasional departures from the optimal interpersonal baseline, this therapist's process is generally friendly, nonhostile, and patient focused. What is missing is a connection between the relational process and decision making about use of techniques to track the patient's interpersonal themes. These missing elements are, in fact, empirically based principles related to the need to follow a clear case formulation.

CROSS-CUTTING PRINCIPLES OF CHANGE: USE OF A CLEAR CASE CONCEPTUALIZATION AND INTERVENTIONS THAT WILL INCREASE ADAPTIVE BEHAVIOR AND DECREASE MALADAPTIVE BEHAVIOR

In addition to the centrality of the therapeutic relationship, several key treatment principles were also identified by the Task Force as shared across treatments and disorders. Several are highlighted here, especially (a) using a case formulation that links patterns of cognition, affect, and behavior to problem maintenance; (b) using a focused, consistent, and theoretically coherent method; and (c) seeking (with sensitivity to pacing and support) to increase adaptive patterns while decreasing maladaptive ones.

The Task Force principles do not specify a theory of pathology or of the change process, instead emphasizing that problems must be addressed in a coherent way that makes sense to the patient. Data suggest that outcomes are improved when therapists make accurate relational interpretations focused on a patient's central interpersonal issues (Crits-Christoph, Cooper, Luborsky, 1988; Crits-Christoph, Gibbons, Temes, Elkin, & Gallop, 2010; Norville, Sampson, & Weiss, 1996). Given a clear formulation, the therapeutic relationship can also be used to steer toward healthy goals. Karpiak and Benjamin (2004) provided sequential data from therapy transcripts showing that when therapists follow either adaptive or maladaptive patient comments with **Affirm**, those behaviors tend to persist and to shape outcomes.

Interpersonal principles are useful for complex interchanges and unusual contexts. The next two case examples show how an interpersonal case formulation, plus a clear sense of the interpersonally defined goal, can be used in concert with principles of complementarity to make specific intervention choices. The first example is interesting in part because the therapeutic goal is the unusual one of needing to cease collaboration and end the relationship. What initially appears to be a friendly announcement and invitation is soon revealed to have another agenda. The goal in this example is not to establish and maintain a therapeutic relationship but to assert a firm boundary and use principles of complementarity to steer the client toward appropriate help without provoking potentially dangerous reactance.

Case Example 1: When the Goal Is Not to Collaborate

Ted entered individual and group treatment with a female trainee supervised by clinic psychology staff as his therapist for a convicted sexual offense. He was a youthful-looking 40-year-old, and his offense involved having sex with a teenage girl he had pursued after seeing her be turned away from a bar. He was of average intelligence with a stable job in finance. He demonstrated strong tendencies toward grandiosity, exertion of control over others, and use of seeming compliance and indirect resistance to demands placed on him, combining features of both narcissistic and passive–aggressive PDs. Ted's interactions with others, particularly women, were often marked by contempt or objectification. During treatment, he began dating a reportedly "young-looking" 18-year-old woman (Heidi), which greatly concerned his probation officer. When confronted in therapy, Ted insisted that his therapist was "making a big deal out of nothing." He received feedback from group therapy members that his choice seemed reckless at best and a return to his major problem pattern at worst. A week later Ted reported to the group that he had told the young woman that he could not see her again. He said he made this decision to make his treatment as smooth as possible, and she was not mentioned again. On his last night in group, Ted told each member what he perceived to be their greatest flaws, and he said to his therapist, "If you weren't my therapist, I would have asked you out a long time ago." He then failed to schedule any of his planned individual follow-up sessions with the clinic director.

Roughly 2 years later, his therapist, who had since left the clinic, received the following text: "Hey, is this still [therapist's] number? This is Ted. You used to be my shrink." Within an hour, a voicemail followed: "Hi, [therapist]. This is Ted. I am married now, and my wife and I wanted to invite you out for coffee or lunch." The former therapist consulted with peers and responded, beginning the sequence of texts shown in Figure 8.2, along with the location of each interpersonal behavior on the SASB model. Ted's initial text and voicemail appear open, inviting, and friendly, although use of the word *shrink* may have been subtly derogatory. The therapist's response was not simply to follow the pull of complementarity (i.e., to happily accept the invitation). Instead, friendliness was returned, but with focus now placed back on the patient (congratulations), coupled with an assertion of interpersonal distance (i.e., refusal of the invitation accompanied by brief explanation of the reason). The hoped-for, complementary response would be for Ted to feel understood and affirmed and no longer to pursue focus on the therapist. The goal was neutral and differentiated interpersonal territory at the top of the SASB model—in other words, a friendly end to the briefly engaged relationship.

The strategy did not work. The next morning, Ted sent a series of text messages, also shown in Figure 8.2. He was blaming and sulking, revealing that he held a strong grudge. What he really wanted from his former therapist was an in-person apology. In other words, the invitation for friendly connection didn't achieve his ends, so Ted next tried to pull his therapist in with a bid toward hostile enmeshment. Given Ted's patterns, concerns grew that he might persist in demands for submission and apology, perhaps escalating to stalking or public confrontation. The trainee consulted her former supervisor, who encouraged her to set firm boundaries, and stated that Ted should direct all further contact to the supervisor.

The trainee used SASB to conceptualize the goal for subsequent relating, complementary pulls involved, and consideration of Ted's likely responses in crafting a response. The chosen medium was by text, in part to emphasize and enforce distance. In SASB terms, the goal was not just to assert a boundary; it was to encourage him to end pursuit of the therapist altogether (i.e., receive from Ted any responses at the top of the model, preferably to simply cease contact and let her go: **Emancipate**). In order to receive this response, a complementary pull was needed from the therapist that involved separation (self-focused, located at the top of the model) and avoided any impression of openness to friendly engagement or enmeshment (i.e., avoiding right and bottom regions of the SASB model). Ted's case formulation predicted that language to avoid included anything paralleling his maladaptive patterns—any form of enmeshed, self-focused language, such as reference to being "supervised," of "trainee status," or "no longer with the clinic"—was

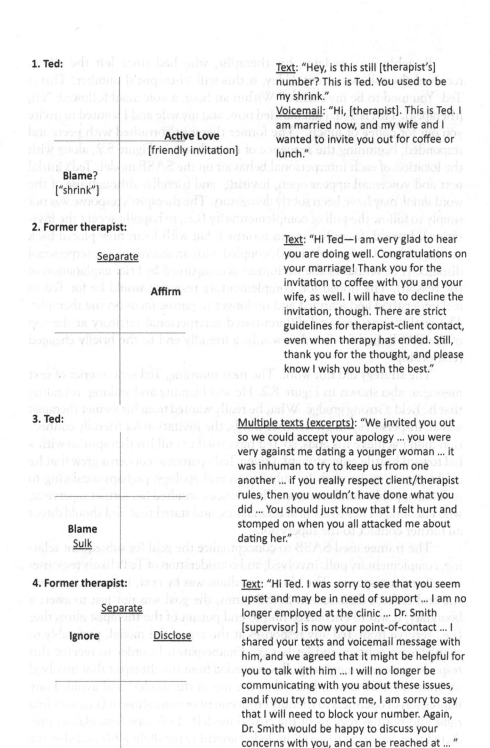

Figure 8.2. Text-based interaction with Ted.

5. Ted:

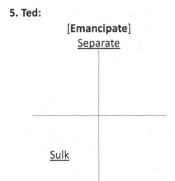

[Emancipate]
Separate

Sulk

Text: "Oh, haha, no I'm not upset at all I was just looking for an apology." **[No further contact]**

potentially hazardous. As seen in Figure 8.2, the therapist's final text emphasized interpersonal distance in several forms but also included interpersonal control worded to further enforce the distance (contact the clinic, not me; if you contact me, I will block your number). Ted's final communication retained a hint of hostile enmeshment but appeared to largely follow the pull of complementarity, and he distanced himself from the entire conversation. Ted has not contacted the therapist again over an interval of several years.

The next example further demonstrates how interpersonal principles of complementarity can be used with a case formulation to enhance adaptive and discourage maladaptive patterns.

Case Example 2: Pursuing Collaboration With the Right "Part" of a Patient

Annie was a 22-year-old woman who worked as an assistant manager at a group home for autistic children, with aspirations to be a singer-songwriter. She was a middle child, with an older brother and two younger sisters. She had a series of treatments, including inpatient hospitalizations for suicide attempts (usually by overdose of prescribed medications), residential treatments, and outpatient treatments, beginning in early adolescence. The major presenting concern was that she was chronically suicidal. Referral to her current therapist was made after two inpatient readmissions within 6 months. Her former therapist of nearly 7 years decided her work was no longer to Annie's benefit and terminated during the last hospitalization, attempting to safely convey her hopes that a different treatment relationship would be more helpful. In formal assessment, Annie qualified for several disorders: major depression; posttraumatic stress disorder; generalized anxiety; anorexia; and a history of polysubstance abuse involving alcohol, marijuana, and amphetamines. She also qualified for avoidant and borderline PDs on formal Structural Clinical Interview for DSM Disorders assessment. In interviews, she conveyed a pervasive pattern of resentful compliance and secret defiance of perceived demands by others, leading to additional diagnosis of passive–aggressive PD.

Annie's case formulation was based on an understanding of her concerns in light of patterns learned in her attachment history. The approach used was interpersonal reconstructive therapy (IRT; Benjamin, 2006), a treatment approach developed in many respects from observations using the SASB model to track patterns from early to adult relationships. Annie's parents were, for most of her childhood, strictly religious and quite authoritarian. Her family appeared as a close, cohesive, and happy unit in their many evangelical church-related functions; her father often held leadership positions in their local parish. However, there were harsh punishments for disobedience. One of her strongest childhood memories was of the "twice-teller," a stick that her father would use to hit her and her siblings, because children "shouldn't have to be told twice." At age 12, Annie returned home to find her father being led away by the police. He was indicted for white-collar felonies and served a several-year prison sentence, and it also emerged that he had had several extramarital affairs. Annie's family's dissolution was sudden and tremendously chaotic; during the process of her parents' divorce, her mother engaged in several new relationships that were supposed to be "kept secret." Both parents began visibly using drugs—cocaine (father) and amphetamines (mother)—after the father was released from prison. The children struggled greatly. Annie and her older brother lived with a family friend for a period of time. Annie was aware that her brother, with whom she was very close, began to slip into a deep depression, but was still surprised when he hanged himself when Annie was 15.

Annie was able to speak at times quite frankly about her own case conceptualization. She identified with both her suicidal brother and her substance-abusing and grief-stricken parents, treating herself as she saw them behave. She also recapitulated the early family experience, expecting and experiencing more instances of betrayal and loss. The suicide attempt that most immediately preceded therapy work was near her brother's birthday, and she stated it was because she felt incredible guilt at becoming older than he lived to be. Annie also carried a great deal of both anger and self-hatred over her process with treatment providers; she felt abandoned by her previous therapist but concluded that she "drives people away" by getting too close and then failing to "get better" when they try to help. This had happened multiple times with family friends, including once immediately prior to her last hospitalization. As she understood it, support from others was wholly contingent on her being different than she was—"pulling herself up by her bootstraps," in her mother's words, and out of the depression.

Given her history of felt betrayal, loss, and the perceived "burnout" of her previous therapist, initial sessions were almost entirely focused around building a stable therapeutic contract and rapport. Annie and her therapist worked explicitly to articulate shared goals, which involved helping her grieve losses and ultimately give herself permission to have a positively defined self. Goals involved positions on the SASB model that, in relation to the self, were the friendly antitheses to her longstanding patterns of self-criticism, self-neglect, and self-destruction. Pacing and accurate empathy were very important: Moving too far or often into her past left her seriously suicidal, but failures to acknowledge the past led her to feel misunderstood, betrayed, and again suicidal.

The course of therapy was tremendously challenging. Annie was often willfully self-harming (including cutting, anorexic behaviors, substance use, reckless sexual encounters, even skydiving with the expressed hope that her parachute would fail to open) and acknowledged these behaviors as partially suicidal and partially to test if her therapist would react as her family did: get mad and attempt to control her or abandon her. Her fear of opening up to her therapist also meant that she was frequently silent and walled-off in session.

A safety contract was in place that involved contact with the therapist to try and forestall crisis and prevent hospitalizations (or to allow collaboration around deciding to hospitalize, when needed). This approach followed another principle identified by the Task Force, unique to PD, recommending increased therapist availability during crisis (Linehan, Davison, Lynch, & Sanderson, 2006). In this spirit, therapist phone numbers were made available to clinic patients. It was made clear that texting was not an acceptable way to communicate suicidality. However, it clearly could still happen at times and needed to be responded to appropriately. The therapist occasionally learned about alliance ruptures in the form of suicidal texts sent after sessions. A series of these texts is shown in Figure 8.3. To fully understand the sequence, a few additional orienting comments about IRT case formulations are needed.

In IRT, the patient is conceptualized as having two basic "parts." One, the Growth Collaborator (GC) is pursuing healthy adaptation. The therapist attempts to engage this part of the patient by supporting and drawing her in while also reinforcing and encouraging her to nurture, care for, and affirm herself. The other, Regressive Loyalist (RL), persists in maladaptive repetition of patterns learned and internalized from close attachment figures. These patterns are articulated by the case formulation that guides treatment. The therapist seeks not to support or reinforce the patient's RL but instead to help the GC recognize where the patterns come from and what they represent (often a persistent loyalty to the perceived rules and values of loved ones)

1. Annie:

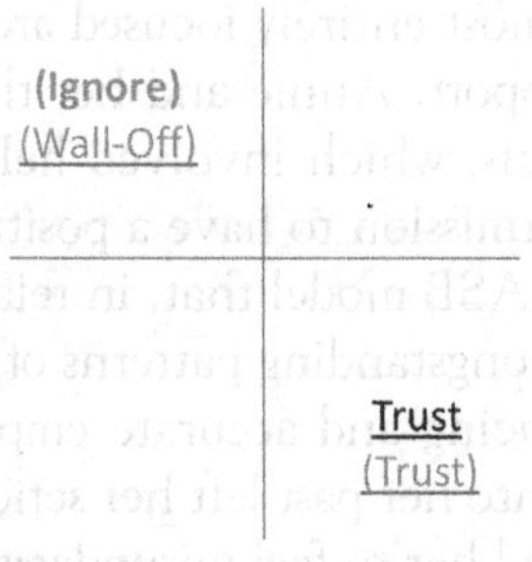

(Ignore)
(Wall-Off)

Trust
(Trust)

2. Therapist:

(Ignore)

Protect

Text: "I'm sorry. I just want to take the easy way out. If someone could just tell me my family would be OK. I don't want to live this life anymore. I don't know why I'm telling you this instead of just going through with it. I guess I just don't want to hurt my sisters, mostly. Why can't I just be grateful with my life? Why can't I just be positive? I hate myself. I truly do. And no, I don't feel like talking, so don't try calling me. I'm sick of people leaving me, I'm sick of people not caring. I'm just fed up. Do you think they'll be OK?"

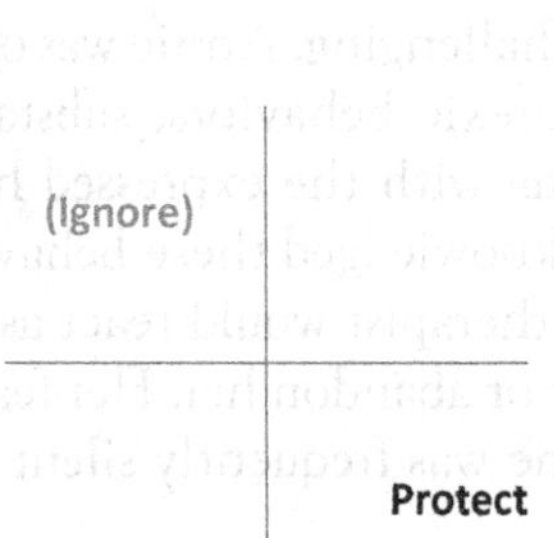

Text: "Message received. I am very concerned—I care, and want to help you through this. Would you call me? Or can I call you? Even if it is just a five minute phone call—if not tonight, then tomorrow morning?"

3. Annie:

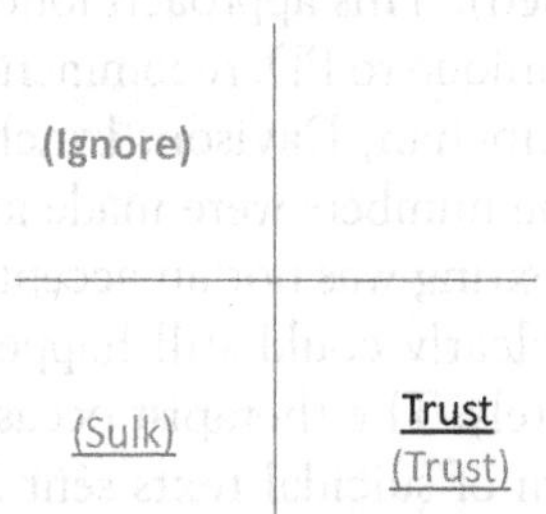

(Ignore)

(Sulk) Trust
(Trust)

4. Therapist:

(Ignore) Affirm

Protect

Texts: "Do you think it [suicide] will hurt my sisters really bad? Please say no...I don't want to be here anymore, I'm so tired," followed by "Sorry, I shouldn't have texted you, I'm just scared of what I'll do and what it will do to my sisters."

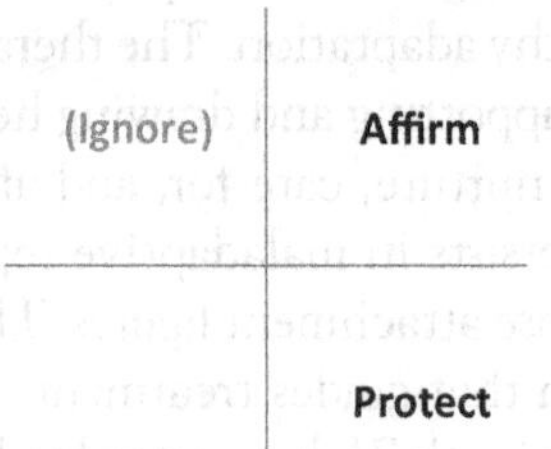

Phone conversation: Collaboratively discussed that part of her feels that suicide is inevitable, and it can be hard to see why not to just "get it over with." Patient agreed that the part of her that is tired is the part of her that has been fighting to live, and cares deeply about her sisters.

Figure 8.3. Interactions with Annie. Behaviors in parentheses show interactions with the Regressive Loyalist (RL) in contrast to interactions with the Growth Collaborator (GC) parts of Annie.

5. Annie:

(Wall Off)

―――――――――
         Trust

Text: "About ready to give up....I can't do this. I might text but I don't want to talk."

6. Therapist:

(Ignore)   **Affirm**
――――――――――
           Protect

Text: "I am very sorry to hear how much you have been struggling - but I am very glad you texted. I would really like to talk with you as soon as you are ready—either by phone or when we meet tomorrow. Would that be okay?"

7. Annie:

(Wall-Off)
――――――――――
(Blame)
(Sulk)

Text: "I don't want to talk. Like anyone cares anyway....Don't plan on me tomorrow either."

8. Therapist:

(Ignore)
――――――――――
           Protect

Phone conversation: Message to patient was that she sent two messages, the first being that she wanted to push help away, but the second that she wanted help; therapist expressed desire to respond specifically to the second.

and make the decision to let them go in favor of healthier ways. The many implications of an IRT approach to treatment is beyond our present scope; primary emphasis here is how relational principles can optimally be used in concert with a clearly articulated case formulation to address severe clinical problems. In IRT, relating with the patient can often be thought of as a relationship not with one unitary patient but two separate persons: one showing RL patterns, another showing GC patterns. Thinking of the patient as having separate parts allows for more targeted use of relational interventions.

Figure 8.3 shows a sample of postsession text exchanges initiated by Annie to her therapist, with the relationship process with the GC in standard text and the relationship with the RL in parentheses. The sequence illustrates how Annie's therapist responded to differentially reinforce adaptive versus maladaptive patterns as defined in Annie's case formulation. Given Annie's strong withdrawal and sense of abandoned alienation, her therapist's struggle is often to simply create and maintain a collaborative alliance in pursuit of a healthy goal; interpersonally, this means to increase friendly forms of enmeshment in the therapeutic relationship (so that the same themes can also be inspected in her self-concept and relationships with others). Annie's old RL pattern, however, is to pull for her therapist to recapitulate her history of abandonment by withdrawing and attempting to frustrate her therapist's attempts to connect and provide help.

In the first text, Annie places her therapist in a bind, expressing suicidality and hopelessness while also requesting that her therapist give permission for suicide and confirm that her family will not be affected by her loss. This is clearly a message from Annie's RL and contains elements of trust in the therapist (albeit maladaptively directed), coupled with neglect of her therapist's feelings and role and clear walling off ("don't try calling me"). Annie's pattern in the past had been simply to implement a suicide attempt, so there is a hint that the GC was also present by the fact of her reaching out to her therapist in any form ("I don't know why I'm telling you this . . ."). Although small, it suggests trust and the potential for greater collaboration in the future.

One relatively common option in crafting a response to the first text in health care settings might be along the lines of: "I'm sorry to hear you are upset. But, it is after hours. If you're suicidal I need you to call the crisis center per our safety contract." Annie had received this sort of response before. It is kind, professional, and appropriate in many respects but would very likely be taken by her as further evidence that she is burdening her therapist and will be abandoned by her sooner or later. The therapist could have responded in an attempt to block suicidality by directly engaging the RL. But any attempt to argue about whether others care for her could be unproductive and even lead to escalation if the healthy GC part perceives it as being told she is "wrong" after reaching out for help. Such "confrontations" are difficult to implement effectively even in the face-to-face setting. Another possibility, simply giving no response (submitting to Annie's stated desire not to interact) would be unacceptably risky and could easily be taken by Annie as further evidence that no one cares, further fueling suicidality.

In this case, the therapist responded by expressing caring and a desire to help, ignoring the request for no further contact to a substantial degree by requesting a follow-up call. On the surface, one could argue that the therapist here has delivered a "mixed message" that involves interpersonal hostility; the patient's clear boundary ("don't try calling me") was ignored. A simple read of the therapy process literature would predict a poor outcome on the basis of this "complex communication." However, looking deeper, the **Ignore** component (moderated by the strategy of asking for permission to talk, rather than immediately calling in response) is directed at the maladaptive pattern of withdrawal and distancing, whereas the friendly and protective part of the message is directed specifically toward the healthier part of Annie in an attempt to engage her in collaboration and sufficient self-protection until their next meeting.

The remaining exchanges are variations of the same pattern. The therapist's intervention is to engage and "draw in" Annie's GC, inviting her away from hostile withdrawal and toward friendly enmeshment using explicit statements and implicitly invoking the principle of complementarity. At the same time, the maladaptive RL component is systematically neglected and set aside. Benjamin (2006) has described other contexts in which forms of interpersonal hostility, carefully directed and contextualized, might also be useful to weaken or confront the RL. Alternatively, there are times when a friendly "cozying up" to the RL may be required to build initial collaboration. In each example with Annie, collaboration was subsequently regained, safety was reestablished, and rehospitalization was avoided.

Annie's therapy ended after 40 sessions, when she decided to move out of state to pursue a better job opportunity. She acknowledged that the decision was partially because the treatment was helpful. She felt that she and her therapist were getting too close, and she feared letting anyone become close enough to care about her if she ultimately killed herself. However, Annie also discussed how improvements in her career options, plus choosing a life separate from close proximity to family, offered increased hope in pursuing her own life and her ability to move on from grief and loss. Annie summarized the therapy by saying that her therapist helped her see that being healthy is both her right and her choice. We believe her conclusion was a result of the therapist's consistent emphasis not just on friendly control (which was especially necessary in crisis and when the RL was poised to take her over) but also on friendly autonomy and the goal of having a self that would be affirmed and nurtured by Annie and no longer defined by internalization of losses, or by loyalty to her family's self-destructive and punitive patterns. For patients like Annie, where the self is a fragile and fragmented thing, the importance of this kind of focus on developing a self (through whatever specific methods may be handy) cannot be underestimated and is largely conveyed through a relationship with a therapist, especially early in the process. To successfully navigate these issues, a case formulation and sense of therapeutic goals need to be clearly articulated at a level of specificity that facilitates decision making about the specific relational approach used at any given moment.

RELATIONALLY BASED PRINCIPLES FOR CASE FORMULATION CAN BE APPLIED COMFORTABLY WITHIN MULTIPLE THEORETICAL FRAMEWORKS

In the interpersonally based approach to case formulation used in IRT, therapists assume that a patient's developmental history includes learning "rules" for interpersonal relatedness and that some of these will be adaptive, whereas others will be maladaptive in the present. As therapists and patients work to uncover and name these rules, the conceptualization comes to include two parts of the patient: the GC, who pursues healthy adaptation, and the RL, who remains loyal to the caregivers with whom the patterns were first learned. These terms have clear corollaries for providers skilled in conceptualizing in different modalities. In CBT, for example, a patient's RL would likely be present in core negative schemas as well as the thoughts, feelings, and behaviors typically engendered by negative schema activation. In dialectical behavior therapy, the maladaptive patterns would likely be captured through behavioral analysis whenever their affect is high and their emotional regulation is taxed to the point of impairment. In psychodynamic treatments, the RL would be captured by defenses and manifestations of old wishes and fears in relation to the self and others. In motivational interviewing (Miller & Rollnick, 2013), the conflict between a patient's GC and RL will appear as ambivalence toward change that tips toward inertia and maintaining the status quo. As we described earlier, SASB principles and IRT make something of a natural pair, but we strongly believe that skilled therapists can operate from their "home orientation" while integrating SASB interpersonal principles to differentially intervene with both adaptive and maladaptive patient patterns.

CONCLUSION

An advanced graduate student therapy trainee recently expressed the following to one of us:

> A patient I'm seeing now doesn't like [the manualized approach I'm using] for specific reasons, and it also hasn't worked for her in the past. But, how can I respond to my patient's needs and still be evidence based? Isn't it unethical to deviate from the manual if it is empirically supported?

Clinicians are often trained to have multiple technical means available to them. Deciding among techniques should not be a matter of fidelity to one school of thought, or even an RCT, nor should it be given over to unbridled eclecticism. Clinical decision making should instead flow from accurate principles related to symptoms, relationships, and change processes. The approach envisioned here emphasizes use of an interpersonal lens on each of these domains.

We believe a principle-based approach will best be served by therapeutic skills and values founded on a commitment to scientific mindedness, critical thinking, integrative capacity, and sensitivity to relational context (Critchfield & Knox, 2010). We also believe the field would be best served by an increased research focus on principles underlying disorders and change processes rather than continuing with our current focus on packages of techniques. In the IRT clinic, recent research has focused directly on measurement of underlying principles of change (Critchfield, 2013). Preliminary results have been promising, showing substantial reductions in rehospitalization rates, symptomatology, and personality dysfunction among patients with severe and comorbid problems that previously had not responded to standard treatment attempts. In particular, and broadly consistent with Task Force findings, there have been observed linkages between outcome and (a) the use of the interpersonal case formulation and (b) interventions that enhance patient will to change. These principles retain potency even after controlling for the more traditional "common factors" principle of therapist empathy. The primary "rule" for clinical decisions in IRT is that any intervention is acceptable so long as it matches the case conceptualization. This rule becomes an easy means of reflection for IRT clinicians: "Does what I am doing make sense for this patient in terms of the case conceptualization?" As illustrated in the examples presented, interpersonal principles can refine options for in-session tailoring of interventions to provide discriminative feedback and differential reinforcement for adaptive versus maladaptive patterns.

REFERENCES

Ahmed, M., Westra, H. A., & Constantino, M. J. (2012). Early therapy interpersonal process differentiating clients high and low in outcome expectations. *Psychotherapy Research, 22,* 731–745. http://dx.doi.org/10.1080/10503307.2012.724538

APA Presidential Task Force on Evidence-Based Practice. (2006). Evidence-based practice in psychology. *American Psychologist, 61,* 271–285. http://dx.doi.org/10.1037/0003-066X.61.4.271

Benjamin, L. S. (1979). Structural analysis of differentiation failure. *Psychiatry, 42,* 1–23.

Benjamin, L. S. (1996). *Interpersonal diagnosis and treatment of personality disorders* (2nd ed.). New York, NY: Guilford Press.

Benjamin, L. S. (2006). *Interpersonal reconstructive therapy: An integrative, personality-based treatment for complex cases.* New York, NY: Guilford Press.

Benjamin, L. S., & Critchfield, K. L. (2010). An interpersonal perspective on therapy alliances and techniques. In J. C. Muran & J. P. Barber (Eds.), *The therapeutic alliance: An evidence-based approach to practice and training* (pp. 123–149). New York, NY: Guilford Press.

Benjamin, L. S., Rothweiler, J. C., & Critchfield, K. L. (2006). The use of structural analysis of social behavior (SASB) as an assessment tool. *Annual Review of Clinical Psychology, 2,* 83–109. http://dx.doi.org/10.1146/annurev.clinpsy.2.022305.095337

Carson, R. C. (1969). *Interaction concepts of personality.* Oxford, England: Aldine.

Castonguay, L. G., & Beutler, L. E. (2006). *Principles of therapeutic change that work.* New York, NY: Oxford University Press.

Chard, K. M., Schuster, J. L., & Resick, P. A. (2012). Empirically supported psychological treatments: Cognitive processing therapy. In J. G. Beck & D. M. Sloan (Eds.), *The Oxford handbook of traumatic stress disorders* (pp. 439–448). New York, NY: Oxford University Press. http://dx.doi.org/10.1093/oxfordhb/9780195399066.013.0030

Cloitre, M., Stovall-McClough, K. C., Miranda, R., & Chemtob, C. M. (2004). Therapeutic alliance, negative mood regulation, and treatment outcome in child abuse-related posttraumatic stress disorder. *Journal of Consulting and Clinical Psychology, 72,* 411–416. http://dx.doi.org/10.1037/0022-006X.72.3.411

Coady, N. F. (1991). The association between client and therapist interpersonal processes and outcomes in psychodynamic psychotherapy. *Research on Social Work Practice, 1,* 122–138. http://dx.doi.org/10.1177/104973159100100202

Critchfield, K. L. (2012). Tailoring common treatment principles to fit individual personalities. *Journal of Personality Disorders, 26,* 108–125. http://dx.doi.org/10.1521/pedi.2012.26.1.108

Critchfield, K. L. (2013, May). *Interpersonal reconstructive therapy: Methods, mechanisms, and findings to date.* Presented at the symposium Interpersonal Foundations of Adjustment, Health, and Change: Current Perspectives on Lorna

S. Benjamin's Structural Analysis of Social Behavior and Interpersonal Reconstructive Therapy, Park City, UT.

Critchfield, K. L., & Benjamin, L. S. (2006). Integration of therapeutic factors in treating personality disorders. In L. G. Castonguay & L. E. Beutler (Eds.), *Principles of therapeutic change that work* (pp. 253–271). New York, NY: Oxford University Press.

Critchfield, K. L., Henry, W. P., Castonguay, L. G., & Borkovec, T. D. (2007). Interpersonal process and outcome in variants of cognitive–behavioral psychotherapy. *Journal of Clinical Psychology, 63,* 31–51.

Critchfield, K. L., & Knox, S. (2010). Conceptual skills needed for evidence-based practice of psychotherapy: A few recommendations. *Psychotherapy Bulletin, 45,* 9–14.

Crits-Christoph, P., Cooper, A., & Luborsky, L. (1988). The accuracy of therapists' interpretations and the outcome of dynamic psychotherapy. *Journal of Consulting and Clinical Psychology, 56,* 490–495. http://dx.doi.org/10.1037/0022-006X.56.4.490

Crits-Christoph, P., Gibbons, M. B. C., Temes, C. M., Elkin, I., & Gallop, R. (2010). Interpersonal accuracy of interventions and the outcome of cognitive and interpersonal therapies for depression. *Journal of Consulting and Clinical Psychology, 78,* 420–428. http://dx.doi.org/10.1037/a0019549

Eubanks-Carter, C., Muran, J. C., Safran, J. D., & Hayes, J. A. (2011). Interpersonal interventions for maintaining an alliance. In L. M. Horowitz & S. Strack (Eds.), *Handbook of interpersonal psychology: Theory, research, assessment, and therapeutic interventions* (pp. 519–531). Hoboken, NJ: Wiley.

Florsheim, P., Henry, W., & Benjamin, L. S. (1996). Integrating individual and interpersonal approaches to diagnosis: The structural analysis of social behavior and attachment theory. In F. Kaslow (Ed.), *Handbook of relational diagnosis* (pp. 81–101). New York, NY: Wiley.

Gallagher, M. W., & Resick, P. A. (2012). Mechanisms of change in cognitive processing therapy and prolonged exposure therapy for PTSD: Preliminary evidence for the differential effects of hopelessness and habituation. *Cognitive Therapy and Research, 36,* 750–755. http://dx.doi.org/10.1007/s10608-011-9423-6

Henry, W. P., Schacht, T. E., & Strupp, H. H. (1986). Structural analysis of social behavior: Application to a study of interpersonal process in differential psychotherapeutic outcome. *Journal of Consulting and Clinical Psychology, 54,* 27–31. http://dx.doi.org/10.1037/0022-006X.54.1.27

Henry, W. P., Schacht, T. E., & Strupp, H. H. (1990). Patient and therapist introject, interpersonal process, and differential psychotherapy outcome. *Journal of Consulting and Clinical Psychology, 58,* 768–774. http://dx.doi.org/10.1037/0022-006X.58.6.768

Holt, H., Beutler, L. E., Castonguay, L. G., Silberschatz, G., Forrester, B., Temkin, R., . . . Miller, T. W. (2013). A critical examination of the movement toward evidence-based mental health treatments in the U.S. Department of Veterans Affairs. *Clinical Psychologist, 66*(4), 8–14.

Karpiak, C. P., & Benjamin, L. S. (2004). Therapist affirmation and the process and outcome of psychotherapy: Two sequential analytic studies. *Journal of Clinical Psychology, 60,* 659–676. http://dx.doi.org/10.1002/jclp.10248

Keller, S. M., Zoellner, L. A., & Feeny, N. C. (2010). Understanding factors associated with early therapeutic alliance in PTSD treatment: Adherence, childhood sexual abuse history, and social support. *Journal of Consulting and Clinical Psychology, 78,* 974–979. http://dx.doi.org/10.1037/a0020758

Keown, P., Holloway, F., & Kuipers, E. (2002). The prevalence of personality disorders, psychotic disorders and affective disorders amongst the patients seen by a community mental health team in London. *Social Psychiatry and Psychiatric Epidemiology, 37,* 225–229. http://dx.doi.org/10.1007/s00127-002-0533-z

Kiesler, D. J. (1996). *Contemporary interpersonal theory and research: Personality, psychopathology, and psychotherapy.* New York, NY: Wiley.

Kinsler, P. J. (2014). Relationships redux: Evidence-based relationships. *Journal of Trauma & Dissociation, 15,* 1–5. http://dx.doi.org/10.1080/15299732.2013.852420

Linehan, M. M. (1993). *Cognitive–behavioral treatment of borderline personality disorder.* New York, NY: Guilford Press.

Linehan, M. M., Davison, G., Lynch, T. R., & Sanderson, C. (2006). Technique factors in treating personality disorders. In L. G. Castonguay & L. E. Beutler (Eds.), *Principles of therapeutic change that work* (pp. 239–252). New York, NY: Oxford University Press.

Macdonald, J., Cartwright, A., & Brown, G. (2007). A quantitative and qualitative exploration of client–therapist interaction and engagement in treatment in an alcohol service. *Psychology and Psychotherapy, 80,* 247–268. http://dx.doi.org/10.1348/147608306X156553

Magnavita, J. J., Levy, K. N., Critchfield, K. L., & Lebow, J. L. (2010). Ethical considerations in treatment of personality dysfunction: Using evidence, principles, and clinical judgment. *Professional Psychology: Research and Practice, 41,* 64–68. http://dx.doi.org/10.1037/a0017733

Miller, W. R., & Rollnick, S. (2013). *Applications of motivational interviewing. Motivational interviewing: Helping people change* (3rd ed.). New York, NY: Guilford Press.

Nayak, N., Powers, M. B., & Foa, E. B. (2012). Empirically supported psychological treatments: Prolonged exposure. In J. G. Beck & D. M. Sloan (Eds.), *The Oxford handbook of traumatic stress disorders* (pp. 427–438). New York, NY: Oxford University Press.

Norcross, J. C. (2002). *Psychotherapy relationships that work: Therapist contributions and responsiveness to patients.* New York, NY: Oxford University Press.

Norville, R., Sampson, H., & Weiss, J. (1996). Accurate interpretations and brief psychotherapy outcome. *Psychotherapy Research, 6,* 16–29. http://dx.doi.org/10.1080/10503309612331331548

Safran, J. D., Muran, J. C., & Eubanks-Carter, C. (2011). Repairing alliance ruptures. *Psychotherapy, 48,* 80–87. http://dx.doi.org/10.1037/a0022140

Samstag, L. W., Muran, J. C., Wachtel, P. L., Slade, A., Safran, J. D., & Winston, A. (2008). Evaluating negative process: A comparison of working alliance, interpersonal behavior, and narrative coherency among three psychotherapy outcome conditions. *American Journal of Psychotherapy, 62,* 165–194.

Schottenbauer, M. A., Glass, C. R., Arnkoff, D. B., & Gray, S. H. (2008). Contributions of psychodynamic approaches to treatment of PTSD and trauma: A review of the empirical treatment and psychopathology literature. *Psychiatry: Interpersonal and Biological Processes, 71,* 13–34. http://dx.doi.org/10.1521/psyc.2008.71.1.13

Schut, A. J., Castonguay, L. G., Flanagan, K. M., Yamasaki, A. S., Barber, J. P., Bedics, J. D., & Smith, T. L. (2005). Therapist interpretation, patient–therapist interpersonal process, and outcome in psychodynamic psychotherapy for avoidant personality disorder. *Psychotherapy: Theory, Research, Practice, Training, 42,* 494–511. http://dx.doi.org/10.1037/0033-3204.42.4.494

Tasca, G. A., Foot, M., Leite, C., Maxwell, H., Balfour, L., & Bissada, H. (2011). Interpersonal processes in psychodynamic–interpersonal and cognitive behavioral group therapy: A systematic case study of two groups. *Psychotherapy, 48,* 260–273. http://dx.doi.org/10.1037/a0023928

Ulberg, R., Amlo, S., Critchfield, K. L., Marble, A., & Høglend, P. (2014). Transference interventions and the process between therapist and patient. [Advance online publication]. *Psychotherapy, 51,* 258–269. http://dx.doi.org/10.1037/a0034708

Von der Lippe, A. L., Monsen, J. T., Rønnestad, M. H., & Eilertsen, D. E. (2008). Treatment failure in psychotherapy: The pull of hostility. *Psychotherapy Research, 18,* 420–432. http://dx.doi.org/10.1080/10503300701810793

Wampold, B. E. (2001). *The great psychotherapy debate: Models, methods, and findings.* Mahwah, NJ: Erlbaum.

Wong, K., & Pos, A. E. (2014). Interpersonal processes affecting early alliance formation in experiential therapy for depression. *Psychotherapy Research, 24,* 1–11. http://dx.doi.org/10.1080/10503307.2012.708794

9

INTEGRATING ONGOING MEASUREMENT INTO THE CLINICAL DECISION-MAKING PROCESS WITH MEASUREMENT FEEDBACK SYSTEMS

THOMAS L. SEXTON AND ADAM R. FISHER

In the search for the best psychological methods, models, and services for helping clients, it has become clear that effective psychological services are those that include the strongest available research evidence delivered with clinical expertise and that are in line with patient values (APA Presidential Task Force, 2006; Hollon et al., 2014; Sackett, Straus, Richardson, Rosenberg, & Haynes, 2000). Yet, debates have continued about the role of research and the mechanisms needed to integrate it into the practice of psychotherapy. These debates are represented in the vibrant series of publications examining the strengths and weaknesses of the research and its potential impact on practice (Hollon et al., 2014; Sexton, Alexander, & Mease, 2003; Sexton & Coop Gordon, 2009; Westen, Novotny, & Thompson-Brenner, 2004). There is considerable outcome and process research that can guide practice in individual, couple, and family treatment (Sexton, Datchi, Evans, LaFollette, & Wright, 2013). However, for many practitioners research remains distant

---

http://dx.doi.org/10.1037/14711-009
Clinical Decision Making in Mental Health Practice, J. J. Magnavita (Editor)
Copyright © 2016 by the American Psychological Association. All rights reserved.

and broad and includes nonspecific findings with clients and problems that are not familiar. It is no surprise that those in practice frequently see research as having little impact on daily clinical decision making. Although both research and clinical experience are important, we still know little about how they can be successfully integrated into the daily practice of clinical professionals.

One thing we do know is that the therapist is a critical element in the delivery of any type of psychological treatment. Growing empirical support shows that treatment outcomes are systematically related to the provider, above and beyond the specific treatment, which suggests the importance of understanding clinical decision making in enhancing positive client outcomes (Crits-Christoph et al., 1991; Huppert et al., 2001; Kim, Wampold, & Bolt, 2006; Wampold & Brown, 2005). These findings should not be a surprise. In a real-life clinical setting it is the clinician who must make the ongoing decisions about adapting treatment on the basis of whether a client is improving, remaining stable, or deteriorating. Sexton (2007) described the role of the therapist as one of a translator between the assumptions and mechanisms of the treatment model and the interactions with the client necessary to promote change. It is through the clinical decision-making process, conducted by the therapist, that the translation of treatment models (whether general or specific) to client occurs. The APA Presidential Task Force on Evidence-Based Practice (APA Presidential Task Force, 2006) suggested that the clinical expertise needed for good decision making is the skillful and flexible delivery of treatment with the highest probability of success. As such, clinical decision making plays an important part of the clinical expertise needed to integrate research, theory, and experience into the complex formula of successful psychological treatments.

Our understanding of the components and processes of clinical decision making is still in its early stages. We do know that effective clinical decision making requires more than clinical experience and individual therapist judgment. When reviewing the relationship between clinician experience (based on years of experience and amount of training) and clinical outcomes, the conclusions of the major reviews are mixed at best (Beutler et al., 2004). Clinicians have not demonstrated high levels of reliability at the tasks of diagnosis, prediction, and case formulation (Garb, 2005). Clinical judgment alone seems vulnerable to the same sources of error that often distort ordinary human judgment, including confirmatory bias, self-enhancement bias, the availability heuristic, and a greater emphasis on personal experience than general information. Clinical decision making requires more than just experience. Shapiro, Friedberg, and Bardenstein (2006) suggested that clinical reasoning consists of therapists' informal analysis, decision making, and planning based on a wide variety of inputs. These include research findings, observations of the client, assessment of etiology, theories considered credible, authors and trainers found to be compelling, graduate education, conversations with colleagues, and past experiences with various techniques.

Magnavita (Chapter 1, this volume) has defined *optimal decision making* as a process involving the gathering of relevant information; consideration and evaluation of alternatives; making judgments that are relatively free of biases; and finally, appraising the outcome of one's decisions. Magnavita suggests that clinical decision making is a dynamic process that requires information beyond the beliefs and judgments of the clinician. One approach to bringing ongoing measurement to clinical decision making is the use of measurement feedback systems (MFS). Bickman, Kelley, and Athay (2012) described MFS as bringing systematic measurement tools and clinically relevant real-time feedback to clinical decision making. MFS integrate reliable and valid measurement of relevant client factors, clinical process, progress, and client improvement with clinically useful "feedback" that can easily be adopted into short- and long-term clinical decision making and case planning. MFS are also a tool to conduct practice-based research by systematically monitoring client status, identifying patients not benefiting from treatment, and providing feedback to clinicians about client progress (Lambert, 2001). Practice-based research can also provide critical data to the clinician for the many within-treatment decisions that go into good clinical decision making and data to the researcher to find trends and common patterns of successful interventions. In fact, with relevant and reliable client information, the clinician can address changes in progress and be flexible in provision of treatment while being able to use client-based information and clinical judgment to adjust and adapt treatment to better fit the client and improve outcomes.

MFS offer clinically relevant information through ongoing measurement of both progress and the process of treatment. The feedback provided enhances clinical decision making through the integration of two essential elements: (a) systematic and theory-based measurement and (b) specific and clinically useful feedback from clients (Sexton, Patterson, & Datchi, 2012). More than a technical tool, MFS represent a dynamic part of providing comprehensive treatment to clients by not only gathering information but also providing a mechanism for translating client and psychotherapy data into clinical feedback using real-time technology. This allows clinicians to focus on interpreting the information delivered by the MFS, examine the effect of treatment session by session, and make decisions about the course of psychotherapy. In addition, the technology of MFS makes it possible to visualize change at both the individual and systemic levels, to assess how each family member or partner is responding to treatment, and to compare their experiences of the family and couple relationships. Clinical feedback from MFS can provide information about what does and does not seem to be working so that clinicians can be more responsive to the needs of their clients by continuing, modifying, or discontinuing treatment plans (Bickman et al., 2012).

In this chapter we define, describe, and illustrate the central role that ongoing measurement and MFS can play as part of effective clinical decision making. We begin with an overview of the role that participant-based data may play. To illustrate the practical uses of MFS we review three specific models that range from systems for common integrative practice and modality-specific practice to evidence-based treatment programs. We focus more specifically on one method used to integrate an evidence-based family treatment (functional family therapy) into a systematic measurement and feedback approach. Within this discussion we illustrate the manner in which MFS can be, when specified to the treatment model being used, a core part of treatment and case planning as well as ongoing within-session decision making. Finally, we suggest some future research directions to further this work.

MEASUREMENT FEEDBACK: USING DATA IN CLINICAL DECISION MAKING

Although experienced as a personal, emotional, and relational interchange between the professional and the client, therapy for the clinician also involves a complex series of thoughtful choices. These choices can either contribute to or detract from finding an effective treatment plan or making useful process choices to facilitate implementation of a successful therapeutic endeavor. The clinical decision making behind the adaptations and adjustments that provide an added and unique benefit above and beyond the treatment type are complex. To adapt treatment successfully, clinicians require sources other than clinical observation to understand the therapeutic process and monitor treatment progress. In fact, the APA Presidential Task Force (2006) suggested that the expertise required for clinical expertise entails the monitoring of patient progress that might suggest the need to make treatment adjustments. As a result, there has been an increased interest in the role of ongoing measurement to systematically gather client-based and reliable evidence to inform clinical decision making.

Using feedback to enhance clinical practice is a relatively new development in the mental health field (Bickman et al., 2012). The importance of feedback can be illustrated by considering the development of any other difficult skill. Sapyta, Riemer, and Bickman (2005) used archery as an example, suggesting that though some archers might be "naturals," it still takes practice, training, and information feedback to hone their skills. Without feedback, the archer never learns to be effective and is unable to adapt to conditions and circumstances even after he or she may demonstrate mastery.

Systematic training, ongoing guidance, and comprehensive information feedback make the difference between trial-and-error learning and an efficient, effective pathway to skills development. MFS are a tool to provide the needed information to fine-tune both the overall skills of a therapist and the ability of the therapist to match the treatment to the unique client, family, or couple context. Adding feedback reduces the time to learn a complex skill and improves the performance of those skills under diverse situations and contexts.

As described by Bickman et al. (2012), MFS have two components. The first is *reliable and clinically sensitive measures* administered regularly throughout treatment to collect information concerning the process and progress of treatment. Assessment in measurement feedback not only requires good psychometric quality but also emphasizes clinical usefulness The second, equally important, component is *timely and clinically useful feedback* about the progress and process of treatment. Typical availability of computers in practice settings now makes it possible to present data-based measurement in engaging, useful, and timely ways that positively impact practice outcomes. MFS use the emerging electronic technology to transform measurement data into information that can influence treatment as it occurs. In other words, information electronically entered into MFS generates automatic feedback that is available to the clinician for immediate use. This immediate information can then be incorporated into the treatment planning for the very next clinical session or even for use in the current session.

The work of Bickman et al. (2012) also has brought attention to the components of MFS that are core and potentially necessary if they are to actually result in clinician behavior change. They have suggested that three principles form the theoretical foundation of an effective MFS: Goal commitment, information relevance, and cognitive dissonance. *Goal commitment* is the amount of interest a person has in accomplishing a goal. To be useful in clinical decision making, *information* relevance is crucial, that is, feedback needs to be related to a goal (e.g., task or outcome) that the clinician finds valuable. According to *cognitive dissonance* theory, the contradiction between what one wants to accomplish and what one has actually accomplished creates dissonance, which is psychologically uncomfortable. It is dissonance that motivates change. When presented with discrepant information, the person either makes changes in his or her behavior to attain the goal or becomes less committed to the goal itself. The clinician must perceive the source of the information as credible and the information must have value (Ilgen, Fisher, & Taylor, 1979). The information value of feedback can be enhanced by attention to the format, time, and type of information received. Feedback should be delivered as promptly as possible after data collection to allow clinicians to perceive the connection of the feedback to their behavior. Feedback should also be given frequently so that changes in processes and outcomes can be observed as they occur and corrective actions can be applied if necessary (Sapyta et al., 2005).

A number of pioneering MFS research approaches are now underway. Bickman et al. (2012) implemented a practical application of the contextualized feedback system (CFS), a model of guided clinician behavior change to enhance effective practice. Their intervention has four major components: (a) organizational assessment, (b) treatment progress measurement, (c) feedback, and (d) training (Bickman et al., 2012). The treatment progress measurement includes assessment of therapy process (e.g., therapeutic alliance, treatment motivation) and of clinical outcomes (i.e., life satisfaction, hope, symptoms, and functioning). Assessment measures are based on a comprehensive common factors–oriented measurement system called the Peabody Measures. Feedback reports summarize treatment measurement information and provide comparisons through data aggregated across clinicians, provider organizations, or types of treatment, and the reports provide suggestions for interventions and training. The CFS is used for professional development and continuous quality improvement and "enables provider organizations to make data-based decisions and transform themselves into learning organizations" (Bickman, 2008, p. 1117).

As MFS begin to develop, research on their potential benefit have also begun to emerge. For example, Anker, Duncan, and Sparks (2009) compared clients randomly assigned to treatment as usual (TAU) with feedback versus TAU without feedback in couples therapy. The couples in the TAU plus feedback had significantly better outcomes. Reese, Toland, Slone, and Norsworthy (2010) replicated this study and also found that the clients in the feedback condition improved more rapidly. Lambert, Harmon, Slade, Whipple, and Hawkins (2005) found positive results from their measurement feedback system built around the Outcome Questionnaire-45: Clinicians who received feedback had clients who decreased in total negative outcomes from 21% to a 5% to 15% range. Lambert et al. concluded that clients of clinicians who are not alerted to the negative responses have "unacceptably high" rates of deterioration. At the same time, it appears that feedback has the greatest benefit with clients who may require changes in their current treatment. This finding is consistent with theories that describe feedback results in therapist changes as the consequence of a discrepancy between the feedback information and some standard (Carver & Scheier, 1981). For example, for clients who were flagged as doing poorly, the effect of feedback effect size was 0.39 (65% of the treatment group was better off than the average of the control group), whereas the effect of feedback on the overall sample was much smaller (0.09; only 54% of the treatment group was better off than the average person in the control group).

Bickman, Kelley, Breda, de Andrade, and Riemer (2011) compared a TAU with feedback with a TAU without feedback, randomly assigned to different centers. They collected data on symptoms from youth clients, therapists, and caregivers at each session. Therapists in the feedback group received weekly computerized reports about clients' functioning, statistically significant change, and notification if clients' scores fell within the most severe quartile of the sample. Bickman et al. (2011) found that clients whose therapists received feedback improved more quickly than control clients. The frequency with which therapists accessed feedback was positively correlated with improvement on two different measures of functioning, and there was a dose–response relationship between feedback viewing and clinical outcomes. Data from the clinician, the youth, and the caregiver showed that the more reports viewed by the clinician, the faster clinical improvement the youth made. MFS have been used successfully to improve outcomes in treatment with couples (Anker, Duncan, & Sparks, 2009), in treatment with families (Bickman et al., 2011), and in general health care (Carlier et al., 2012).

Thus, it appears there is growing evidence that MFS may add to successful outcomes above and beyond that attributed to the treatment or therapist. We view MFS as a technology that brings unique and needed evidence to therapists' clinical decision-making processes. As such, these systems have the potential to aid in general TAU and in specific evidence-based treatments (Sexton, Datchi, Evans, LaFollette, & Wright, 2013). In fact, as Pinsof, Goldsmith, and Latta (2012) noted,

> The good news is that as the result of developments in psychotherapy research and information technology, we have arrived at the point where it is possible to diminish if not eliminate the scientist-practitioner gap. The psychotherapy research development is the emergence "patient focused," "progress" or "feedback" research." (p. 254)

ILLUSTRATIVE EXAMPLES

We present here a number of illustrative examples of MFS that are currently in use. Each demonstrates the critical role of reliable measurement and feedback that are incorporated into the workflow of clinicians in a way that adds to their ability to adapt and adjust treatment to specific clients.

OQ-Analyst

The OQ-Analyst (OQ-A) is a computer-based system designed to monitor and feed back progress information about clinical treatment (Lambert, 2012) and to alert therapists to cases that are at a high risk for failing prior to early termination (Lambert et al., 2005). The OQ-A utilizes two main measures, depending on the client being seen: the Outcome Questionnaire 45

(OQ-45; Lambert, 2004) and the Youth Outcome Questionnaire (Y-OQ; Burlingame, Wells, Lambert, & Cox, 2004). The OQ-A is utilized every week and prior to each session, with clients entering their responses on a computer, handheld device, or hard copy (Lambert, 2012).

The OQ-45 provides information every week on the client's progress in therapy, specifically addressing areas such as symptoms of anxiety and depression, interpersonal relationships, and quality of life (Lambert et al., 2005). There is also a shorter version, the OQ-30, available for adult populations. The Y-OQ consists of 64 items related to parent or guardian report of how a child (ages 4–17) is progressing in treatment across subscales such as Interpersonal Distress, Social Problems, and Behavioral Dysfunction. (Lambert, 2012). A Y-OQ self-report measure is also available for youth ages 12 to 17, as is a shorter, 30-question version of the Y-OQ (Lambert, 2012). Finally, the OQ-A also includes a 40-item therapeutic alliance measure when feedback suggests that it may be necessary (Lambert, 2012). After a client takes a questionnaire, a report is generated for the therapist on the progress of the client in graph form, which includes all of the weekly scores to date (Lambert et al., 2005). This report also clearly alerts the therapist on whether the client is progressing, deteriorating, or stagnating (Lambert et al., 2005). For ease of use, alerts are color-coded as white (functioning in normal range, consider termination), green (rate of change adequate, no change of treatment plan is needed), yellow (rate of change is not adequate, consider modifying the treatment plan), and red (early termination likely, and therapist should consider new course of action). This information can assist a therapist's decision-making process. The therapist has the option of sharing these data with the client (Lambert, 2012).

Systemic Therapy Inventory of Change

The Systemic Therapy Inventory of Change (STIC), developed at the Family Institute at Northwestern University, is a multisystemic and multidimensional measurement feedback system designed for monitoring alliance and client progress in individual, couple, and family therapy (Pinsof et al., 2009, 2012). The creators of the STIC view therapy as an intervention not only with an individual client but also with a system that includes anyone involved in the presenting problem (Pinsof et al., 2012). The STIC system includes sets of questionnaires completed by clients before the intake (STIC INITIAL), and before each session (STIC INTERSESSION).

The STIC INITIAL forms begin with demographic questions, followed by anywhere from two to six systems scales, based on a client's demographics. These systems scales address individual problems and strengths, recollections regarding family of origin, relationship with romantic partner, family and household issues, parental perception of child functioning, and the quality of the parent–child relationship. As an example, a client with a romantic partner and children would fill out all six scales, whereas an adolescent would complete two (individual problems and strengths; family and household). All six take about 45 minutes to complete. Based on these initial results, primary targets of change become the first to be focused on in therapy. Before each subsequent session, clients complete the shorter STIC INTERSESSION forms, in addition to alliance measures fit to the modality of therapy (Pinsof et al., 2012). All of the data becomes part of the Clinical Profile, provided online. The Clinical Profile provides graphs and an outcome analysis and guides the clinician in the decision-making process through highlighting the primary targets of change. These targets typically include six key factors per case (Pinsof et al., 2012). The feedback from the STIC also facilities treatment plans throughout the course of therapy in a collaborative manner (Pinsof et al., 2012). Pinsof et al. (2012) viewed the STIC as being empowering for clients through the facilitation of collaboration with therapists and providing clients with opportunities for recognition of problem areas in their relationships. For example, the STIC is able to show a client their own and their partner's ongoing data, and gives the client a key role in how they are interpreted and used in therapy.

Partners for Change Outcome Management System

The Partners for Change Outcome Management System (PCOMS) was designed for clinicians to identify clients who are not progressing in treatment and to guide therapists in addressing this in a collaborative manner (Duncan, 2012). Because of its atheoretical nature and general framework, PCOMS is a measurement feedback system that can be integrated with any model of clinical practice (Duncan, 2012). PCOMS consists of two four-item measures completed by clients: the Outcome Rating Scale (ORS), which assesses client progress, and the Session Rating Scale (SRS), which assesses therapeutic alliance (Miller, Duncan, Sorrell, & Brown, 2005).

The ORS assess the dimensions of individual well-being, including distress from symptoms, relationships, work or school satisfaction and an overall sense of well-being (Duncan, 2012). When scores on the ORS are decreasing, clinicians can utilize this information in their decision-making process in a collaborative manner with the client, including whether to continue therapy (Duncan, 2012). Problems in the alliance are also discussed if they arise (Duncan, 2012). Miller et al. (2005) noted that clients often drop out of therapy before bringing up issues in the relationship with the therapist, hence the need for the SRS. PCOMS monitors the alliance through the SRS at every session, as opposed to Lambert's MFS, which only addresses alliance in cases of a lack of progress (Duncan, 2012).

INTEGRATING PATIENT INFORMATION INTO CLINICAL DECISION MAKING WITHIN AN EVIDENCE-BASED FAMILY TREATMENT

Evidence-based treatment models provide a useful example to illustrate the potential of MFS in clinical decision making. Evidence-based models provide a useful illustration because they are specific in the description of the treatment, allowing for measures of specific treatment goals as well as ongoing measurement of phase and session-based therapeutic process that are hypothesized to contribute to positive change. Functional family therapy (FFT) is an evidence-based treatment model for youth and families with behavior problems (Alexander, Robbins, & Sexton, 2000; Sexton, 2010). Like many evidence based treatments, FFT has a number of efficacy and effectiveness trials showing its success in reducing youth behavior problems, improving family functioning, and reducing family conflict (Sexton, 2010). The most recent FFT outcome study found that in community-based settings, FFT was most successful when practiced by therapists who followed the model (Sexton & Turner, 2010). Thus, it became clear that in order to maximize potential outcomes in complex community settings, therapists needed help in implementing the model with fidelity and adherence (Sexton & Turner, 2010). The FFT–Clinical Feedback System (FFT-CFS; Sexton, 2010) is a product of that effort and the work of Bickman, Sexton and Kelly (NIMH: RO 1 MH087814; Bickman, Sexton, & Kelly, 2010).

FFT-CFS uses a state-of-the art web-based computer system to administer and collect information using brief questionnaires completed by the clinician, caregiver, youth, and teacher. Using electronic data entry, user-friendly feedback reports are immediately available to the clinicians and their supervisors. The FFT-CFS system is unique in that it is a single system that provides real-time information to therapists, supervisors, administrators, evaluators, and researchers regarding model fidelity, client outcomes, and service delivery profiles. The specificity of the FFT model allows for the monitoring of treatment, training, and clinician model adherence in a systematic manner that is not possible with other, less specific treatment interventions. The FFT-CFS system is, therefore, both a clinical decision-making and a participant-based research tool.

As recommended by Bickman (2008), the FFT-CFS has both a measurement core and a systematic feedback system. The FFT Clinical Measurement Inventory (FFT CMI) is the measurement core and is built on the assumption that continuously measuring the major domains of clinical practice will improve the quality of FFT if it is done in a relevant way (Sexton, 2010). The FFT CMI consists of brief and psychometrically sound measures to be completed by clients, therapists, and supervisors. These measures can be taken electronically or on paper (to be put in the system manually) and inform four central domains of clinical decision making: Treatment Planning (service delivery, case conceptualization, and session planning), Treatment Progress and Process (family relational factors, alliance, phase-specific progress, general improvement, and symptom level), Model Fidelity (therapist model fidelity from supervisor–client perspective), and Client Outcomes (family and symptom changes).

The clinical feedback is designed to inform the clinical decision making of the therapist by providing information that leads to actionable model-specific adaptations in a way that incorporates an understanding of how cognitive processes influence responses to feedback (Cannon & Witherspoon, 2005). There are three primary domains of clinical feedback in the FFT-CFS. First, measures target the *symptom level* of youth functioning, which is central given the primary goal of youth behavior change in FFT. In addition, because of the phasic nature of FFT, the CFS design includes the *impact* of session on the accomplishment of phase goals that are the change mechanisms of the treatment model. Finally, the system has a central feature for client report phase and overall *progress*. Because FFT is a conjoint family therapy, both measurement and feedback are based on individual perspectives (youth, caregiver, etc.), increasing the complexity and utility of the system.

There are also four specific mechanisms through which feedback in these areas is delivered. First, *status* feedback, which is where the client–family are in the present with regard to how they view progress, the impact of the treatment, and the symptom level of their youth. Status feedback is designed so that merely glancing at the feedback report can offer a useful interpretation. At-a-glance clinical feedback indicates broad levels of current status in a way that does not require significant attention or resources. The FFT-CFS also provides feedback on symptoms, impact, and progress over time, or *trend-based* feedback. This information allows therapists to make judgments regarding changes in treatment plans and interventions. Feedback is also provided in more extensive ways if needed by the clinician. A Comprehensive Feedback Report provides information at the level of each question on each measure. This level of analysis allows for a greater understanding of the meaning of the broad status indicators, further improving clinical decision making. Finally, the system provides clinical *alerts* in response to high scores on critical items, high overall scores, or other indicators of dropout and clinical importance. Figure 9.1 illustrates the four domains of clinical feedback.

Figure 9.2 illustrates the three domains of information in the FFT-CFS system. Scheduling appointments is the major mechanism through which client contacts, measurement scheduling, and case planning is built. An appointment produces the designated case planning tools and the measure designed for that particular session and adds them automatically to the to-do

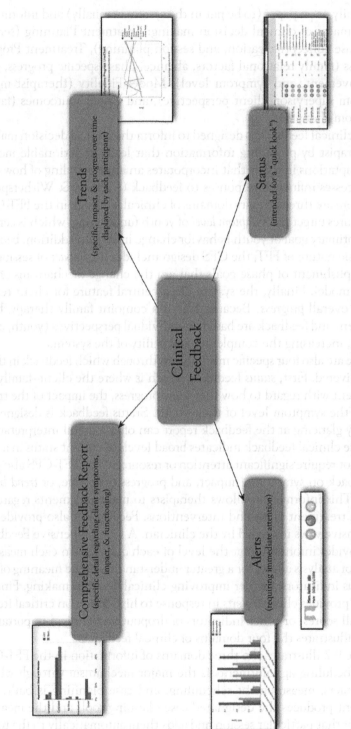

Figure 9.1. Information domains in the functional family therapy–clinical feedback system.

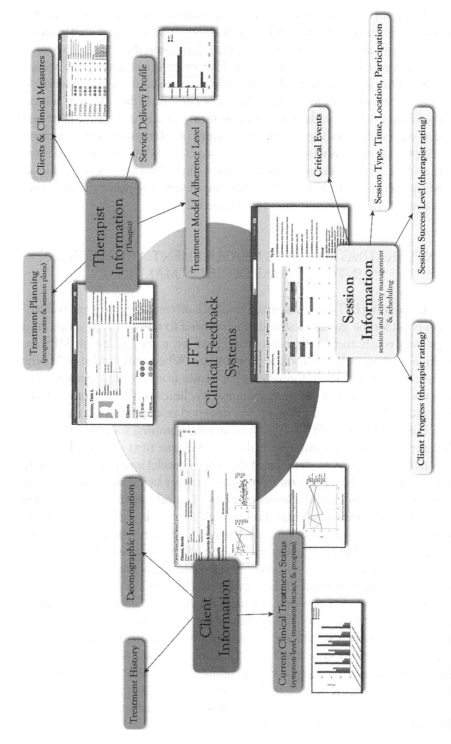

Figure 9.2. Domains of the functional family therapy (FFT)–clinical feedback system.

list. This prompts clinicians, in a very user-friendly way, to complete the needed material in a timely manner. The Therapist Information section includes adherence rates, which consist of service delivery information that can be compared with other cases within the therapist caseload, or to others in the same agency or to the entire FFT database. These comparisons give content to the feedback. Session Information includes basic data about sessions (date, length, session goals, focus, critical incidents) as well as rating of client improvement and session success. Integrating these three domains of information into a platform for the primary work functions of the clinicians (scheduling, therapist information, and session information) allow for these major functions of the clinician to be represented so that the FFT-CFS is thus designed to move the MFS into the center of all clinical activities (see Figure 9.2).

INTEGRATING ONGOING MEASUREMENT AND FEEDBACK INTO CLINICAL DECISION MAKING

Combining FFT with systematic feedback on treatment progress and processes provides the guidance that therapists need to tailor FFT to youth, thus improving youth and family outcomes. However, to be successful, MFS are much more than technical tools to provide data. When only "added on" to the treatment provided, the information that comes from ongoing measurement does not become part of the treatment, and its clinical utility decreases. To be relevant to clinicians, the FFT-CFS was designed be central to the user workflow. For the therapist, FFT-CFS is a treatment-planning tool used to record the events of each encounter with the family, make next session plans, and integrate each of the core elements of the clinical model into practice. As such, it was designed to be a platform to engage therapists by moving case planning into a system in which client feedback plays a central role in decision making to help keep the therapist focused on the relevant goals, skills, and interventions for each phase of FFT. It was also designed to identify when cases are going poorly, when families are not responding, and when a service delivery profile is not model adherent. It helps supervisors with specific, focused, and session-by-session information that reflects how therapists think, the decisions they make, and the outcomes of their work. Agencies use it as an outcome measurement and program evaluation tool. Researchers use it to gather participant-based research data, which is integrated into training, treatment, clinical consultation, and supervision to focus clinical work, facilitate accountability, and improve outcomes. In this approach, ongoing measurement is an integral part of treatment occurring at each therapeutic encounter.

It is the treatment session that initiates measurement and case planning. As illustrated in Figure 9.3, session information can include both descriptive

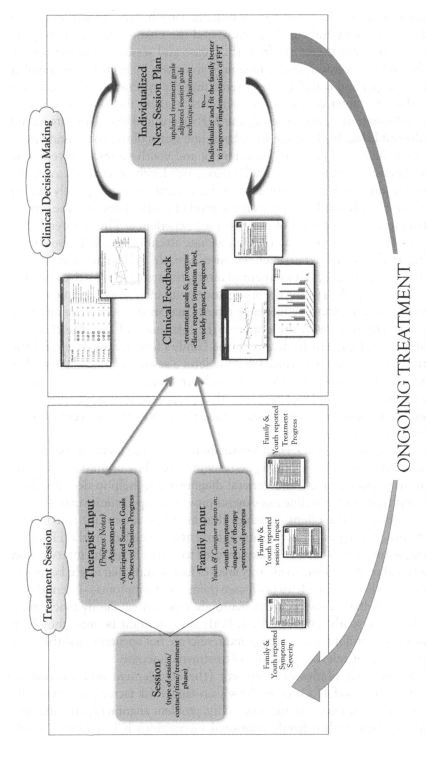

Figure 9.3. Clinical decision-making process in functional family therapy (FFT)–clinical feedback system.

information about the session itself (e.g., its length, type, focus) and information from clients (about their status and the change trajectory they are experiencing) and therapist (from their case and session planning notes). At the end of a session, client measures are taken by each family member either by paper and pencil (to be entered into the system later) or electronically through tablet or computer devices that allow the client to directly enter information. Once entered, the MFS translates the data into useful and digestible feedback on the initial baseline status of the youth and family based on their level of family functioning and youth symptom levels. The multidimensional nature of this MFS makes two levels of feedback available to review after each treatment session. First, clinicians can quickly review the status of each family member on the level of youth symptoms, the impact of treatment, and the level of progress they experience. This is intended to alert the clinician to areas that need immediate attention. There is also client-specific feedback that details each measure, subscale, and question answer for detailed case planning. In treatment planning the system allows the clinician to look broadly at data (using the at-a-glance status indicators) or more specifically through the extensive feedback reports that show client score and how that score compares with the norms of the instrument. Once the clinician has reviewed the client feedback on the family's functioning level and the youth symptom level, the clinician completes a session planning guide that integrates client feedback on level of youth symptom and family functioning into the next session plan. Over time that process continues, resulting in a focused and tailored approach to matching the treatment intervention with the specific client.

Client, therapy, and session information can also be useful at the specific phases of treatment. For example, assessment at baseline or intake allows the clinician to gather broad and general diagnostics to help in deciding how to deliver treatment. Baseline assessments provide an opportunity to systematically understand the client variables that might be important to consider in planning the types of therapeutic interventions needed. In the FFT-CFS system, there are two baseline measures used to ensure fit for the intervention (family and symptom) and to identify areas of functioning that might be targets of understanding the problems or change (family and symptoms—internalizing and externalizing). Two specific domains are represented: family functioning and the other youth symptom level. Both are important because they help adjust treatment if it is not working and results are not apparent, and they also serve as clinically relevant measures of treatment outcome.

In the early phases of treatment (the engagement and motivation phase) the FFT model focuses on the within-family risk factors, systematically addressing within-family blame, negativity, problem alignment, and alliance. Changing these within-family relational interactions is intended to result in improvement in youth behavior. Process and progress measures are integrated into each treatment encounter. These measures represent the degree of engagement and improvement in family functioning. In the middle phase of treatment (the behavior change phase) the focus is on identifying and implementing specific behavior changes within the family that result in building within-family protective factors. To accomplish the goal, the family needs to know what to do, and the therapist needs to monitor the family attempts at implementing the changes. The clinician is helped by knowing how to make ongoing adaptations to overcome barriers.

In the final phase of treatment (generalization phase), the primary goals are to generalize, support, and maintain the changes made in treatment. To accomplish this, the family needs to demonstrate the ability to apply skills to other areas within the family, use existing community resources to support them, and overcome barriers to prevent relapse. As symptoms improve, treatment termination is planned. Using the FFT-CFS, initial clinical hypotheses are measured and delivered by client feedback, which leads to revised session and treatment plans.

WHAT IS NEXT: CREATIVITY, CLIENT DATA, AND CLINICAL DECISION MAKING

MFS bring an important element to clinical decision making: client real-time data for use in both the macro (which treatment to use) and micro (how to respond to an event in a single session) clinical decisions. When integrated into the workflow of the clinician, MFS can become the golden thread that ties together good treatment, quality improvement, and ongoing evaluation and research (Kelley & Bickman, 2009). MFS also give patients a voice in treatment. In implementing clinical treatments for individual clients, MFS bring a source of information and perspective that adds to the therapist experience to result in therapeutic and helpful clinical decisions. In a recent review of psychotherapy research, Newnham and Page (2010) concluded that "use of patient monitoring and feedback in routine practice is imperative. The focus on the individual rather than the average patient empowers the patient and encourages dialogue about progress, the direction of treatment and achievement of treatment goals" (p. 136).

In many ways MFS have the potential to become an essential component of treatment. "Much like manuals added specificity, MFS bring specificity to the actual delivery of therapy which is dependent on the contributions and interactions that take place between . . . people" (Koss & Shiang, 1994, p. 675). In this way MFS are interventions that stand alongside treatments and the interventionists as core components of treatment because they bring information that cannot be generated by clinical experts alone or the efficacy of the treatment model being used. MFS bring research-informed evidence that becomes part of the structure within which the expert develops systematic and complex case conceptualizations by providing a reliable and clinically relevant way to understand clients, problems, and context. It is this scaffolding that forms the structure within which cases are conceptualized, forms the foundation of how "in the room" decisions are made, and provides a road map of the steps to take to promote successful change process. It is also the information that helps treatments stay relevant by helping specify, tailor, and focus on effective interventions of treatment by providing "context" to the case.

MFS also represent an important future research tool. In addition to providing the clinical decision-making assistance described in this chapter, MFS are also a platform upon which systematic research data can be gathered for participant-based research on clinical practice. Whether for individual therapist, organization, or model-specific analysis, the ongoing measurement of MFS provides a useful slice of evidence about treatments in real-life contexts. Because data will be gathered on a routine basis, clinical practitioners may actually be best situated to conduct systematic inquiry into the outcomes and processes at the center of clinical intervention research. Stricker and Trierweiler (1995) coined the term "local clinical scientist" to describe an approach for clinicians to move research into their practice by studying their own practices and profiles of service delivery, types of interventions, outcomes, and even process measures, which over time accumulate to produce a "local" set of "evidence" for that practitioner in that setting.

SUMMARY

Growing empirical support shows treatment outcomes are systematically related to the provider, above and beyond the specific treatment, which suggests the importance of understanding clinical decision making in enhancing positive client outcomes (Crits-Christoph et al., 1991; Huppert et al., 2001; Kim et al., 2006; Wampold & Brown, 2005). These findings should not be a surprise. In a real-life clinical setting, it is the clinician who must make the ongoing decisions about adapting treatment based on whether a client is improving, remaining stable, or deteriorating. It is through the clinical decision-making process, conducted by the therapist, that the translation of treatment models (whether general or specific) to client occurs. Clinical decision making is a complex process requiring more than clinical judgment alone.

Understanding the components and processes of clinical decision making is still in its early stages. One approach to bringing ongoing measurement to clinical decision making is MFS. MFS integrate reliable and valid measurement of relevant client factors, clinical process, progress, and client improvement with clinically useful feedback that can easily be adopted into short- and long-term clinical decision making and case planning. MFS are also a tool to conduct practice-based research by systematically monitoring client status, identifying patients not benefiting from treatment, and providing feedback to clinicians about client progress. Practice-based research can also provide critical data to the clinician for the many within-treatment decisions that go into good clinical decision making and data to the researcher to find trends and common patterns of successful interventions. When integrated into the workflow of the clinician, MFS can become the golden thread that ties together good treatment, quality improvement, and ongoing evaluation and research (Kelley & Bickman, 2009) and gives patients a voice in treatment while providing information that adds to the therapist experience to result in therapeutic and helpful clinical decisions.

REFERENCES

Alexander, J. F., Robbins, M. S., & Sexton, T. L. (2000). Family-based interventions with older, at-risk youth: From promise to proof to practice. *The Journal of Primary Prevention, 21*, 185–205. http://dx.doi.org/10.1023/A:1007031219209

Anker, M. G., Duncan, B. L., & Sparks, J. A. (2009). Using client feedback to improve couple therapy outcomes: A randomized clinical trial in a naturalistic setting. *Journal of Consulting and Clinical Psychology, 77*, 693–704. http://dx.doi.org/10.1037/a0016062

APA Presidential Task Force on Evidence-Based Practice. (2006). Evidence-based practice in psychology. *American Psychologist, 61*, 271–285. http://dx.doi.org/10.1037/0003-066X.61.4.271

Beutler, L. E., Malik, M., Alimohamed, S., Harwood, T. M., Talebi, H., Noble, S., & Wong, E. (2004). Therapist variables. In M. J. Lambert (Ed.), *Bergin and Garfield's handbook of psychotherapy and behavior change* (5th ed., pp. 227–306). New York, NY: Wiley.

Bickman, L. (2008). A measurement feedback system (MFS) is necessary to improve mental health outcomes. *Journal of the American Academy of Child and Adolescent Psychiatry, 47*, 1114–1119. http://dx.doi.org/10.1097/CHI.0b013e3181825af8

Bickman, L., Kelley, S. D., & Athay, M. (2012). The technology of measurement feedback systems. *Couple and Family Psychology: Research and Practice, 1*, 274–284. http://dx.doi.org/10.1037/a0031022

Bickman, L., Kelley, S. D., Breda, C., de Andrade, A. R., & Riemer, M. (2011). Effects of routine feedback to clinicians on mental health outcomes of youths: Results of a randomized trial. *Psychiatric Services, 62*, 1423–1429. http://dx.doi.org/10.1176/appi.ps.002052011

Bickman, L., Sexton, T. L., & Kelly, S. (2010). *The synergistic effects of FFT and a computer-based monitoring system*. National Institute of Mental Health (RO 1 MH087814).

Burlingame, G. M., Wells, M. G., Lambert, M. J., & Cox, J. C. (2004). Youth Outcome Questionnaire (Y-OQ). In M. E. Maruish (Ed.), *The use of psychological testing for treatment planning and outcome assessment* (3rd ed., Vol. 2, pp. 235–274). Mahwah, NJ: Erlbaum.

Cannon, M. D., & Witherspoon, R. (2005). Actionable feedback: Unlocking the power of learning and performance improvement. *The Academy of Management Executive, 19*, 120–134. http://dx.doi.org/10.5465/AME.2005.16965107

Carlier, I. V. E., Meuldijk, D., Van Vliet, I. M., Van Fenema, E., Van, D. W., & Zitman, F. G. (2012). Routine outcome monitoring and feedback on physical or mental health status: Evidence and theory. *Journal of Evaluation in Clinical Practice, 18*, 104–110. doi:10.1111/j.1365-2753.2010.01543.x

Carver, C. S., & Scheier, M. F. (1981). *Attention and self-regulation: A control-theory approach to human behavior*. New York, NY: Springer-Verlag.

Crits-Christoph, P., Baranackie, K., Kurcias, J. S., Beck, A. T., Carroll, K., Perry, K., . . . Zitrin, C. (1991). Meta-analysis of therapist effects in psychotherapy outcome studies. *Psychotherapy Research, 1*, 81–91. http://dx.doi.org/10.1080/10503309112331335511

Duncan, B. L. (2012). The Partners for Change Outcome Management System (PCOMS): The Heart and Soul of Change Project. *Canadian Psychology/Psychologie canadienne, 53*, 93–104. http://dx.doi.org/10.1037/a0027762

Garb, H. N. (2005). Clinical judgment and decision making. *Annual Review of Clinical Psychology, 1*, 67–89. http://dx.doi.org/10.1146/annurev.clinpsy.1.102803.143810

Hollon, S. D., Areán, P., Craske, M. G., Crawford, K. C, Kivlahan, D. R., Magnavita, J, . . . Kurtzman, H. (2014). Developing clinical practice guidelines. *Annual Review of Clinical Psychology, 10*, 213–241.

Huppert, J. D., Bufka, L. F., Barlow, D. H., Gorman, J. M., Shear, M. K., & Woods, S. W. (2001). Therapists, therapist variables, and cognitive–behavioral therapy outcome in a multicenter trial for panic disorder. *Journal of Consulting and Clinical Psychology, 69*, 747–755. http://dx.doi.org/10.1037/0022-006X.69.5.747

Ilgen, D. R., Fisher, C. D., & Taylor, M. S. (1979). Consequences of individual feedback on behavior in organizations. *Journal of Applied Psychology, 64*, 349–371.

Kelley, S. D., & Bickman, L. (2009). Beyond outcomes monitoring: Measurement feedback systems in child and adolescent clinical practice. *Current Opinion in Psychiatry, 22*, 363–368. http://dx.doi.org/10.1097/YCO.0b013e32832c9162

Kim, D. M., Wampold, B. E., & Bolt, D. M. (2006). Therapist effects in psychotherapy: A random-effects modeling of the National Institute of Mental Health Treatment of Depression Collaborative Research Program data. *Psychotherapy Research, 16*, 161–172. http://dx.doi.org/10.1080/10503300500264911

Koss, M. P., & Shiang, J. (1994). Research on brief psychotherapy. In A. E. Bergin & S. L. Garfield (Eds.), *Handbook of psychotherapy and behavior change* (4th ed., pp. 664–700). New York, NY: Wiley.

Lambert, M. J. (2001). Psychotherapy outcome and quality improvement: Introduction to the special section on patient-focused research. *Journal of Consulting and Clinical Psychology, 69*, 147–149. doi:10.1037/0022-006X.69.2.147

Lambert, M. J. (Ed.). (2004). *Bergin and Garfield's handbook of psychotherapy and behavior change* (4th ed.). New York, NY: Wiley.

Lambert, M. J. (2012). Helping clinicians to use and learn from research-based systems: The OQ-analyst. *Psychotherapy, 49*, 109–114. http://dx.doi.org/10.1037/a0027110

Lambert, M. J., Harmon, C., Slade, K., Whipple, J. L., & Hawkins, E. J. (2005). Providing feedback to psychotherapists on their patients' progress: Clinical results and practice suggestions. *Journal of Clinical Psychology, 61*, 165–174. http://dx.doi.org/10.1002/jclp.20113

Miller, S. D., Duncan, B. L., Sorrell, R., & Brown, G. S. (2005). The Partners for Change Outcome Management System. *Journal of Clinical Psychology, 61*, 199–208. http://dx.doi.org/10.1002/jclp.20111

Newnham, E. A., & Page, A. C. (2010). Bridging the gap between best evidence and best practice in mental health. *Clinical Psychology Review, 30*, 127–142. http://dx.doi.org/10.1016/j.cpr.2009.10.004

Pinsof, W. M., Goldsmith, J. Z., & Latta, T. A. (2012). Information technology and feedback research can bridge the scientist-practitioner gap: A couple therapy example. *Couple and Family Psychology: Research and Practice, 1*, 253–273. http://dx.doi.org/10.1037/a0031023

Pinsof, W. M., Zinbarg, R. E., Lebow, J. L., Knobloch-Fedders, L. M., Durbin, E., Chambers, A., . . . Friedman, G. (2009). Laying the foundation for progress research in family, couple, and individual therapy: The development and psychometric features of the initial systemic therapy inventory of change. *Psychotherapy Research, 19*, 143–156. http://dx.doi.org/10.1080/10503300802669973

Reese, R. J., Toland, M. D., Slone, N. C., & Norsworthy, L. A. (2010). Effect of client feedback on couple psychotherapy outcomes. *Psychotherapy, 47*, 616–630. http://dx.doi.org/10.1037/a0021182

Sackett, D. L., Straus, S., Richardson, S., Rosenberg, W., & Haynes, R. B. (2000). *Evidence-based medicine: How to practice and teach EBM* (2nd ed.). London, England: Churchill Livingstone.

Sapyta, J., Riemer, M., & Bickman, L. (2005). Feedback to clinicians: Theory, research, and practice. *Journal of Clinical Psychology, 61*, 145–153. http://dx.doi.org/10.1002/jclp.20107

Sexton, T., & Turner, C. W. (2010). The effectiveness of functional family therapy for youth with behavioral problems in a community practice setting. *Journal of Family Psychology, 24*, 339–348. http://dx.doi.org/10.1037/a0019406

Sexton, T. L. (2007). The therapist as a moderator and mediator in successful therapeutic change. *Journal of Family Therapy, 29,* 104–108. http://dx.doi.org/10.1111/j.1467-6427.2007.00374.x

Sexton, T. L. (2010). *Functional family therapy in clinical practice: An evidence-based treatment model for working with troubled adolescents.* New York, NY: Routledge.

Sexton, T. L., Alexander, J. F., & Mease, A. C. (2003). Levels of evidence for the models and mechanisms of therapeutic change in couple and family therapy. In M. Lambert (Ed.), *Handbook of psychotherapy and behavior change* (pp. 690–743). New York, NY: Wiley.

Sexton, T. L., & Coop Gordon, K. (2009). Science, practice, and evidence-based treatments in the clinical practice of family psychology. In J. H. Bray & M. Stanton (Eds.), *The Wiley-Blackwell handbook of family psychology* (pp. 314–326). Oxford, England: Wiley-Blackwell. http://dx.doi.org/10.1002/9781444310238.ch21

Sexton, T. L., Datchi, C., Evans, L. E., LaFollette, J., & Wright, L. (2013). The effectiveness of couple and family therapy interventions. In M. Lambert (Ed.), *Bergin and Garfield's handbook of psychotherapy and behavior change* (6th ed., pp. 587–639). New York, NY: Wiley.

Sexton, T. L., Patterson, T., & Datchi, C. C. (2012). Technological innovations of systematic measurement and clinical feedback: A virtual leap into the future of couple and family psychology. *Couple and Family Psychology: Research and Practice, 1,* 285–293. http://dx.doi.org/10.1037/cfp0000001

Shapiro, J. P., Friedberg, R. D., & Bardenstein, K. K. (2006). *Child and adolescent therapy: Science and art.* New York, NY: Wiley.

Stricker, G., & Trierweiler, S. J. (1995). The local clinical scientist. A bridge between science and practice. *American Psychologist, 50,* 995–1002. http://dx.doi.org/10.1037/0003-066X.50.12.995

Wampold, B. E., & Brown, G. S. (2005). Estimating variability in outcomes attributable to therapists: A naturalistic study of outcomes in managed care. *Journal of Consulting and Clinical Psychology, 73,* 914–923. http://dx.doi.org/10.1037/0022-006X.73.5.914

Westen, D., Novotny, C. M., & Thompson-Brenner, H. (2004). The empirical status of empirically supported psychotherapies: Assumptions, findings, and reporting in controlled clinical trials. *Psychological Bulletin, 130,* 631–663. http://dx.doi.org/10.1037/0033-2909.130.4.631

10

CLINICAL DECISION MAKING AND RISK MANAGEMENT

STEVEN A. SOBELMAN AND JEFFREY N. YOUNGGREN

Any letter, e-mail, or contact from your licensing board certainly grabs your attention. For most, the contact is generally associated with license renewal. However, receiving notification from your licensing board that a complaint by a current or former patient or client has been filed against you surely gets the heart pumping at near panic rate. Making good clinical decisions and using good judgment, providing good standards of care, and using sound risk management procedures will keep those latter types of letters either to a minimum or nonexistent. Obviously, some patient populations who are seen in a psychotherapy practice—such as those involved with custody issues and evaluations, parent coordination, and forensic evaluations as well as high-risk mental health patients/clients (those with personality disorders)—may involve more contentious interactions. These patient population groups have a higher risk of licensing board complaints than others. However, most psychologists, especially those in private practice, adhere to ethical and professional standards of care and have an understanding of proper risk management. If the standards are followed, the potential of interacting with a licensing board in a negative way becomes greatly reduced.

There are many reasons why we chose to become psychologists. Those of us who have chosen to go into private practice, whether independent or group, have dedicated ourselves to providing high-quality care to those we serve. But there are events (external or internal stressors) that seem to close the door to good judgment and decision making. So, let's jump into the deep end of the pool right at the outset of this chapter with a case study to begin illustrating what we mean by clinical decision making and risk management.

> A well-known and well-liked psychologist (Dr. A.) accepted a new patient into his practice. The 37-year-old woman (Ms. Z.) presented on time for her appointment, was appropriately attired, was pleasant in mood, and seemed comfortable in the office as she engaged in small talk about the amount of rain they were having during the first few moments of the intake session. As the patient and psychologist settled in for the intake session, the psychologist followed his normal procedure of providing written information on the Health Insurance Portability and Accountability Act (HIPAA), his office policies (to include confidentiality, emergencies, and even social networking), and his fees, and then he verbally explained issues related to confidentiality and further explained his "fee for service" policy, which included some narrative on how he does not belong to any insurance panels but would be happy to provide the patient with an invoice or statement of office visits that she could submit for possible reimbursement. Ms. Z. then told him that she would check with her husband's insurance carrier although she didn't believe her insurance carrier provided for "out of network" providers and therefore her sessions with him would not be covered. She indicated that she would pay by check or credit card for each session. When she was asked whether she had any questions, the patient, who worked in a hospital setting, indicated that she was well aware of HIPAA and issues related to confidentiality, billing, and so on and signed an informed consent form.
>
> After the paperwork and business of psychology was put behind him, Dr. A. began the task of developing a therapeutic alliance as he carefully and empathically listened to what brought the patient to his office. At the end of the first session, Dr. A. summarized what he had heard and developed a treatment plan with the patient for future sessions. They both agreed that his understanding of her situation and his approach for working with her seemed appropriate.
>
> Dr. A. and Ms. Z. for all intents and purposes were engaged in an appropriate therapeutic relationship. The good news is that they seemed well suited for each other in that he felt very comfortable dealing with her issues and she was active in responding to new insights and perspective on

her situation. After five sessions, Ms. Z. told Dr. A. that she had always been skeptical of psychotherapy but was seeing the benefits as she now knew that she would gain some control of the distress that had brought her to his office.

At the seventh office visit, Ms. Z. said, "My husband informed me that our insurance has changed and my sessions will now be covered. He said that you would need to fill out a treatment plan." Dr. A. said he was familiar with treatment plans and that he'd be willing to do so since she would now have coverage. She thanked him, and they continued discussing issues related to her psychotherapy.

In the next session, Ms. Z. said the following:

> My husband asked me to ask you two things. Would you be okay if he referred one of his colleagues to you? And, as I mentioned last week, we have new insurance. My husband also wanted to know if there is any way you could help us out with our insurance and your bill. I began seeing you on February 15th and had two sessions in February. Our new insurance started on March 1st. So, would it be possible for you to rebill my new insurance company for the February sessions as though I saw you in March? It would save us a lot of money as they are paying 70% of your fee. Is there any way you could do that? You know, it is weird, but if I had waited just 2 weeks to see you in March, we wouldn't be having this conversation.

Dr. A., who had purchased a practice management software system, did his own billing and record keeping, so it was easy to comply with Ms. Z.'s request. And at the end of the day, he went into his billing system and changed the dates on the February sessions.

Dr. A. and Ms. Z. had a positive next 6 months of psychotherapy as she examined issues related to her self-worth, lack of assertiveness, and being the adult child of an alcoholic; she related that "both my parents were alcoholics, and I had to take care of them from middle school through high school." And Ms. Z.'s husband referred not one patient but two to Dr. A. It appeared that psychotherapy was assisting Ms. Z. in her efforts to feel better about herself, and Dr. A. had a new referral source.

In August, Dr. A. received a frantic phone call from Ms. Z., who was crying. Through her tears she said, "My husband has been having an affair at work for years and now he wants to leave us. He is going to pack his clothes, tell the kids, and just move out. I need to see you today, if possible." Dr. A. made arrangements to see Ms. Z. later in the day and helped calm her down—or at least as reasonably as one could do given the circumstances.

In the next month, Mr. Z. moved out and told Ms. Z. that now that money was tight, he would not be paying for her "frivolous spending," which included her psychotherapy sessions with Dr. A., who he now believed was one of the problems with their marriage. Ms. Z. reported that Mr. Z. said, "All of the crap you're being told by Dr. A. has caused you to be a different person. He has brainwashed you into believing you're somebody you're not." However, Ms. Z. was still on his insurance plan and told him that she would continue to see Dr. A.

In November of that year, Dr. A. received notification from his licensing board that a complaint had been filed against him. The complaint alleged that Dr. A. had (a) "brainwashed Ms. Z.," which was described in a Google search description as Dr. A. causing "alienation of affection," and (b) perpetrated insurance fraud for billing two sessions to an insurance carrier that actually took place during a prior time period. And two cancelled checks were submitted as evidence.

In the end, Dr. A. was sanctioned by his licensing board, not for the allegation of brainwashing Ms. Z. but for insurance fraud. Dr. A. spent a lot of money on attorney fees in addition to having to collect all the information the licensing board required regarding his private psychotherapy practice. Additionally, there is no way of measuring the wear and tear on Dr. A.'s emotional system because he knew he was guilty, knew he was wrong, and yet he could not control the outcome. He only hoped that his livelihood would not be taken from him by the licensing board suspending or revoking his license.

Oops! Now if you were thinking "no good deed goes unpunished," you are not thinking clearly about this situation.

When initially confronted with the option to bill February sessions in March (after all, it was just 14 days difference between having no insurance coverage and having great insurance coverage for the patient), Dr. A. stopped using critical thinking, which led him down the path of making a poor clinical decision. Dr. A.'s emotional decision and possible countertransference created a risky situation that ended poorly for him. So no, this wasn't really about "no good deed goes unpunished" but was instead about poor clinical decisions leading, in this case, to licensing board sanctions.

We hope reading this case study gets your attention and spurs you to read further and that the information we provide in this chapter will make you think about your role as a psychologist. Just having the title by virtue of one's academic studies (classroom and internships) and passing the requirements of a licensing board does not fully ensure that one has the ability to manage the responsibilities of maintaining a high standard of care. Just like most relationships in life, the relationship we have with our profession and those we serve requires a certain level of continued work.

What does "continued work" mean? In the context of this chapter we discuss two areas: (a) the work involved in making good clinical decisions and (b) the work involved in reducing one's risk when working with clients–patients.

CRITICAL THINKING

Although we understand the words *clinical decision making*, we don't always understand what components serve as its foundation or basis. Before delving into a discussion of clinical decision making, it is important to remember that the process for making good clinical decisions rests on our ability to use critical thinking. Critical thinking in society and education is not a new concept. Somewhere in our studies, usually in an Introduction to Psychology course, we learned that Socrates (469–399 BC) taught his students how to analyze their critical thinking processes. Even the word *critical* comes from the Greek word *kritikos*, which means to question or to analyze.

W. G. Sumner (1940) provided the generally accepted foundational definition of critical thinking when he stated that it is "the examination and test of propositions of any kind which are offered for acceptance, in order to find out whether they correspond to reality or not" (p. 632).

Definitions of critical thinking were sharpened to encompass other elements of skills and thought:

> Critical thinking is that mode of thinking—about any subject, content, or problem—in which the thinker improves the quality of his or her thinking by skillfully analyzing, assessing, and reconstructing it. Critical thinking is self-directed, self-disciplined, self-monitored, and self-corrective thinking. It presupposes assent to rigorous standards of excellence and mindful command of their use. It entails effective communication and problem-solving abilities, as well as a commitment to overcome our native egocentrism and sociocentrism. (Scriven & Paul, 2008)

> In layperson's terms, critical thinking consists of seeing both sides of an issue, being open to new evidence that disconfirms your ideas, reasoning dispassionately, demanding that claims be backed by evidence, deducing and inferring conclusions from available facts, solving problems, and so forth. (Willingham, 2007, p. 8)

In short, the purpose of critical thinking is to weed out prejudice and bias to allow well-reasoned views to take root in order to motivate proper action. Many have studied the characteristics of a critical thinker, and these include being a self-directed, active learner (Browne & Keeley, 2011; Duckworth & Seligman, 2005); being open and fair minded about other points of view (Paul & Elder, 2006; Stanovich, 2009); being keenly aware of one's own biases and assumptions (Browne & Keeley, 2011; Paul & Elder, 2006); respecting evidence and reasoning (Nickerson, 1986; Paul & Elder, 2006); and learning to tolerate uncertainty (Nickerson, 1986; Paul & Elder, 2006). The Foundation for Critical Thinking (2014) proposed the following "valuable intellectual traits" associated with critical thinking, and they strongly suggested that all who use critical thinking learn to embrace the following:

- *Intellectual humility*: Having a consciousness of the limits of one's knowledge, including sensitivity to circumstances in which one's native egocentrism is likely to function self-deceptively; to bias and prejudice; and to limitations of one's viewpoint. Intellectual humility depends on recognizing that one should not claim more than one actually knows. Intellectual humility does not imply spinelessness or submissiveness. It implies the lack of intellectual pretentiousness, boastfulness, or conceit, combined with insight into the logical foundations, or lack of such foundations, of one's beliefs.
- *Intellectual courage*: Having a consciousness of the need to face and fairly address ideas, beliefs, or viewpoints toward which one has strong negative emotions and to which one has not given a serious hearing. This courage is connected with the recognition that ideas considered dangerous or absurd are sometimes rationally justified (in whole or in part) and that conclusions and beliefs inculcated in us are sometimes false or misleading. To determine for ourselves which is which, we must not passively and uncritically "accept" what we have "learned." Intellectual courage comes into play here because, inevitably, we will come to see some truth in some ideas considered dangerous and absurd and distortion or falsity in some ideas strongly held in our social group. We need courage to be true to our own thinking in such circumstances. The penalties for nonconformity can be severe.
- *Intellectual empathy*: Having a consciousness of the need to imaginatively put oneself in the place of others in order to genuinely understand them, which requires the consciousness of people's egocentric tendency to identify truth with their immediate perceptions of longstanding thought or belief. This trait correlates with the ability to reconstruct accurately the viewpoints and reasoning of others and to reason from premises, assumptions, and ideas other than our own. This trait also correlates with the willingness to remember occasions when we were wrong in the past despite an intense conviction that we were right and with the ability to imagine our being similarly deceived in a case at hand.
- *Intellectual integrity*: Recognition of the need to be true to one's own thinking, to be consistent in the intellectual standards one applies, to hold oneself to the same rigorous standards of evidence and proof to which one holds one's antagonists, to

practice what one advocates for others, and to honestly admit discrepancies and inconsistencies in one's own thoughts and actions.

- *Intellectual perseverance*: Having a consciousness of the need to use intellectual insights and truths in spite of difficulties, obstacles, and frustrations; firm adherence to rational principles despite the irrational opposition of others; and a sense of the need to struggle with confusion and unsettled questions over an extended period of time to achieve deeper understanding or insight.
- *Faith in reason*: Confidence that in the long run, one's own higher interests and those of humankind at large will be best served by giving the freest play to reason and by encouraging people to come to their own conclusions by developing their own rational faculties. This also means having faith that with proper encouragement and cultivation, people can learn to think for themselves, form rational viewpoints, draw reasonable conclusions, think coherently and logically, persuade each other by reason, and become reasonable persons despite the deep-seated obstacles in the native character of the human mind and in society as we know it.
- *Fair-mindedness*: Having consciousness of the need to treat all viewpoints alike, without reference to one's own feelings or vested interests or the feelings or vested interests of one's friends, community or nation. This implies adherence to intellectual standards without reference to one's own advantage or the advantage of one's group.

Critical thinking, whether one is seeing a patient for individual psychotherapy or evaluating a patient for a learning disability, creates a paradigm for understanding the complexities of patient treatment or rendering an opinion about the patient. Many—it is hoped most—but probably not all, psychologists are taught to use critical thinking while engaging in their academic studies. What was learned in the classroom should be applied to professional world, too.

The following summarizes the steps for critical thinking:

1. Determine the facts of a new situation or subject without prejudice;
2. place these facts and information in a pattern so that you can understand them; and
3. accept or reject the source values and conclusions on the basis of your knowledge, experience, judgment, and beliefs.

Wade and Tavris (2005) expanded on these points when they defined critical thinking as "the ability and willingness to assess claims and make objective judgments on the basis of well-supported reasons and evidence rather than emotion or anecdote" (p. 12). In their analysis, critical thinking has eight premises, as they have clearly detailed (pp. 13–17):

1. *Ask questions; be willing to wonder.* Always be on the lookout for questions that have not been answered in the textbooks, by the experts in the field, or by the media. Asking "What's wrong here?" and/or "Why is this the way it is, and how did it come to be that way?" leads to the identification of problems and challenges.
2. *Define the problem.* An inadequate formulation of a question can produce misleading or incomplete answers. Ask neutral questions that don't presuppose answers. Be very concrete and very absolute in defining terms because vague or poorly defined terms can lead to misinformation, misleading conclusions, and incomplete answers.
3. *Examine the evidence.* Ask yourself, "What evidence supports or refutes this argument and its opposition?" Just because many people believe, including so-called experts, it doesn't make it so. How *reliable* is the evidence? If checking the reliability of the evidence directly is not possible, the person should consider whether it came from a reliable *source*.
4. *Analyze assumptions and biases.* All of us are subject to *biases*, beliefs that prevent us from being impartial. Evaluate the assumptions and biases that lie behind arguments, including your own. Researchers, for example, put their own assumptions to the test by stating a hypothesis in such a way that it can be refuted or disproved by counterevidence.
5. *Avoid emotional reasoning:* "If I feel this way, it must be true." Passionate commitment to a view can motivate a person to think boldly without fear of what others will say, but when "gut feelings" replace clear thinking, the results can be disastrous. Making sound, reasoned decisions and being very emotional when a decision is made are incompatible; you can't be reasonable and completely rational if you're very emotional about something.
6. *Don't oversimplify.* Critical thinkers avoid either–or reasoning because life—and science—is rarely that simple. Look beyond the obvious, resist easy generalizations, and reject either–or thinking. Don't argue by anecdote.

7. *Consider other interpretations.* A crucial aspect of critical thinking is not to limit oneself to only one or two possibilities. Before settling on an explanation of some behavior, however, critical thinkers are careful not to shut out alternative possibilities. They generate as many interpretations of the evidence as they can before choosing the one that is most likely. Formulate hypotheses that offer reasonable explanations of characteristics, behavior, and events.
8. *Tolerate uncertainty.* Sometimes there is little or no evidence available to examine. Sometimes the evidence permits only tentative conclusions. Sometimes the evidence seems strong enough to permit strong conclusions—until, exasperatingly, new evidence throws our beliefs into disarray. Critical thinkers are willing to accept this state of uncertainty. They are not afraid to say "I don't know" or "I'm not sure."

Through our understanding of how to think "critically" we can now embark on a journey of learning to navigate the world of clinical decision making. As such, clinical decision making consists of a core process (what decisions are made about a patient's mental health problems or concerns, the appropriate therapeutic intervention strategy to use, what are the optimal modes of interaction, and what methods of evaluation will I use) that is dependent on attributes of the task such as difficulty, complexity, and uncertainty.

CLINICAL DECISION MAKING

Once critical thinking is learned and understand, as well as accepted, the foundation for clinical decision making begins. Decision-making research in the field of behavioral and mental health has established that attributes of individuals influence decision making, with particular reference to decision-making biases. This is important information because confounding variables interfere with our abilities to make sound decisions. More specifically, our own capabilities, confidence, self-efficacy, emotions, frames of reference, and degree of expertise will influence our decision making. Thus, we, as decision makers, may deviate systematically from normative models of decision making. Such deviations are referred to as *biases* in decision making (Keren & Teigen, 2004). Thus, we, as psychologists, seem to be the problem. Some examples of reasoning biases include misinterpreting findings as confirming a hypothesis when they indicate that an alternate finding should be considered (Elstein & Schwartz 2000); overemphasizing the likelihood of rare conditions (Dowie & Elstein 1988); and making different decisions for individuals than for groups of people, even though they have the same condition (Chapman, 2004).

This becomes problematic because quality decision making is an essential component of good clinical practice. Believing that just understanding the concerns that brought the patient through your office door will open the door for effectively resolving those issues is myopic. Remember Dr. A. in our example? If Dr. A. were truly to understand, critique, and improve his clinical decision making, then it would be imperative for him, in addition to understanding the elements of the immediate clinical problem or concern that Ms. Z. brought to him, to make explicit the contextual factors (his cognitive, metacognitive, emotional, and social capabilities) that should have been taken into account when he made his clinical decision to change the dates of the insurance billing form.

Because contextual factors play such a salient and key role in the clinical decision making process, Smith, Higgs, and Ellis (2008) proposed the following delineation:

1. *Cognitive capabilities.* Capability to (a) identify and collect relevant information (task and contextual) and process these data in order to make decisions in the focal areas of problems, intervention, interaction and evaluation; (b) form relevant mental representations of decision-making situations; (c) predict the consequences of decisions; (d) process and interpret a multitude of decision inputs (task and contextual) to make ethical and justified decisions; (e) make pragmatic decisions in the face of uncertainty and/or under-resourcing; and (f) adapt practice decisions to new and changing circumstances.
2. *Metacognitive/reflexive capabilities.* (a) Awareness of the process of decision making and factors that influence one's decision making; (b) capability to monitor and evaluate decision making throughout the process of making decisions; and (c) capability to self-critique experience of and effectiveness of decision making and use this critique in the development of knowledge structure to inform future decision making.
3. *Emotional capabilities.* (a) Awareness of emotions and when they are having an impact on decision making, particularly awareness of self-efficacy; (b) capability to deal with problematic emotions in order to make difficult decisions required for patient management; (c) motivation to learn and improve quality of decision making in the face of potentially conflicting emotions that impact on decision making; and (d) capability to establish and maintain effective relationships in the workplace, if applicable, with patients, caregivers, and work colleagues by managing the emotions of others.

4. *Social capabilities*. Capability to (a) interact effectively with others in the decision-making context; (b) critically learn from others; (c) manage relationships where differentials in power exist and to achieve effective decision making autonomy; and (d) involve others meaningfully and appropriately in collaborative decision making (including team members and at times patients).

As mentioned previously, the "continued work" of being a psychologist involves a fairly consistent review of all the previously mentioned factors. One way of engaging in the review process is for the psychologist (you) to participate in one (or more) of the suggested following activities: (a) self-reflection; (b) personal psychotherapy; (c) professional supervision; (d) peer consultation; and (e) remaining informed of current research trends in the field through continuing education activities, seminars, additional training, or other forms of staying abreast of research findings. If we're committed to providing a quality service to our patients, then we need to ensure that we are also committed to being a quality service provider.

Dr. A. would have avoided his troubles with the licensing board and everything that went along with that process if he simply had consulted with a peer, quite aside from following a preventive model involved in making a good clinical decision with his patient.

STANDARD OF CARE

Many would advocate that an evidence-based practice is a means for improving the quality of one's clinical practice. Many treatment protocols that adhere to the strict guidelines required for being designated as evidence-based treatment also need to be integrated with many other influences on one's practice. More specifically, and as already mentioned in the previous pages, consideration of critical thinking and social and organizational dimensions of context (contextual factors) associated with critical thinking will determine the quality of clinical decision making. Each psychologist must remain open to understanding and recognizing that the immediate clinical decisions involved in first making a diagnosis and then selecting an intervention strategy come only as a result of managing the multiplicity of factors that influence them, starting with the critical thinking process.

There is no doubt that what puts us, as mental health practitioners, in the best position to make sound clinical decisions is our understanding (and practice) of high-quality standards of care. It is probably sound thinking to accept that the standard of care is one of the most important constructs in mental health and psychotherapy practice. In a very generic sense, the *standard of care* can be defined as the usual and customary professional standard practice in the community. Zur (2010) described standard of care as "the qualities and conditions which prevail, or should prevail, in a particular mental health service, and that a reasonable and prudent practitioner follows." Zur further stated that the standard is based on "community and professional standards" (Caudill, 2004; Doverspike, 1999; Woody, 1998; Zur, 2007). Zur (2010) asserted the following:

> Compliance with the standard of care means that therapists have acted in a prudent and reasonable manner and followed community and professional standards as have others of the same profession or discipline with comparable qualification in similar localities. Demonstrating compliance with the standard of care is done primarily via documentation in the clinical records.

Caudill (2004), Doverspike (1999), Reid (1998), Williams (1997, 2003), Zur (2010), and others have concluded that standard of care measures are derived from the following six elements:

1. *Statutes*: Individual state laws—This is the "what" the law says.
2. *Licensing boards' regulations*: Individual state licensing board regulations that govern the state laws—In other words, this is the "how" the law is imposed.
3. *Case law*: You should see this as an important element of standard of care, to include your knowledge of HIPAA regulations.
4. *Ethical codes of professional associations*: These are guidelines proposed by American Psychological Association (APA) and generally adopted by many states as part of their ethics codes in their regulations.
5. *Consensus of the professionals*: This is established by expert witnesses about the consensus of other professionals practicing in the same discipline and is more oriented toward forensic psychology or within the context of charging documents at the state or federal level.
6. *Consensus in the community*: This standard of care might be different across various contexts such as working with specific religious groups or cultures, practicing in the military environment or Veterans Affairs facilities, and services in a rural area.

As was just mentioned, the standard of care is the usual and customary standard of practice in the community for the same profession or discipline (Caudill, 2004; Doverspike, 1999; Williams, 2003). Many psychologists don't understand the concept even though it is important when dealing with liability claims and issues as well as concepts that should be used to guide one's psychotherapy practice. This is further discussed when risk management issues are addressed later in this chapter.

In the end, however, the standard of care is a legal concept that is used to evaluate whether a professional's activities meet the "standard." More specifically, this is also what licensing boards address when a complaint is made against a psychologist. All professions have standards, and if you meet the standards of care, there is a low likelihood that you'll hear from a licensing board. Thus, the standard of care is what most reasonable psychologists under similar circumstances do. To put it another way, if you do what most of your colleagues do, you are meeting the standard of care. It is important to note that this isn't what most of your colleagues think they should do or what an expert has identified as a "best practice," and some would not see that as an aspirational standard. For example, if all psychologists invited their patients to lunch in order to assess their social skills, then that would be considered a "standard of care," but it wouldn't be considered a "best practice." In other words, there are probably many other ways of assessing a patient's social skills rather than having lunch with a patient. Thus, the standard of care is what most of your colleagues are actually doing.

When thinking about a definition of standard of care, there isn't one particular set of specifics one should follow as much as trying to determine what ingredients make up the standard of care recipe. Reid (1998) suggested that much like the way in which words that were obsolete 50 years ago are now accepted and in the dictionary, standard of care "is usually correlated with professionally accepted clinical texts, clinical journal articles, clinical training programs, and what real doctors do across the country" (p. 1). Thus, it appears that we are responsible for recognizing and knowing the current laws (and trends) within our own profession. As we've learned throughout our training and throughout lessons learned in life, *ignorantia legis neminem excusat*, or ignorance of the law excuses no one.

In further understanding the issues related to standard of care, it is best to have the mind-set that a standard of care is a minimum (and sometimes aspirational) standard as opposed to something concrete, specific, and perfect. Mental health practitioners are not expected to be perfect, nor are patients–clients guaranteed positive or desired results (Caudill, 2004). It is important to note that licensing boards more traditionally may sanction a psychologist if the board finds that the psychologist worked below the standard of care, which again is defined as a minimal standard.

CLINICAL JUDGMENT

Understanding what is being written in this chapter—that is, the issues related to critical thinking, standards of care, and clinical decision making, all important keys to providing quality services to our patients—is well and good as long as it is followed in one's practice. But there are times when understanding evidence-based practice, for example, doesn't guarantee that a psychologist will follow the tenets of the data in her or his practice of psychology. Why would a psychologist who is bright, well versed in the research of a particular psychological intervention strategy, and well respected in the community, "choose" (consciously or unconsciously) to violate professional and ethical standards?

What we do know is that there is a power differential between the therapist and patient–client. Lammers, Stapel, and Galinsky's (2010) research revealed that power and influence can cause a severe disconnect between public judgment and private behavior, and as a result, the powerful are stricter in their judgment of others while being more lenient toward their own actions, whereas the powerless collaborate in reproducing social inequality because they don't feel the same entitlement. "Ultimately, patterns of hypocrisy perpetuate social inequality" (p. 737).

Licensing boards continue to receive complaints regarding boundary and ethical violations that reveal the power differential between the seemingly powerful and the vulnerable. Examples include "My psychologist asked me to walk her dog"; "My psychologist hired me as her secretary to help me build my self-confidence while continuing my on-going psychotherapy sessions with her"; "I was sent letters and cards, we prayed together, and eventually we engaged in sexual relations"; and "The psychologist invited several patients to her apartment, which included consumption of alcohol and sexual activities." (These excerpts were taken from public orders.)

Using critical thinking as a core base on which to build clinical decision making is a first step in providing quality treatment to your psychotherapy patients. Your understanding and adherence to the elements of high standards of care further ensures that your patients will be safe and secure. The APA (2010) *Ethical Principles of Psychologists and Code of Conduct* provides five general principles to guide and inspire psychologists toward the very highest ethical ideals of the profession. Principle A, Beneficence and Nonmaleficence, is most pertinent to this chapter because *nonmaleficence* is related to *primum non nocere*, commonly translated as "first, do no harm."

Good risk management and good clinical decision-making thinking would remind us to be mindful to "first, do no harm" by using evidence-based or empirically based practices to ensure that standards of care are kept within minimally accepted standards. However, the issue of evidence-based or empirically based practice has recently received a great deal of attention in the mental health literature, and policy statements from a variety of professional and governmental organizations have been formulated on this subject. This issue has stimulated discussion and debate about how to define "best treatment practices" within the health and mental health professions. In the end, there is no universal consensus on what constitutes "evidence" in evidence-based practice (e.g., case-based vs. experimental studies; evidence from efficacy trials vs. clinical experience and expertise; process therapies that emphasize practitioner competency–skills–qualities; therapeutic alliance vs. specific techniques). All types of evidence may be important in making professional decisions.

RISK MANAGEMENT

The Trust, a major malpractice carrier for psychologists, has defined *risk management* as "prospective assessment of retrospective evaluation" (Knapp, Younggren, VandeCreek, Harris, & Martin, 2013, p. 34). Although to some this might be seen as just another cliché, the guidance it gives is actually the essence of good risk management. Effective risk management requires practicing psychologists to be aware of how their conduct today might be evaluated at a later date by another person or entity, like a licensing board, that has full knowledge of the outcome of that past conduct. What is key here is that when the decision was made by the psychologist to do what he or she did, that psychologist did not know what the outcome of that service was going to be. Yet, when the appropriateness of that professional service or conduct is later evaluated retrospectively, the outcome will be a part of the evaluative process. Consequently, it is very easy for the evaluator to engage in hindsight bias when determining not only what could have been done to avoid the outcome in question but, and more dangerously so, to determine what should have been done. This retrospective analysis, often a key component of licensing investigations and civil actions against psychologists, clearly runs risk of falling prey to this hindsight bias, making the whole process potentially unfair.

Because of their fears about being sued or having a licensing board complaint filed against them, practicing psychologists have dealt with the realities of professional risk in both maladaptive and adaptive ways. Maladaptive solutions to reduce risk can be found among those who simply refuse to treat populations of people who present a risk to them. Psychologists who do this can frequently be heard saying, "I just don't treat people who . . ." Other maladaptive solutions include those who have adopted a series of "rules" that they believe will protect them and, consequently, reduce their risk. Psychologists who do this can frequently be heard saying, "You never . . . with a patient." Both of these risk management styles are, in reality, bad and reflect a black-and-white approach to a world that is filled with gray. In addition, each of these is a least-common-denominator solution to risk management that is designed only to protect the professional, with little focus on patients and their needs. Psychologists who utilize either of these approaches can be termed *risk-averse psychologists* and differentiated from what we call *risk-managed psychologists*.

THE RISK-AVERSE PSYCHOLOGIST

As previously stated, the risk-averse psychologist will frequently operate in a world of absolutes and find safety in doing so. For example, they say that they do not see patients who have certain disorders or who present with certain kinds of problems simply because of the risk. Although they might be more than capable of assisting these people, they avoid doing so because they see potential danger ahead for them professionally if they do. As a result, they deny the patients the care that they need and fail to provide care that they are qualified to do. Examples of this style of risk management abound. Many capable psychologists avoid treating children whose parents are involved in a divorce because of the risk that they might become involved in litigation related to the child or become involved in the parents' dispute in some way. Other capable psychologists refuse to see depressed patients who have a history of suicidal risk because of the fear that the patient might be successful in committing suicide and that this could later involve the psychologist in a legal action alleging that the psychologist had a role in causing the suicide and seeking damages for this. Finally, some psychologists avoid treating patients who are concurrently involved in a legal action that involves the condition for which the patient is seeking care. Although not a single one of these decisions may be in the best interests of the consumer in need, the goal of professional protection is all that is important in this approach to risk management.

The risk-averse psychologist is also rule bound. He or she avoids engaging in boundary crossings because of the fear that others might allege that this conduct was a violation of some standard of practice, even though they know that these boundary crossings, in and of themselves, might be appropriate and even therapeutic. Examples of this type of conduct include taking gifts, hugging, touching, engaging in out-of-office services, and self-disclosure (Zur, 2007). They fail to demonstrate insight into the reality that although a boundary crossing on the part of the psychologist could be problematic, it is not the act itself that makes the boundary crossing a problem, it is the purpose of the crossing that creates the risk. The risk-averse psychologist, however, does not approach the problem in this way. This psychologist finds comfort and safety in the rule and lacks understanding of the fundamental principles that create the rule. For example, it is not the hugging of a patient that is, in and of itself, a violation of professional conduct, it is why a psychologist would hug a patient and whom they hug. Whereas hugging a patient who has suffered a serious loss, like the death of a child, and with whom the psychologist has had a good alliance might be seen as an appropriate act of empathy, it would not be appropriate to hug a patient who had been the victim of sexual assault. The difference is key. Because of his or her lack of understanding regarding the fundamental differences between these two examples, the risk-averse psychologist simply does not hug. Consequently, he or she is willing to sacrifice the benefits of honest empathy in order to avoid any allegation, no matter how remote, of inappropriate conduct on his or her part.

THE RISK-MANAGED PSYCHOLOGIST

The risk-managed psychologist approaches professional decisions differently than does the risk-averse psychologist. This psychologist has an understanding of the fundamentals of professional ethics and conduct (APA, 2010) and knows how to apply this knowledge to a specific question being asked or a problem being faced. There are few absolutes for this professional, who manages risk by evaluating ethical dilemmas in a thoughtful, conceptual, and thorough way. This psychologist makes decisions on the basis of the needs of both the professional and the consumer. To this professional, risk management is a part of good therapy, an approach that is much more effective than the rule-based approach used by his or her risk-averse colleague. Finally, this professional not only makes use of the many rational models of risk management that are available (Cottone, 2012) but also is in touch with the feeling component of good and ethical decision making (Rogerson, Gottlieb, Handelsman, Knapp, & Younggren, 2011).

In 1956, psychologist and educator Benjamin Bloom developed a tiered taxonomy that reflects a classification of thinking according to six cognitive levels of complexity. The goal of this conceptual model was to lead people away from simple thinking and problem solving into more complex styles of thinking that reflect creativity and thoughtfulness and not just a rote understanding of information. According to Bloom and his colleagues, the lowest three levels of thinking are knowledge, comprehension, and application. Simply put, if you know something, understand it, and apply it, you have accomplished the lowest level of thinking. Creative thinkers, however, make use of higher levels of thinking, which include analysis, synthesis, and evaluation. These thinkers analyze and integrate information into new concepts and evaluate the outcome of that process (Bloom & Krathwohl, 1956).

This taxonomy was later modified and updated in order to make it more useful (Anderson & Krathwohl, 2001). The revised taxonomy, still tiered in six conceptual levels, is composed of remembering, understanding, applying, analyzing, evaluating, and creating. The lowest levels of thinking are found in remembering, understanding, and applying. That is, if a person remembers something, understands it, and applies it, they have accomplished the lowest level of thinking. This process does reflect learning and understanding, but key here is that it is not creative; it is not higher order thinking. To be creative, the learner must learn to engage in analyzing what has been learned, evaluating the results of that process and creating something new from that synthesis. According to the models proposed by Bloom and his colleagues, higher order thinking requires this integration of information in order to arrive at the right decision—the decision that is unique to all of the information involved in the process. This is exactly what the risk-managed psychologist does.

For the risk-managed psychologist, a decision about what to do is not simply based on the avoidance of risk or knowledge about a rule but also on an understanding of that risk and how it applies to a specific and unique circumstance. The risk-managed psychologist knows how to make unique decisions based on these unique circumstances. Good risk management is not simply professionally protective conduct but is done in the best interests of both the psychologist and the patient. It is based on the specifics of the circumstance, an understanding of the principles that are the foundation of the rules of professional conduct, and knowledge about how to integrate this understanding into a decision about what to do. It is not reflexive nor is it rote. It is good thinking. However, it is not easy thinking; it takes time and an understanding of the ethics of professional conduct and the law.

As pointed out already, good risk management makes use of the unique nature of the circumstance within which the psychologist finds him- or herself. It does not focus just on the conduct of the professional but requires an understanding of patient characteristics, the psychologist's skills, the setting within which the psychologist finds him- or herself, and the potential disciplinary consequences of the conduct in question (Knapp et al., 2013). An understanding of patient characteristics reflects respect for the unique nature of those we treat, including their individual and social realities. Risk is a variable that changes with each one of these variables. For example, if a patient is a self-pay, choices regarding interventions to be used and goals that can be achieved are different than are those for patients who have a managed care insurance benefit, the latter requiring decisions made with an understanding of how the insurance company's oversight might affect the provider's professional choices. The patient's psychological condition also drives the direction of risk management choices. If the patient is highly disturbed with a history of erratic and unpredictable emotion and behavior, the therapist's choices would be vastly different than those made for a patient with a more stable and predictable emotional style.

The skills of the therapist are another factor driving risk management decisions. Psychologists providing services to individuals must always be able to answer the following questions: "Am I qualified to do this by my education, training and/or experience?" and "Could I defend my qualifications to do this if I were asked to do so on a witness stand?" If the answer to these questions is either "no" or "maybe," then the psychologist should reconsider what he or she is doing. Only under emergent or unusual circumstances can a psychologist provide services they are only questionably qualified to provide through education, training, and/or experience (APA, 2010).

Risk changes with both setting and circumstance, so the setting in which the service is being provided also warrants careful evaluation when making a risk management decision. For example, a psychologist providing recommendations to parents regarding custody of children in a forensic matter runs substantially more risk of an allegation of unprofessional conduct than does one who is involved in helping those same parents learn how to manage a the same child within a stable parental family system. The former forensic matter obviously requires significantly higher levels of structure and consistency than does the latter, where all parties are likely to be cooperating and sharing a common therapeutic goal.

The potential for disciplinary action being taken against the psychologist is the final factor that must be weighed when making a risk management decision. This requires that a psychologist know ethics, the law, and the nature of the licensing board that regulates their professional conduct. In addition, it requires a respect for the conduct of entities that might also be involved. For example, seeing a patient who pays out of pocket for sessions removes the oversight of a third-party payer regarding the appropriateness of conduct of the psychologist. Those who treat patients covered by insurance companies always run the risk of having to deal with audits and recoupment of fees if the company disagrees with the service provided in some way. Conversely, the psychologist who only sees self-pay cases does not have to be concerned about any of this. Finally, a lack of understanding of the law and specifically issues regarding consent, confidentiality, and privilege, to name only a few, can drive risk through the ceiling.

The risk-managed psychologist also intuitively makes use of what have been termed the "three keys to effective risk management" (Knapp et al., 2013). She or he engages in a formal informed consent process at the outset of any professional relationship. This informed consent process informs the patient about not only the state and federal laws that affect the profession of psychology and the professional relationship being established but also the specific policies by which the psychologist operates. It outlines payment responsibilities and requirements, the psychologist's relationship with any insurance company, consent issues, and confidentiality policies. For example, this policy might include the statement that the psychologist reserves the right to contact others, to include family members, if the patient becomes suicidal or dangerous. It also might outline the need to keep some things confidential when treating a minor and solicits the agreement of the parents to do so. If the patient agrees to these conditions, the psychologist has the freedom to enforce them without worries about exceptions to law that might allow this. He or she has an agreement with the patient that this is exactly what will happen.

The risk-managed psychologist also makes use of informed consent throughout the treatment process (Pope & Vasquez, 2007). Given that therapy is an ever-changing dynamic, informed consent must change as therapy changes. These changes and agreements are reflected in the patient's chart, and significant changes in original agreements need to be formally executed.

Record keeping is key to the risk-managed practice, and poor record keeping is directly related to an increase in professional liability claims (Gallegos, 2013). The risk-managed psychologist understands the federal and state laws that impact record keeping and incorporates these requirements into his or her professional record keeping style. This psychologist understands that record keeping is a dynamic that changes with treatment, such that some sessions require detailed record keeping whereas others require much less, all the time bearing in mind that incomplete records are the most common error made by health care professionals (Gallegos, 2013). This professional also knows what should be written down in a chart and what should not. Because confidentiality is always a risk, this professional knows that excessive detail in a chart is as risky as inadequate detail and is comfortable operating in the midst of this. Finally, this professional knows that because the information in the record almost always belongs to the patient and there is always the likelihood that the patient will see the record, nothing should be written in a chart that should not be read by the patient.

The risk-managed psychologist also makes effective use of consultation as a tool to reduce risk. He or she consults with others whenever necessary and sees consultation as key to the treatment process. Not only does this increase the likelihood that the psychologist will glean new ideas on how to deal with an issue, but consultation assists with meeting the judicial standard of conduct, that being what other practitioners would do under similar circumstances. Finally, the risk-managed psychologist uses the law of parsimony when doing consultations because these are likely not privileged, and information related to a specific consultation on a patient could be discovered if identities were revealed as a part of this process. The risk-managed psychologist welcomes input from other psychologists in assisting him or her in treatment.

RISK MANAGEMENT IN ACTION

No specific area of professional conduct is more professionally risky than that which brings the psychologist into the forensic setting. Whether the psychologist is providing clinical services within that setting or is operating as an expert providing guidance to the court, the psychologist's risk exponentially rises with increased forensic involvement. As is clear from the thesis of this chapter, this increase in risk does not mean that psychologists should avoid providing these services but that they should do so and, in the process, make use of a risk management strategy that is protective of their conduct.

Perhaps good risk management is best taught through real examples of bad risk management. The following are three examples of patients who are seen in a psychologist's practice.

The Divorcing Family

Psychologists must be very careful when treating children whose parents are divorcing. Not only is this almost always something that is quite painful to the minor being treated, but the parents, with the best of intentions, frequently become lost in disputes that revolve around their children. Consequently, the risk-managed psychologist establishes the rules for involvement in legal proceedings at the outset of treatment. The treatment plan clearly states what the psychologist will and will not do, and the psychologist seeks legally binding stipulated agreements with the parents regarding that plan. Frequently, psychologists can even obtain stipulations that prevent either parent from pulling them into their disputes. Although their involvement in the treatment of a minor whose parents are divorcing is positive for the child, their involvement in the legal proceeding may not be and is, at a minimum, fraught with professional risk. Under these circumstances it is vital for the psychologist to establish the rules at the outset of therapy and then to act to enforce them throughout the process. This also requires cautious conduct on the part of the professional to avoid anything that might appear to be "choosing sides" in the case. This includes notifying parties when requests are made for the records and to respect the roles that others, such as a guardian ad litem, play in the case.

Too often psychologists involved in the treatment of minors whose parents are divorcing choose to become advocates for the children at the expense of themselves. This also is bad risk management because this can only result in a decrease of therapeutic effectiveness on the part of therapist and an increase in the risk of a legal action taken against the therapist.

The Toxic Therapeutic Relationship

Few areas of professional conduct are more confusing to psychologists than the areas of termination and abandonment. In spite of the clear evidence that clinicians have rights to stop seeing any patient (Younggren, Fisher, Foote, & Hjelt, 2011), many therapists maintain nonproductive alliances with patients out of a fear that if they stop seeing them, they will have to deal with charges of abandonment or wrongful termination. They do this out of a fear that if they terminate the patient against their wishes, they will be charged with abandonment. This view is simply wrong and is reflective of terrible risk management.

Heather Ensworth was a California psychologist, and Cynthia Mullvain was her patient from November 1982 until September 1984 (*Ensworth v. Mullvain*, 1990), when Ensworth terminated the treatment. The record indicates that Mullvain did not accept the termination very well, and Ensworth decided to see her again for a period of time to "resolve the termination issues to help her disengage from Ensworth." Subsequently, a series of harassing incidents occurred, including Mullvain following Ensworth's car, trying to stop her car in the middle of the street, circling around her office building, keeping her house under surveillance, driving repeatedly around her house, making numerous phone calls, sending threatening letters to Ensworth, and making phone calls to other professionals in the community in an effort to harm Ensworth's reputation. She also wrote a letter to Ensworth alluding to committing suicide in her presence. Consequently, Ensworth was forced to terminate contact with Mullvain again, and this time she stuck to it.

In May 1987, after the second termination, Ensworth sought a restraining order against Mullvain. The restraining order was granted from May 29, 1987, until November 29, 1988. Mullvain objected to the restraining order and testified to the court that she had business contacts at a local library, which is located approximately 150 feet from Ensworth's home. Those "contacts" included doing research at the library for movie productions and teaching calligraphy classes, not as a library employee but on a community service basis. She also used the library "for time in between seeing clients to do some research or do studying or write papers or to use the bathroom facilities and computer there." She also mentioned three different door-to-door sales jobs she had in the area. Mullvain testified that as a result of the restraining order sought by Ensworth, she had not gone to the Altadena Library, not contacted her photography clients, and not conducted research for her film projects. As a result, she lost money and referrals. Although her arguments were strong and direct, they failed to convince the court that they had merit in light of the evidence about Mullvain's behavior and Ensworth's testimony, which Mullvain did not refute.

In *Ensworth v. Mullvain*, it is clear how serious a toxic treatment relationship can become. The records of this case demonstrate clearly that Mullvain was willing to do whatever she could do to stay in contact with Ensworth. This included not only the lengthy list of inappropriate conduct on her part but also incurring substantial legal expenses to overcome her therapist's wishes to be left alone. Although no risk management strategy can guarantee this would never occur, it is best for the therapist who decides on an adversarial termination to maintain that decision and discontinue any interactions with the client. To do otherwise can only further confuse the client and drive emotional levels higher. In addition, it is important to bear in mind that when patients behave in ways that are inconsistent with any claim of confidentiality, psychologists can take action, to include legal actions, to protect their rights.

The Unnecessary Multiple Relationship

Multiple relationship violations are a much written about subject area in psychological ethics. Views on what constitutes a multiple relationship violation extend from those that are very liberal (Zur, 2007) to those that are quite conservative. Theoretical debate aside, what the risk-managed psychologist knows is that it is not the existence of the multiple relationship on its own that is problematic, it is the "why" of the relationship and what impact it has on treatment and the patient. Although not all multiple relationships can be avoided, because they occur naturally, unnecessary ones can and should be avoided (Gottlieb, 1993; Younggren & Gottlieb, 2004). The multiple relationships that cannot be avoided need to be addressed and solved in an ethically responsible way. If they cannot be resolved in this fashion, and if they interfere with treatment, solutions like termination and transfer need to be considered.

In 1999, psychologist Tom Spencer Allison was found in an administrative law hearing to have been grossly negligent in his practice and treatment of two patients with whom he formed multiple relationships (*Board of Psychology v. Tom Spencer Allison*, 1999). Among other allegations, it was proven at the hearing that Allison involved a husband and wife couple, as patients, in his Amway multilevel marketing business and also became personally involved with them, paying for personal travel and other activities deemed patient boundary violations. His defense was that these activities were therapeutic. The administrative law judge and the California Board of Psychology rejected this argument. Allison's license was revoked, the revocation stayed, and a term of probation imposed.

With respect to Allison's case, one might ask, "Why was it necessary to involve patients in an Amway business as part of their treatment?" Clearly, the logic that this was part of effective therapy was not compelling to the administrative law judge who heard the case. What is clear from the ruling is that the judge felt that the secondary relationship was unprofessional, unnecessary, and exploited the therapeutic alliance the psychologist had with his patients.

SUMMARY

It should be apparent that the business of psychology is not easy, and it seems to become more complex with each passing year. Even so, the risk of some type of adverse action happening to a psychologist because of his or her professional conduct is actually rather low. For example, recent research shows that even among the high-risk population of child custody evaluators, out of complaints filed the actual likelihood that a board would sanction a psychologist is less than 2% (Bow, Gottlieb, Siegel, & Noble, 2010), which is consistent with other research done in this area (Van Horne, 2004). Coupled with the reality that civil actions are a far less likely occurrence (Knapp et al., 2013), this makes psychology a relatively safe, if not perfectly safe, profession to be a part of from a legal perspective.

Psychologists must remain in touch with their competence and make sure they have a thorough understanding of both the law and the standards of professional practice. This is probably best done by being a part of the profession in some way or making the review of "what is happening in psychology" a regular activity. One important risk management skill that psychologists need to develop is conceptual decision making in which theoretical concepts are tied to specific legal and risk management questions. Finally, psychologists should avoid finding safety in concrete rules because it is the reality of professional life that any rule will have an exception.

Further, we make the following suggestions to the reader:

- Remember, it is not the existence of a legal action that is professionally dangerous; it is losing a legal action that is professionally dangerous. People always have the right to question.
- At some time in your career, someone will complain about you. That is to be expected considering the populations with which we work. That complaint, however, does not mean you did anything wrong.
- If you do not know what to do when a dilemma surfaces, do not do anything. Guidance will surface or be found.
- Make sure that your records are complete and are an accurate reflection of what you did and what happened.

- Consult frequently with colleagues, and make regular consultation a part of your standard practice.
- Make sure that your informed consent forms reflect what you do, are consistent with the law, and clearly state your policy.
- If you are not a lawyer, do not practice law.

REFERENCES

American Psychological Association. (2010). *Ethical principles of psychologists and code of conduct (2002, Amended June 1, 2010)*. Retrieved from http://www.apa.org/ethics/code/index.aspx

Anderson, L. W., & Krathwohl, D. R. (Eds.). (2001). *A taxonomy for learning, teaching and assessing: A revision of Bloom's taxonomy of educational objectives: Complete edition*. New York, NY: Longman.

Bloom, B. S., & Krathwohl, D. R. (1956). *Taxonomy of educational objectives: The classification of educational goals, by a committee of college and university examiners. Handbook 1: Cognitive domain*. New York, NY: Longman.

Board of Psychology v. Tom Spencer Allison, Ph.D., CA Board of Psychology Case No. 1F1995053156, eff. Oct. 21, 1999.

Bow, J. N., Gottlieb, M. C., Siegel, J. C., & Noble, G. S. (2010). Licensing board complaints. *Journal of Forensic Psychology Practice, 10*, 403–418. http://dx.doi.org/10.1080/15228932.2010.489851

Browne, N., & Keeley, S. (2011). *Asking the right questions: A guide to critical thinking*. Saddle River, NJ: Pearson.

Caudill, C. O. (2004). *Therapists under fire*. Retrieved from http://www.cphins.com/Default.aspx?tabid=75

Chapman, G. B. (2004). The psychology of medical decision making. In D. J. Koehler & N. Harvey (Eds.), *Blackwell handbook of judgment and decision making* (pp. 585–604). Malden, MA: Blackwell. http://dx.doi.org/10.1002/9780470752937.ch29

Cottone, R. R. (2012). Ethical decision making in mental health contexts: Representative models and an organizational framework. In S. J. Knapp, M. C. Gottlieb, M. M. Handelsman, & L. D. VandeCreek, *APA handbook of ethics in psychology: Vol.1. Moral foundations and common themes* (pp. 99–121). Washington, DC: American Psychological Association.

Doverspike, W. (1999). *Ethical risk management: Guidelines for practice: A practical ethics handbook*. Sarasota, FL: Professional Resource Press.

Dowie, J., & Elstein, A. (Eds.). (1988). *Professional judgment: A reader in clinical decision making*. New York, NY: Cambridge University Press.

Duckworth, A. L., & Seligman, M. E. P. (2005). Self-discipline outdoes IQ in predicting academic performance of adolescents. *Psychological Science, 16*, 939–944. http://dx.doi.org/10.1111/j.1467-9280.2005.01641.x

Elstein, A. S., & Schwartz, A. (2000). Clinical reasoning in medicine. In J. Higgs & M. Jones (Eds.), *Clinical reasoning in the health professions* (2nd ed., pp. 95–106). Oxford, England: Butterworth-Heinemann.

Ensworth v. Mullvain (1990). 224 Cal. App. 3d 1105 [274 Cal. Rptr. 447].

Foundation for Critical Thinking. (2014, September). *Valuable intellectual virtues*. Retrieved from http://www.criticalthinking.org/pages/valuable-intellectual-traits/528

Gallegos, A. (2013, March 25). *Medical charting errors can drive up liability suits*. Retrieved from http://www.amednews.com/article/20130325/profession/130329979/5/

Gottlieb, M. C. (1993). Avoiding exploitative dual relationships: A decision making model. *Psychotherapy, 30*, 41–48.

Keren, G., & Teigen, K. H. (2004). Yet another look at the heuristics and biases approach. In D. J. Koehler & N. Harvey (Eds.), *Blackwell handbook of judgment and decision making* (pp. 89–109). Malden, MA: Blackwell. http://dx.doi.org/10.1002/9780470752937.ch5

Knapp, S., Younggren, J. N., VandeCreek, L., Harris, E., & Martin, J. (2013). *Assessing and managing risk in psychological practice: An individualized approach* (2nd ed.). Washington, DC: APAIT.

Lammers, J., Stapel, D. A., & Galinsky, A. D. (2010). Power increases hypocrisy: Moralizing in reasoning, immorality in behavior. *Psychological Science, 21*, 737–744.

Nickerson, R. S. (1986). *Reflections on reasoning*. Hillsdale, NJ: Erlbaum.

Paul, R., & Elder, L. (2006). *The art of Socratic questioning*. Dillon Beach, CA: Foundation for Critical Thinking.

Pope, K., & Vasquez, M. (2007). *Ethics in psychotherapy and counseling: A practical guide* (3rd ed.). San Francisco, CA: Jossey-Bass.

Reid, W. H. (1998). Standard of care and patient need. *The Journal of Psychiatric Practice*. Retrieved from http://www.reidpsychiatry.com/columns/Reid05-98.pdf

Rogerson, M. D., Gottlieb, M. C., Handelsman, M. M., Knapp, S., & Younggren, J. (2011). Nonrational processes in ethical decision making. *American Psychologist, 66*, 614–623. http://dx.doi.org/10.1037/a0025215

Scriven, M. & Paul, R. (2008) *Our concept of critical thinking*. Available at http://www.criticalthinking.org/aboutCT/ourConceptCT.cfm

Smith, M., Higgs, J., & Ellis, E. (2008). *Clinical reasoning in the health professions*. New York, NY: Elsevier, Churchill Livingstone.

Stanovich, K. E. (2009, November/December). The thinking that IQ tests miss. *Scientific American Mind, 20*(6), 34–39. http://dx.doi.org/10.1038/scientificamericanmind1109-34

Sumner, W. G. (1940). *Folkways: A study of the sociological importance of usages, manners, customs, mores, and morals*. New York, NY: Ginn.

Van Horne, B. A. (2004). Psychology licensing board disciplinary actions: The realities. *Professional Psychology: Research and Practice, 35*, 170–178. http://dx.doi.org/10.1037/0735-7028.35.2.170

Wade, C., & Tavris, C. (2005). *Invitation to psychology* (3rd ed., pp. 12–17). Upper Saddle River, NJ: Pearson Education.

Williams, M. H. (1997). Boundary violations: Do some contended standards of care fail to encompass commonplace procedures of humanistic, behavioral, and eclectic psychotherapies? *Psychotherapy, 34,* 238–249.

Williams, M. H., (2003). The curse of risk management. *The Independent Practitioner, 23,* 202–205.

Willingham, D. T. (2007, Summer). Can critical thinking be taught? *American Educator,* pp. 8–19.

Woody, R. H. (1998). *Fifty ways to avoid malpractice.* Sarasota, FL: Professional Resource Exchange.

Younggren, J. N., Fisher, M. A., Foote, W. E., & Hjelt, S. E. (2011). A legal and ethical review of patient responsibilities and psychotherapist duties. *Professional Psychology: Research and Practice, 42,* 160–168. http://dx.doi.org/10.1037/a0023142

Younggren, J. N., & Gottlieb, M. C. (2004). Managing risk when contemplating multiple relationships. *Professional Psychology: Research and Practice, 35,* 255–260. http://dx.doi.org/10.1037/0735-7028.35.3.255

Zur, O. (2007). *Boundaries in psychotherapy: Ethical and clinical explorations.* Washington, DC: American Psychological Association. http://dx.doi.org/10.1037/11563-000

Zur, O. (2010). *The standard of care in psychotherapy and counseling: Bringing clarity to an illusive standard.* Retrieved from http://www.zurinstitute.com/standardofcaretherapy.html

11

TEACHING CLINICAL DECISION MAKING

GREGG HENRIQUES

When you look for it, it is everywhere—it permeates almost every aspect of professional practice. Whether one is setting up one's office, consulting on a referral, deciding what assessment instrument to use, meeting a client for the first time, reviewing and assessing the literature, or advocating for a particular treatment approach for a particular case, one is engaged in a form of it. The "it" can be termed *clinical decision making*, and it's not too much of a stretch to say that the fundamental goal of doctoral training in professional psychology or training in any advanced mental health discipline is to produce budding clinicians who have the knowledge, skills, and attitudes that enable them to make and carry out good clinical decisions.

Despite the centrality of this concept, professional psychologists are generally less likely than some other health professionals, such as nurses and physicians, to deliberately frame their work and teach their craft in terms of clinical decision making, although there are exceptions (e.g., O'Donohue &

Henderson, 1999). The failure to explicitly frame our training in this manner may be a function of the old debate about clinical versus empirical judgment or the fact that "clinical" is still used to denote one of the three broad practice areas (with "counseling" and "school" being the other two) or the fact that conflict remains between the romantic and empirical visions of professional psychology. Whatever the reasons, it is my hope that this volume will change the current state of affairs. Emphasizing clinical decision making is apt because it encourages a deliberate, reflective, and intentional stance with regard to how to go about one's work as a professional psychologist.

Because *clinical decision making* is such a broad term, it has, not surprisingly, many facets and can be approached from many different angles. For example, Magnavita and Lilienfield (Chapter 2, this volume) offer a powerful analysis that deconstructs the key elements of the clinical decision-making process from the vantage point of cognitive psychology (Kahneman, 2011). Part of that analysis includes a review of how people make decisions in general. Perhaps most central to understanding general decision making is that human's process information via two related but separable streams of mentation. The first stream is a fast, relatively automatic, perceptual, holistic, affective system of processing that sizes up a situation via "thin slicing" (Gladwell, 2005) and forms quick, intuitive judgments. The second system is a slower, more explicitly self-conscious and deliberate form of thought, mediated largely by processes of verbal justification. From an educator's perspective, this is a basic and central feature of the human mind of which students of professional psychology should be very aware. For example, a training exercise that I find useful when the class is viewing video is to stop the tape as soon as the patient (or client) appears on the screen and ask students for their report of their immediate perceptions, feelings, and intuitions about the client. Often trainees are initially reticent to say anything, generally because they don't want to appear as though they "judge a book by its cover." But once they are given permission, the associations flow, and we see that many impressions are formed almost instantaneously. They first notice the obvious demographics of the patient. Then they will notice how attractive they perceive the client to be and the manner of dress, hygiene, and body position, all which serve as indicators of socioeconomic status. Following that, a host of more imaginative wonderings will begin. These impressions are examples of thin slicing, an inevitable aspect of being human, and students need to be aware that they will then begin to form narratives and expectations on the basis of this very brief exposure.

Building on this basic formulation of the human mind, Magnavita and Lilienfeld (Chapter 2, this volume) further articulate how individuals develop *heuristics*, the general rules of thumb that are acquired over time that help consolidate the massive amounts of incoming information into relatively reliable interpretations and guides. Although heuristics are necessary and central features of our cognitive system that enable us to get along in our everyday lives, it is also the case that they can be characterized as "lazy" and "miserly," meaning that in the service of efficiency they frequently result in inaccurate and misinformed judgments. Because the biases and traps are so easy to fall into, it is essential to teach clinical trainees about these cognitive mechanisms. Students should be shown explicit examples of how such biases and traps can lead practitioners astray and should be given training opportunities that allow them to build self-reflective awareness regarding their own heuristic processing tendencies that might result in them deviating from best practice.

Because the mechanics of clinical decision making are well examined elsewhere in this volume, I do not review them in detail here. From a training perspective such processes can be subsumed within a broader context—that is, within the identity and conceptual framework employed by the professional practitioner. The foundational elements that ground the more microlevel and situation-dependent cognitive processes can be considered, from the vantage point of decision making, as the "frame" of the practitioner. The *frame* of the practitioner refers to his or her worldview and practice orientation, and it is of tremendous importance in clinical decision making.

Magnavita and Lilienfeld (Chapter 2, this volume) offer the example that a psychoanalytic therapist will hear and respond to a patient's symptoms in a very different way than a psychopharmacologist. This gives rise to the question "What is the appropriate frame for a professional psychologist?" My position as an educator and scholar of the field is that practitioners should operate from the most coherent and comprehensive frame possible for understanding the key elements of a particular situation that requires clinical decision making. Unfortunately, this is difficult because the field of psychology is rife with competing, conflicting, overlapping, and somewhat redundant models and paradigms that attempt to offer practitioners a frame for understanding their patients or clients. This chapter introduces a framework that emphasizes key elements of the training of professional psychologists that enable them to make good clinical decisions. This framework is grounded in what is known as a *combined–integrated* approach to training professional psychologists (Shealy, 2004) and a more unified approach to the field of psychology as a whole (Henriques, 2011).

The first section of this chapter describes the general scientific humanistic philosophical approach and key values that we attempt to instill in our students, followed by a discussion regarding the implications for decision making. The second section provides a brief overview of the field and articulates why decision making needs to be grounded in a conceptual knowledge base. Following that an integrative approach to conceptualizing people is offered that directly informs budding clinicians in a wide variety of different contexts, including consulting and assessing patients. The fourth section addresses what is perhaps the most well-known and important frame of the clinical decision making of professional psychologists, the position of the American Psychological Association (APA) on evidence-based practice (EBP; APA Presidential Task Force, 2006). The history of EBP is reviewed, highlighting some of the major historical tensions that went into the emergence of EBP and how we train our students to approach the issue. Finally, an overview of a new unified approach to psychotherapy is offered that sets the stage for a heuristic that we train our students to use to frame their decision making in psychotherapy, called "TEST RePP."

CORE VALUES AND A SCIENTIFIC HUMANISTIC PHILOSOPHY

One of the most perplexing challenges for the field of professional psychology has been its struggle to navigate the tensions between the cold logic of science and the moral necessities of humanism. Indeed, in a seminal article, Kimble (1984) empirically documented the split between science and humanism in the broader field. It is the obligation of professional psychologists to understand the historical and epistemological issues that have contributed to this split and to be informed by both scientific and humanistic lenses when engaged in professional practice. First, by virtue of a core institutional identity, professional psychology is grounded in science, which means that it embraces the epistemic values and methods associated with science (Henriques & Sternberg, 2004). As such, it is crucial that a scientific attitude is instilled in budding professional psychologists. Some of the key ingredients of this attitude are skepticism and critical thought, a worldview that frames cause and effect with certain assumptions based on scientific plausibility, and reliance on evidence acquired in a systematic way (see Lilienfeld & O'Donohue, 2012).

Although a scientific attitude is crucial, it is not all there is to being a professional psychologist. Indeed, the primary identity of professional psychology is as an applied health service profession, and this means that the primary charge of professional psychology is prescriptive (Henriques & Sternberg, 2004). Ultimately, the function of professional psychologists is to change an existing state. This can be conceived as having the goal to move individuals or systems toward more valued states of being, which requires having a broadly philosophical—some might say metaphysical (O'Donohue, 1989)—position regarding the values that are guiding one's actions. The ethical code offered by the APA prescribes some of the key values that all psychologists need to consider in their professional behavior but, although essential, leaves much ambiguity in the details of how to be an ethical, values-driven practitioner. Because an individual psychologist has the potential for great influence over others, and because much clinical work and professional practice can be inherently subjective, it is essential that students be willing and able to understand and critically explore who they are; what they believe and why; and what they must do—personally and professionally—to become highly knowledgeable, skilled, and competent scientific practitioners. Thus, it is incumbent on the practitioner to be self-reflective and aware of the assumptions and the broader worldview that guides their actions. And there must be a narrative associated with that view that ties together core moral values, such as promoting human dignity and well-being with integrity (Henriques, 2011). These ingredients are fundamentally humanistic in nature.

To understand how training in a broad scientific humanistic philosophy has implications for clinical decision making, consider the following case: A 19-year-old college freshman is referred by the office of disability of her university for an evaluation because she believes she might have attention-deficit/hyperactivity disorder (ADHD). The scientific methodological perspective should inform the clinician to approach this case in a number of different ways. Specifically, a clinician should be informed regarding the empirical research that discriminates this disorder from other possible presenting conditions and be aware of the most reliable and valid assessment measures. Thus, a scientifically informed clinician would know that impressions formed in the course of a brief interview are a poor way to diagnose ADHD. Instead, what is needed is a detailed history of prior behavior patterns such as impulsivity, inattention, hyperactivity, poor organization, and poor academic performance relative to intellectual potential, supplemented via perspectives of an informant such as a parent, coupled with records from past school performance. In addition, reliable symptom inventories, both self- and observer report, a cognitive and academic profile suggesting difficulties with attention and processing speed, clinical observations, and a detailed interview assessing the nature and trajectory of the symptoms are all essential to make a diagnosis that would be "scientifically" valid.

But a scientifically informed methodological approach to assessment, although crucial, is not enough. Indeed, from the vantage point of a larger metaphysical humanistic philosophical approach, a pristine application of the scientific method that results in reliable diagnoses and points to evidence-based interventions might be seriously problematic when viewed from a broader perspective. Why? Because diagnostic entities such as ADHD have huge sociological implications. It carries meaning for how individuals understand their very natures, and there are good reasons to be extremely concerned about the "medicalization" of human experience. Indeed, the rising epidemic of mental health concerns (i.e., depression, anxiety, ADHD, etc.) has been linked by some scholars to the rise of the "disease–pill" model of human experience (Whitaker, 2010). Because humans are meaning-making entities, a professional psychologist in this context would be obligated to understand the personal significance of this diagnosis and its meaning in the context of this individual's social system. It is also the obligation of the professional psychologist to consider his or her role in the context of a system that creates policies that have broad social implications. There are no simple decision-making algorithms that can be applied at this level of analysis. However, if we are teaching leaders in mental health who will attempt to guide the system toward wise policies, it is incumbent on us to instill in our students a broad awareness of the implications of our actions beyond the narrow application of the scientific method to develop reliable, evidence-based answers in specific situations.

IS SCIENTIFICALLY INFORMED DECISION MAKING GROUNDED IN A METHOD OR A CONCEPTUAL KNOWLEDGE BASE?

When asked how he defined *science*, Robyn Dawes, well known for his work on fostering empirically based decision making, answered,

> I would define it as testing hypotheses through the systematic collection and analysis of data whether via what are called "randomized trials," where we randomly assign people to be given a vaccine or not or to a placebo group, all the way to informed observation. These are really the two essences of science. (Gambrill & Dawes, 2003; cited in Lilienfeld & O'Donohue, 2012, p. 59)

Dawes captured the methodological view of science. This view is embraced by many psychologists, both researchers and practitioners alike. Indeed, some argue that grounding psychology in the scientific method is the defining and unifying feature of the discipline (see, e.g., Stam, 2004). However, from the vantage point of a broad scientific humanistic philosophy, the purely methodological view of science is inadequate. In isolation, the scientific method (i.e., generating hypotheses and conducting studies) yields data and information. However, the professional psychologist needs to operate first from knowledge and wisdom. The incompleteness of method is obvious on reflection. Consider the question of why we engage in the scientific method in the first place. It generally is not solely for the specific data it yields about the specific phenomena under investigation. Indeed, if the data gathered were not generalizable at all, they would be largely irrelevant because scientific findings from specific studies—in the absence of a nomological network of scientific understanding—are essentially meaningless. The data and information from scientific studies become meaningful only when they are linked with data from other investigations and then placed within a network of understanding. Thus, science must include attention to the conceptually grounded meaning-making schema that organizes scientific knowledge.

A bit of probing of even the most committed methodologists reveals this necessity. Consider, for example, the spirited call for the "clinical scientist" model of training in professional psychology offered by Baker, McFall, and Shoham (2009). Like Dawes, these authors have strongly equated science with the scientific method. Yet they acknowledged that the information gathered from science must be assessed for its external validity and generalizability. How do we accomplish this? The authors proclaimed that the "scientific plausibility" of the information gleaned from the scientific method must be considered. Consider, for example, that on the basis of the authors' articulation of scientific plausibility, it seems highly likely that they would dismiss empirical data derived via the scientific method that pointed to the existence of parapsychological phenomena (see, e.g., Radin, 2011) or the utility of energy psychology methods in reducing psychological distress (Feinstein, 2008).

All of this, of course, raises the question "What is 'scientifically plausible'?" We must have a way of answering this question or else we will simply generate a mountain of data and information without genuine understanding. To be a mature science, psychology must have an answer to the following: Is there a scientifically grounded conception of the human condition that is rich enough to speak to the complexities of the human experience while also assimilating and integrating major lines of information gleaned from various empirical investigations? To the extent that the answer is no, the field of professional psychology is destined to be deeply divided. Those who are impressed with the advances in the natural sciences will lean more toward the epistemic values of accuracy, objectivity, and reliability of knowledge and will emphasize the scientific method. In contrast, those who question the extent to which the natural sciences have effectively elucidated the nature of the human condition and who value meaning, relationships, subjectivity, and the unique and idiographic nature of the human experience will view the empirical commitment as sacrificing too much and missing the essence of what it means to be human. This is the fundamental reason the field has been pulled into two cultures.

The argument here is that the field of professional psychology needs to evolve from a conception of "science" as consisting solely of the method of hypothesis testing and data collection as Dawes described it to thinking about science as a knowledge system that provides a map of the human condition and our place in the universe. To be a credible system, the map must make sense out of the field of scientific psychology and point to a way of thinking about human behavior that offers a sophisticated guide to the practitioner. The construction of just such a formulation has been the focus of my efforts over the past decade (Henriques, 2003, 2004, 2008, 2011, 2013a).

Consider that it is not uncommon for students, in the course of their professional training, to be exposed to approaches such as person-centered therapy, cognitive–behavioral and emotion-focused therapy, family systems, and psychodynamic frameworks. Each of these perspectives has "data" supporting its views, yet they all have quite different fundamental assumptions that can overwhelm a student (or even a seasoned practitioner!). In addition, the conceptual connection between the various therapeutic paradigms and the science of human psychology as articulated by major domains of scientific inquiry, such as evolutionary, personality, developmental, cognitive, social, and cultural psychology, can easily result in contradictory messages and confusion.

For example, many ideas in evolutionary psychology seem to conflict with a cultural psychological perspective (Henriques, 2011). Even domains that seem like they should be obviously connected frequently are not. Consider that as a graduate student I took a personality theories class that was followed by a personality assessment class, and I found that the two courses were largely independent from one another. This was so even though they were taught by the same instructor! The main personality assessment instrument covered was the Minnesota Multiphasic Personality Inventory—2, and that seemed to introduce a whole different set of concepts than those that were covered in the personality theories class, which itself consisted of a series of schools of thought that were different and often disconnected and contradictory (e.g., radical behavioral, psychodynamic, humanistic, social cognitive). And when I was taught psychotherapy, the perspectives I was introduced to there were only loosely related to concepts in personality or personality assessment.

Given the enormous diversity, pluralism, and conceptual fragmentation in the field of psychology, I became deeply concerned that psychology in general and psychotherapy in particular were producing vast amounts of information but little cumulative knowledge (Henriques, 2011). In the 1990s, I began work on a project that sought to remedy this problem with a framework that would ultimately become known as the *unified theory* (Henriques, 2003, 2008). Because the term *unified theory* might sound to some like an all-encompassing idea that explains everything and makes precise predictions about how humans behave, it can also be characterized as a *unified approach*, which refers to an integrative metatheoretical framework that can define the field of psychology; integrate key insights from the major paradigms; and resolve long-standing philosophical disputes, such as the debates between mentalists and behaviorists (Henriques, 2004).

The unified approach works via the introduction of several new broad ideas (the tree of knowledge system, behavioral investment theory, the influence matrix, and the justification hypothesis) that allow for the key ideas of the major domains of psychological inquiry (e.g., evolutionary, cognitive, personality, social, cultural, developmental) and the major therapy paradigms (e.g., psychodynamic and cognitive–behavioral therapy perspectives) to be effectively assimilated and integrated into a more coherent whole. In short, the unified theory allows for both the "vertical" integration of the biological, psychological, and sociocultural dimensions of human functioning and the "horizontal" integration of perspectives on the human mind and behavior at the level of the individual (Henriques, 2013b).

The specific details of the unified approach are beyond the scope of this chapter, and the reader is referred elsewhere for an overview of the ideas that make up the system (see, e.g., Henriques, 2011, 2013a). What it offers in terms of teaching good clinical decision making is the position that it is both possible and useful to pull together, in a conceptually sound way, the primary lenses that are offered from the major perspectives in psychotherapy (i.e., behavioral, cognitive, existential, humanistic, psychodynamic, and family systems). In addition, it allows a foothold for organizing the vast data that researchers have gathered about human nature under the broad heading of psychology and the more specific research on psychotherapy such that those data can be brought to bear on real-life clinical situations in a holistic, nuanced, and effective way (see also Melchert, 2014).

AN INTEGRATIVE MODEL FOR CONCEPTUALIZING PEOPLE THAT INFORMS CLINICAL DECISION MAKING

In this approach, concepts and theories are the bridges that link data and information gleaned from the scientific method to wise practice. Consequently, a major goal I have as a trainer of budding clinicians is to provide them with a broad framework that effectively maps the discipline, clears up the current psychotherapy tower of Babel, and allows the key insights from myriad perspectives and traditions to be coherently integrated into a whole. Directly related to clinical decision making in a wide variety of contexts is the approach to conceptualizing people based on analyzing five systems of character adaptation and the biological, learning and developmental, and sociocultural contexts in which the individual is immersed (Henriques, 2011; see Figure 11.1). The systems of character adaptation refer to the hierarchical arrangement of mental systems that enable an individual to respond to the current situation. The character adaptation system theory (CAST) approach refers to the hierarchical arrangement of mental systems that enable an individual to respond to the current situation. From the most basic to the most advanced, the five systems are as follows: (a) the *habit system*, which refers to the basic procedural processes shaped by learning and stimulus control; (b) the *experiential system*, which refers to the core of experiential consciousness that is organized by the flow of perception, motivation, and emotional reactions; (c) the *relationship system*, which is an outgrowth of the experiential system

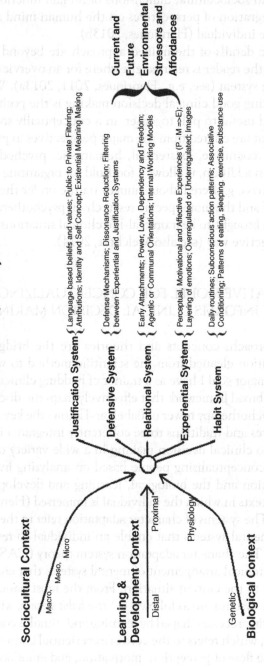

Figure 11.1. The five systems of character adaptation. From *A New Unified Theory of Psychology* (p. 230), by G. Henriques, 2011, New York, NY: Springer Science+Business Media. Copyright 2011 by Springer Science+Business Media. Reprinted with permission.

that tracks self–other exchanges in an intuitive way on the dimension of relational value and social influence; (d) the *defensive system*, which refers to the ways the individual manages psychic equilibrium in the form of experiential avoidance, dissonance reduction, and defense mechanisms; and (e) the *justification system*, which refers to the verbally mediated explicit beliefs, values, and attributions people use to make sense of themselves and others.

As articulated by Henriques and Stout (2012), the five systems of character adaptation provide a framework for assimilating and integrating the key insights from major traditions in psychotherapy, placed in a biopsychosocial context. For example, behaviorists have historically tended to think and focus on habits, whereas humanistic and experiential practitioners have focused on core emotions and experiences; psychodynamic practitioners have focused on underlying relationship patterns and psychological defenses, and cognitive and narrative therapists have emphasized semantic meaning making in various ways. The CAST approach provides a way to understand how these are all component systems of adaptation that can be effectively woven together in to a more coherent whole.

How does this system influence clinical decision making? As O'Donohue and Henderson (1999; cited in Lilienfeld & O'Donohue, 2012) pointed out, "choosing appropriate treatment methods involves knowing and instantiating causal relations" (p. 51). To do this, a clinician needs to be able to understand the key variables and their hypothesized causal relations, and the CAST approach guides students on how to accomplish this. To see this, let's continue with the example that was introduced earlier, that of a college student who receives a referral for assessing the presence of ADHD and possible accommodations. Let's add the following background to the formulation and then apply the CAST approach to fostering a conceptualization:

> Tina is a 19-year-old college freshman. She grew up in a small rural town in southwestern Virginia. She is a first-generation college student and entered college with hopes of being a physician. She did extremely well in high school and has always been very driven and conscientious. However, her first semester at college did not go very well. She experienced difficulty making friends, and she was uncomfortable with the drinking and party atmosphere. She focused a lot on her studies and studied several hours a day, but she struggled to get the As she expected (her first semester grade point average was 3.2). Now she is reporting problems taking tests and staying focused and is worried that she has ADHD. She is starting to have trouble sleeping; she can't fall asleep because she is constantly worrying about what she needs to do the next day. She is also having nightmares about failing out of school. She also is reporting frequent stomachaches, and she is now considering whether she should transfer to a different college because it is closer to home.

As O'Donohue and Henderson (1999) pointed out, people consult psychologists because they possess a form of specialized expertise. Specifically, they are able to understand key psychological variables and causal processes that contribute to the situation, have knowledge about what might foster adaptive change, and have a skill set that enables them assist with this process. Yet, exactly what scientific and professional information is considered relevant, and how psychologists are to maintain a reasonable level of awareness so that they understand people's presenting problems and make epistemologically informed and ecologically valid clinical decisions, remain extremely difficult and contentious. The volume of information and the markedly disparate lines of thought within our field makes this issue particularly daunting, and the CAST approach offers a heuristic to delineate key psychological variables that will enable the effective conceptualization of psychological problems. Here is an example of a formulation that might emerge if one was to apply the CAST approach:

> Tina is at a key developmental time in her life and is experiencing significant distress and psychological dysfunction due to a host of interrelated variables. Perhaps most salient issue is that Tina seems to be struggling with her identity and her sense of competence (Justification System), which is generating significant levels of negative affect, especially anxiety (Experiential System). It seems that her confusion is tied to her difficulties in adjustment associated with the change in her social context, from a rural setting to a university setting (Social Context). In the former context, she likely shared many of the social values and was able to perform in a way that was both personally and relationally affirming (i.e., she achieved academically and had friends—Justification and Relationship Systems). However, at college, the social values are deviating from hers in a way that leaves her more likely to feel isolated and uncomfortable (Experiential and Relational Systems). In addition, she is finding academic success more challenging than she expected. Thus, compared with high school, she is having trouble in two key life domains, academic and social. It seems that in an attempt to cope with her difficulties and control what she could (Defensive System), she has tried to increase her academic performance and has isolated herself a bit from her social connections. Unfortunately, it seems likely that the intense pressure she has placed on herself to succeed (Defense and Justification Systems) likely created additional problems because her anxious arousal (Experiential System) probably had the function of impairing her ability to perform in high-stakes situations like taking tests, thus creating a vicious, anxiety-producing cycle. As her general stress level increases, it seems likely that her basic biological and habitual patterns (e.g., eating and sleeping) have become disrupted, which will likely contribute to a dysfunctional spiral. It will be crucial to assess Tina's family history (past Social and Learning and Developmental Contexts) and what her status as a first-generation

college student and desire to be a physician means in that context (Justification System). It would also be important to assess for any history of illnesses (in Tina or her family), especially for anxiety or depressive disorders (Biological Context). From the vantage point of diagnosis, it does not appear Tina has problems indicative of ADHD, but depending on additional information, she might meet criteria for a generalized anxiety disorder or an adjustment disorder with anxious features.

The CAST approach is a useful heuristic that is justified by its utility, parsimony, and conceptual coherence and is based on the argument that clinicians need to be guided by rationally coherent systems, which brings us to the point of exploring existing systems of decision making. It is helpful to review the history of the concept of EBP and then offer a framework that extends it on the basis of a metatheoretical approach to the field grounded in a scientific humanistic philosophy.

A BRIEF HISTORY OF EVIDENCE-BASED PRACTICE

Professional psychology has long been torn between two visions, the practice of psychology as an art versus an empirically based science. The artistic vision promotes the image of the master clinician as a wise and insightful healer guided by a deep intuitive knowledge. A prototype of such a clinician was offered by Caldwell (2004; cited in Garb, 2005), who, on receiving an award for his work in personality assessment, gave the following example of successfully interpreting a Minnesota Multiphasic Personality Inventory:

> We got a severe 4-6-8 profile on a young woman. I looked at the tortured implications of the pattern and somehow said, "She will have something like cigarette burn scars on her hands, where her father prepared her to steel herself to the suffering of life." The round burn marks were on her hands and extended a little way up her arms. (Caldwell, 2004, p. 9)

In contrast to the vision of the master practitioner as a wise artisan, the empiricist vision cautions psychologists against such ideals (Garb, 2005) and emphasizes judgments and decision making based not on intuition and the like but on existing empirical evidence. The practitioner's skill is in knowing how to acquire, interpret, and apply good empirical data to the question at hand. Empirically trained practitioners tend to dismiss with skepticism anecdotes like the one in the previous paragraph and point out the incredible biases of the human mind in seeing spurious patterns in nature. As a consequence, proponents of the empirical tradition argue that there is a great need to ground assessments and treatments in those validated by the scientific method. As alluded to earlier, the empirical tradition is now explicitly represented in "clinical science" training programs (Baker et al., 2009) that define clinical psychology solely as a science and generally reject the notion that clinical practice is in any way an art form.

Historically, these two traditions have been framed as the competition between the empirical and romantic visions of professional practice (Garb, 2005), but I believe this is an unfortunate way to characterize the split. In philosophy, there are two broad positions on the mechanisms humans use to achieve knowledge. The empirical tradition, epitomized by individuals like John Locke and David Hume, posits that the most fundamental and reliable way to achieve knowledge comes from systematic observations and data collection. This accords very well with the methodological view of science articulated by Dawes. The rationalist tradition, epitomized by individuals like René Descartes and Immanuel Kant, argues that the best approach to knowledge is achieved by using reason to arrive at conclusions about the most justifiable claims. Whereas empiricists emphasize "show me the evidence," rationalists emphasize "show me the logic and rationale." Consistent with my emphasis on approaching human psychology and the profession from the vantage point of conceptual coherence (Henriques, 2013a), my view is that the rationalist position has not received enough attention in the identity of professional psychology. This chapter can be characterized as a call for how to teach clinical decision making grounded in a rationalist approach. Of course, empirical data and the honed, artistic skills of the practitioner are valued, but from this perspective, the central guiding key to wisdom that informs best practice is a comprehensive system of justification.

Returning to the history of EBP, the competition for the core identity of practitioners and for the conceptual groundwork for making clinical decisions in psychotherapy reached a fever pitch in the 1990s. Much of it centered on the debate about the role and place of empirically supported treatments (ESTs) in psychological practice. For a host of reasons—managed care being a primary one—pressure was mounting on the field in the 1980s to demonstrate the effectiveness of psychotherapy interventions. At the same time, there emerged interventions that offered models and manuals for treatment that could be tested empirically relatively easily. For example, A. T. Beck produced a model and treatment for depression, the effectiveness of which he and his colleagues were able to test using a randomized controlled design. Studies began to emerge that suggested that cognitive therapy (or cognitive–behavioral therapy) was more effective in reducing symptoms than either no treatment or control conditions like supportive therapy. From the empirical–methodological perspective such findings were exactly the kind of data needed to ground the field in science. Many academics began to promote the idea that students of psychotherapy must be taught empirical approaches and that such interventions ought to be the first line of treatment in practice.

Given that virtually all agree that by virtue of its history and identity, professional psychology is tied in some way or another to science, one might think at first glance that the EST movement would not inspire much controversy. It seems to represent a straightforward scientific advance, and indeed, from a pure methodological view of science and practice, ESTs are a straightforward advance. However, from the vantage point of a rationalist informed by a broad scientific humanistic view of the field, the issues are enormously complicated. I offer a brief discussion of just a few of them and refer the reader to Marquis and Douthit (2006) and Wachtel (2010) for more detailed critiques. The overall point here is that from a broad scientific, humanistic, philosophically informed view, it is naive and a form of scientism (i.e., an overreliance on power of the procedures and methods of science) to believe that data and information derived from studies emphasizing sound scientific methodology should be the sole guide in clinical decision making.

We can start unpacking the debate surrounding ESTs by considering that virtually all ESTs are grounded in concepts from the *Diagnostic and Statistical Manual of Mental Disorders* (*DSM*). Many have criticized the *DSM*, which was produced largely by the field of psychiatry, as offering an overly simplistic, medicalized descriptive categorization of psychopathology that ignores psychosocial etiology and, as such, does not lead to effective treatment plans because it is blind to the dimensions of functioning that are crucial to understand in psychotherapy. Psychodynamically oriented clinicians were so frustrated by what the *DSM* failed to capture that they developed their own *Psychodynamic Diagnostic Manual* to guide practitioners in assessment and case formulation (PDM Task Force, 2006). Humanistic, critical, and positive psychologists have all been critical of the *DSM* system in various ways. Even biologically oriented scientists who study mental disorders have started to abandon the *DSM* (including researchers at the National Institute of Mental Health; see, e.g., Insel, 2013). The fact that the major mental health research institution in the United States is abandoning the *DSM* must raise a host of questions about the foundational validity of so many EST research projects.

The conceptual structure of the EST movement does not implicitly endorse just the *DSM* but also the medical model of treatment. By that I mean that the EST model of psychotherapy assumes that psychological disorders exist within individuals, are of a specific identifiable type, and are amenable to specific interventions that result in helpful change. Conceptually, the medical model places the disorder as the "figure" to be analyzed, along with the impact of the specified and generalizable intervention. In the traditional medical model of researching disorder–intervention match, the personality of both the individual and the treating professional and the nature of their relationship become the "ground" and are generally treated as error or noise, both in the way the interventions are presented and the way data are analyzed in randomized controlled trials.

The potential problem with this framing is that many view psychotherapy as a psychosocial or human relational process. In this view, the personality of both individuals in the therapy room and the nature of their healing relationship are front and center. In his now classic work, *The Great Psychotherapy Debate*, Bruce Wampold (2001) argued that the scientific data were clear on the best way to conceptualize psychotherapy: It should be considered a human relational process rather than a depersonalized medical intervention. Why? According to Wampold, the scientific data strongly support the notion that it is the quality of the therapeutic alliance that is more closely associated with good outcomes than is the process of specifically matching particular techniques to *DSM*-type problems.

To understand the differences between the two perspectives, consider an individual diagnosed with clinical depression being treated with a behavioral activation intervention (e.g., Martell, Dimidjian, & Herman-Dunn, 2010). The EST approach focuses on the nature of depression as a state of behavioral shutdown, and the key ingredient of change is considered increases in mastery, pleasure, and rewarding activity. Randomized controlled trials focus on comparing whether those in a behavioral activation condition show more symptom relief than those in a different condition. The specific personalities of the individual and the therapist and their relationship might be examined as moderating influences but generally are not considered central. In contrast, the process approach emphasizes that the key ingredient is not the specific intervention but the extent to which the therapist and client form a positive, trusting relationship; agree on the formulation; and are able to set tasks that foster change. This angle on psychotherapy research points out that widely different approaches to thinking about conditions like depression (e.g., behavioral, cognitive–behavioral, emotion focused, interpersonal, modern psychodynamic) tend to get very similar results. The key ingredients, according to Wampold and other outcome-informed therapists (e.g., Duncan, 2013), are not the model of the disorder or intervention per se. Instead, these scholars have argued that as long as the model is credible, the key ingredients are whether the healing relationship is strong, the formulation of the problem is shared, and the work leads to change-oriented tasks in which both individuals are invested. Thus, in this case, the key ingredients are whether the individual is at a stage of change that makes him or her receptive to the conceptualization of depression offered by behavioral activation, whether the therapist is seen as trustworthy and knowledgeable, and whether the individual is motivated to comply with the tasks designed to change the current state of affairs. Wampold pointed out that if these ingredients are present, the data suggest the outcomes are the same for all the credible kinds of therapy, which raises serious questions about a host of issues.

In addition to debates about how to think about psychotherapy in general (i.e., whether we approach it via a medical model or a psychosocial process), there are many theoretical approaches to psychological treatment, and when one takes a broad view of the field it must be noted that the EST debate has been deeply entangled with the competition between the schools of thought on the various ways to conceptualize people in general and psychopathology and psychotherapy in particular. Compared with psychodynamic and humanistic approaches, cognitive and behavioral approaches were more closely connected with empirical traditions in academic psychology and were structured in a way to be more readily examined via traditional research methods. Thus, historically, support for ESTs basically translated into support for behavioral or cognitive approaches over psychodynamic and humanistic ones. All these forces set the stage for a deep and complicated debate, which, as is evident from the growth of "clinical science" programs, has yet to be settled.

Largely in response to the conflict the EST debate sparked in the field, the APA developed a broad framework for clinical decision making with its position on EBP (APA Presidential Task Force, 2006). EBP is defined as approaching practice via "the integration of the best available research with clinical expertise in the context of patient characteristics, culture and preferences" (p. 273). Sometimes conceptualized as a three-legged stool, EBP thus has three predominant elements that should go into considerations of best practice: (a) the available research evidence applicable to the current situation, (b) the professional expertise of the practitioner, and (c) the values of the client in the given cultural context. The EBP concept is broader than the focus of ESTs and was issued in part by APA to provide a form of conceptual rapprochement between the various factions in the debate over the relevance and power of ESTs to influence practice. For example, the acknowledgement of both available research and professional expertise in the unique context of the specific client and culture attempts to speak to both sides of the issue. The basic framing of EBP provides a generally useful heuristic to guide practitioners in the key elements that should go into the decisions surrounding assessments, interventions, and consultations. However, despite its usefulness as a general framework, I have found as an educator that EBP requires more clarification to serve as an effective guide.

Grounded in the same integrative metatheoretical approach that generated the CAST approach for conceptualizing individuals, we have developed TEST RePP to provide students in behavioral and mental health programs with a heuristic that informs them of how to make effective, holistic, clinical decisions in a wide variety of professional contexts. It is a framework that is embedded in a course on integrative psychotherapy for adults, although it could extend to other related domains of practice, such as consultation and assessment. To apply it, we must first articulate a how a broad and general view of psychotherapy can set the stage for resolving the great psychotherapy debate and allow practitioners a truly comprehensive framework for rationally integrating research, professional wisdom, and unique contextual elements and client values into effective practice.

A GENERAL, UNIFIED VIEW OF PSYCHOTHERAPY

The argument laid out so far is that if students are going to be informed consumers of scientific research applied to professional practice, they must operate from a broad scientific humanistic philosophy of the field. Such a view will enable them to consolidate findings into meaningful information that guides their decision making. Without such a framework, the field and its practitioners are destined to endless debates because of foundational disputes about assumptions that are not resolvable at the level of scientific data gathering. Earlier I described how a broad scientific humanistic philosophy is necessary to reflect on and make decisions about diagnoses and develop holistic conceptualizations that elucidate key variables and their causal interrelations in a way that leads to informed clinical decision making. In this section of this chapter, the focus turns to therapy and how the unified system offers a new way to approach the field of psychotherapy, one that is quite different from other approaches.

The field of psychology in general and the practice of psychotherapy in particular have been "pre-paradigmatic," meaning that there was no available broad framework from which professional psychologists could operate. This is apparent when one considers that the emergence of the major schools of thought were generally through a master practitioner gaining insights based on useful techniques in the therapy room. Although they were all students of human nature, the founders of the great therapy endeavors like Freud, Rogers, and Beck largely started with observations about the therapeutic process and generalized from there about insights for the field of psychology. These gurus then generated a following of individuals who tried to apply their insights and argue for the best approach to psychotherapy on the basis of this process.

The unified approach advocated for here works in the opposite direction. It specifically concerns itself with the construction of an integrative metatheoretical framework that then can be used to assimilate and integrate key insights and findings from both the science of human psychology (e.g., personality, cognitive, affective, developmental, neuroscience, social, abnormal) and psychotherapy from a multitude of perspectives (e.g., cognitive–behavioral therapy, psychodynamic). Thus, the unified approach enables the psychotherapist to move beyond specific paradigms and toward a general model of psychotherapy that is grounded in the science of human psychology (Henriques & Stout, 2012; Magnavita & Anchin, 2014; Melchert, 2014).

Because the unified framework enables us to take a broad view of the field, it is well positioned to advance the search for a more effective way to approach psychotherapy integration. First, it can offer a general conception of psychotherapy, one that other perspectives cannot do because they are not tied to a coherent conception of human psychology. Via the unified view, psychotherapy can be defined as a professional relationship between a patient (or client) and a professional psychologist who is trained in applying psychological knowledge toward improving human well-being. In addition, the integrative metatheoretical perspective can also serve as a way to unify the various approaches to psychotherapy integration. One such perspective that has been quite influential has been the *common factors* approach, which is based on the early work of Jerome Frank. This view, supported strongly by Wampold's (2001) analysis of the field, emphasizes the fact that generally speaking, the different bona fide treatments yield very similar outcomes (the so-called dodo bird effect) and thus the primary curative agents are likely in the "common factors" of the various treatment protocols. One of the most robust findings in the research on psychotherapy has been the association between a strong working or therapeutic alliance and good outcomes. Consistent with Bordin's (1979) early formulation and much subsequent research, the working alliance consists of three primary components: (a) the bond or quality of the therapeutic relationship; (b) the shared goals of the therapy, which emerge out of a shared conceptualization of the problems; and (c) the tasks, which are the changes and interventions that are hopefully going to take place to achieve the stated goals. In accordance with this view, students can be taught to think about general psychotherapy as consisting of the three elements that together make up the concept of the therapeutic alliance.

Although some tend to think about the therapeutic alliance only in terms of the process and quality of the relationship, it is, of course, much more than that. In addition to the human bond, it also involves developing an effective, shared narrative of the problem and useful tasks that foster reaching specified therapeutic goals. This is where the CAST approach to conceptualizing is placed in the system because it attempts to ensure that a comprehensive, holistic picture of the individual can be formed and in a way that is both systematic and that can be shared with clients (Henriques & Stout, 2012). If successful, the conceptualization results in the collaborative weaving together of the key forces and domains that tell a story of how the person got to where they are and what will influence their trajectory in an adaptive as opposed to maladaptive way. The CAST approach is integrative because, as mentioned earlier, the five systems of character adaptation align with the dominant perspectives in individual psychotherapy. The conceptual foundations that drive behavioral, experiential, modern, psychodynamic, cognitive, and narrative approaches can now be integrated into a holistic biopsychosocial formulation. Thus, students can now effectively transcend the competing insights from these grand traditions and coherently integrate them into a more cohesive framework.

If this is done well, the case formulation gives rise to the goals of the therapy, which can be framed as a description of what would influence the ultimate outcome to be desirable and adaptive (e.g., if an individual could be less negative in their self-talk, be more assertive in their relationships, become aware of ways they defend against certain feelings). In this light, the goals of therapy can be now framed as decreasing distress and dysfunction and increasing valued states of being. Finally, these goals can then be matched with the empirical literature in psychotherapy, and a series of therapeutic tasks can be developed that can be expected to have a positive impact on the stated goals. In short, for the first time there is now a model of psychotherapy that can be effectively corresponded with the science of human psychology, allowing for much more unity and synergy between these two branches of our field.

A FRAMEWORK FOR CLINICAL DECISION MAKING IN PSYCHOTHERAPY

The three broad domains of a general psychotherapy (relationship, case formulation, and intervention assessed via clear outcomes) grounded in the conceptual map provided by the unified theory enables students to disentangle the complicated process of psychotherapy into more discrete, but clearly related, parts. To foster a deliberate working conception of the kinds of thought processes that ought to be guiding them in their clinical decision making, students are introduced to the mnemonic TEST RePP, which stands for "Theoretically and Empirically Supported Treatment and Relationship Processes and Principles." It provides a heuristic that captures the key elements that evidence-based practitioners ought to be aware of and adhering to. It is specifically organized in a way that allows the field to transcend the current "midlevel" paradigms, build bridges between psychotherapy research and meaningful practice, and move toward resolving the great psychotherapy debate by holding both the "disorder–intervention" and "healing relational process" perspectives in complementary relation to one another.

TEST REPP APPLIED TO THE CASE OF TINA

Each element of TEST RePP is described in greater detail in the subsections that follow. To help see how its elements have implications for clinical decision making, it is applied to Tina, with the context being that she has come to see a staff psychologist at a college counseling center, seeking guidance on what she should do and greatly desiring to reduce her distress. Note that TEST RePP guides the clinician within the context of an appropriate, ethical, and professional therapeutic relationship, and the assumption is made here that the proper considerations have been taken in setting up the frame for the relationship.

Theoretically Supported Treatment

A basic principle stemming from the argument thus far is that, as philosophers often point out, "facts are theory laden." Professional psychologists must be aware that humans do not perceive the world directly as it truly is (whatever that might mean), but we have perceptual and conceptual categories that enable us to actively make meaning out of the patterns in the world. This is the first meaning of the word theory here. Because the background conceptual structure "frames" what the practitioner sees in making decisions, it is crucial that the practitioner be as fully aware of those structures as possible. This starts at the level of broad philosophy and worldview and includes the views the professional psychologist has for how the world works, his or her religious and political perspectives, beliefs about the nature of human nature, and beliefs about humanity's place in the universe at large. If these sound deeply philosophical, they are. This is central because we relate to our clients at the level of meaning and inevitably hear their stories through a particular lens defined by our worldview.

Applied to Tina, consider how a Christian psychological practitioner might hear and respond to her story differently than a secular skeptical practitioner. To do so, let's make the reasonable assumption, on the basis of Tina's story and the demographics of southern rural Virginia, that she was raised in a socially conservative, Christian home. If so, it follows that some of her current anxiety and confusion likely would stem from the potentially conflicting messages she has received in the context of her transition from a socially and religiously conservative environment where she felt comfortable to one that is more secular and has looser mores regarding drinking and sexual activity. If so, then it is highly likely that a socially conservative Christian psychological practitioner will hear Tina's story differently than a purely secular practitioner. This is the case even when both practitioners are engaged in "secular" psychotherapy and are appropriately ethical and sensitive about imposing their own personal beliefs on the therapy practice. The issue here regarding clinical decision making is one of awareness as opposed to explicit formulations regarding what one ought to do. Because these deep structures will have a profound impact on how we practice, a foundational pillar of good practice is to have strong self-reflective awareness of one's identity, deep-seated beliefs, and values and the capacity to clearly identify the ways in which those frames influence how one hears and responds to a client's presentation.

The second meaning of the term *theory* refers to the practitioner's knowledge of human psychology. This consists of the biological, developmental, and social understanding of personality, psychopathology, relational, and human change processes through which both the individual and the process of intervention will be understood. Professional psychologists should have basic knowledge of elements such as behavioral genetics and their influence on mental illnesses; personality traits (e.g., neuroticism and conscientiousness); emotions and motivations; social psychological processes of first impressions, stereotypes, attitudes, and attributions; and general knowledge of intelligence and academic aptitude, along with categories and classification of mental disorders (i.e., the *DSM*).

This second level of theory, knowledge of human psychology, is usually organized around and telescoped into the primary paradigm of practice that the professional operates from (e.g., third wave cognitive–behavioral therapy, eclectic therapy, emotion-focused therapy). A humanistic psychologist operating from a person-centered approach would likely emphasize the external pressures that Tina is experiencing that "force" her to feel compelled to fit into a specific socialized mode. The assumption that she has within her an organizing growth force will position the humanistic practitioner to make choices in the therapy room to focus on Tina's internal emotional experience and create a relational context of empathy, congruence, and positive regard in which she can begin to discover and give voice to her "true" self, which is seen as central to healthy development from the vantage point of the humanistic tradition. In contrast, from a traditional cognitive–behavioral perspective, a psychological practitioner will attend to the interpretations and beliefs that Tina has about herself, others, and her situation. These beliefs will be seen to be the key to understanding the negative emotions and maladaptive behaviors that follow. Here the therapist will listen for how Tina's story indicates the presence of beliefs that she is incompetent or that she must get all As in order to be successful. From the current perspective, it is the obligation of the practitioner to be able to identify the general paradigm from which he or she is operating in understanding Tina and explain how it is consistent with the body of human psychological knowledge in general. This is deemed to be a basic requirement of doing psychological therapy.

One of the distinguishing features of the unified approach that fosters advances in this area is that because its starting point is a holistic view of human psychology, it sets the stage for a much greater correspondence between the body of psychological knowledge and the conceptual understanding of the current situation. For example, as articulated when describing how Tina might be conceptualized, lenses from a wide variety of different domains were combined in a holistic picture, including biology and behavioral genetics, learning and development, interpersonal and sociological, behavioral (habits), experiential and emotion focused, psychodynamic (i.e., defenses and relational schema), and cognitive–narrative perspectives.

In short, to effectively decide how to frame the therapy with Tina, the professional psychologist must be clear about his or her theoretical and conceptual frame. The reason for this is that it guides how the psychologist sees Tina, conceptualizes her problems, and inquires about and deciphers Tina's valued states of being. It also informs the psychologist of how to think about the current condition, the key causal variables that led up to it, and the proposed mechanisms of change. The argument here is that the more coherent, clear, and comprehensive one's approach is and the more it aligns with our knowledge of human psychology, the better the decision making that will ensue about a particular case. That said, I am not advocating for a "purely" rationalist approach to intervention. Coherent and comprehensive formulations must be buttressed and informed by the empirical literature that has been done on cases similar, and that brings us to the next piece of TEST RePP, the EST.

Empirically Supported Treatment

As valuable as theory is, it needs to connect to and correspond with empirical research. Indeed, research and theory are complementary ingredients to growing our scientific knowledge. In this context, we can be reminded of Eysenck's (1952) famous early challenge to the field of psychotherapy, which was an important motivator to examine whether psychotherapy is actually helpful. Decades of empirical research have since demonstrated that, generally speaking, psychotherapy is an effective health intervention (Lambert & Bergin, 1994). In addition, much has been learned about the elements that are effective and associated with positive outcomes, and practitioners have an obligation to be aware of the research on the validity of the assessment instruments and treatment interventions they use. In addition, psychologists should be aware of their personal biases and seek to check their beliefs against objective research, be cognizant of the way motives and needs influence one's beliefs and perceptions, and be aware of alternative perspectives. They should also be aware of the way the research they are interpreting was conducted, be able to critique issues of methodology that might raise questions of internal validity, and have a conceptual map that allows them to consider issues of generalizability.

More concretely, practitioners operating in well-researched domains, as when working with anxious adults like Tina, should be aware of empirical findings associated with different treatment interventions, such as cognitive–behavioral and psychodynamic approaches, as well as common medications. Intervention principles that have consistent connections with good outcomes, such as those involving exposure with response prevention, should be at least acknowledged and seriously considered in a case like Tina's. Indeed, if there is a clear desire by the patient to reduce his or her anxious symptoms and there is good reason to believe that the levels of anxiety are contributing to dysfunction in important areas (as in Tina's case), it is the obligation of the practitioner to provide guidance toward interventions that have been empirically shown to be effective at reducing anxiety and improving performance.

In the case of Tina, for example, it seems that the minimum a professional psychologist should be aware of in terms of the broad empirical literature on reducing anxiety is summed up well by the renowned cognitive–behavioral psychotherapy researcher David Barlow. Reviewing a large literature on ESTs, Barlow and his colleagues have suggested that practitioners be able to view depressive and anxiety disorders from the general perspective of negative affect (Barlow, Allen, & Choate, 2004). From this, he argued that research has demonstrated three broad principles that foster effective treatment: (a) reducing catastrophic or overly pessimistic expectations for future events, (b) reducing avoidance patterns and increasing the capacity to stay with aversive emotions, and (c) training individuals to develop antithetical emotional responses to their dominant response style (e.g., fostering general relaxation skills for anxious individuals). Thus, high on the decision-making list of the clinician working with Tina are the following questions: When should Tina's anxiety symptoms become the focus of the intervention, how should they be conceptualized with her, how should she be motivated to engage in interventions known to be effective, and how can the utility of these interventions be tracked?

Generally speaking, the term *treatment* here evokes a "medical model" conception, in which the individual is thought of as having an identifiable problem that can be matched with a set of interventions that will alleviate the difficulty. This model is the dominant frame of thinking in cognitive–behavioral literatures, and from our broad scientific humanistic view of human psychology and psychotherapy, it is a useful framework. But it is limited in scope. It often fails to consider deeply other issues of personality, especially identity and relational functioning. And it frames psychotherapy in a particular way that can blind practitioners to equally important aspects of treatment. As mentioned earlier, referencing the great psychotherapy debate, the other major perspective is to consider the process of psychotherapy as a psychosocial or relational one, whereby two individuals enter into a meaningful professional relationship with the intent of relieving distress and improving functioning. Students should be taught and professionals should be able to think about the psychotherapeutic process both as matching a presentation to an intervention and as a unique human relationship process that unfolds between two individuals. This brings us to the "Re" in TEST RePP.

Relationship

Whereas the "EST" stands for thinking about systematic interventions that might reduce suffering and improve functioning, with "relationship" the focus shifts to the nature of the exchange between the practitioner and client and their personalities as well as the broader social variables at play. At a basic descriptive level, this would include attention to the gender, age, and socioeconomic and ethnic background of both parties. But it is much more than that. Every psychotherapy encounter consists of two unique individuals experiencing one another at a unique moment in time. The individual uniqueness of both the therapist and the client tend to be considered either error or noise in traditional treatment research. That is, for research purposes, the treatment is standardized, a set of inclusion and exclusion criteria are developed based on symptoms, and then the results are reported in aggregate form, averaging across groups.

Humanistic and psychodynamic thinkers have done the most developed systematic work on the therapeutic relationship and how it can be used to foster healing. As noted previously, a strong empirical claim can be made that the effectiveness of psychotherapy is related to and dependent on the quality of the therapeutic relationship. There are several crucial key relationship variables. First, it is important that the therapist be seen as competent, trustworthy, and someone who has the best interests of the client at heart. The client must experience positive regard from the therapist as well as empathy and warmth. Moreover, therapists are expected to have interpersonal grace and be able to understand how they feel about their clients and maintain a helpful, professional stance.

Second, the unique interpersonal relationship provides a wonderful opportunity for psychosocial learning. Thus, the therapist ought to be skilled in the art of interpersonal process, and should be dialoguing, when appropriate, about the way the exchange is unfolding and eliciting narrative from the client about how his or her experience of the therapist relates to past experiences. The opportunity for this kind of conversation should be present in all meaningful therapy, certainly not just analytic therapies that emphasize working with transference.

Third, the therapist should be effective at tracking the nature of the relationship and pacing it appropriately. Interpersonal process comments need to be timed appropriately relative to the nature and development of the relationship. For example, strong feelings toward the therapist are much less likely to be present very early in the process. In addition, recognizing potential ruptures and subtle changes in the patient's attitudes about either the therapy or therapist is crucial to maintaining an effective working alliance.

With regard to Tina, the relationship factors will likely be central in a successful intervention. They are also likely to be complicated. It is reasonable to surmise that Tina is both feeling extremely vulnerable and at the same time desperately seeking guidance. In addition, given the context of her emergence into the therapy system via a referral for ADHD, it is highly likely that Tina will already feel frustrated with the system. If she wanted a label, a pill, and accommodations to foster her academic performance and she gets referred for the reflective work of psychotherapy, then there already is a mismatch between what she anticipated and what she is receiving. And, given that her anxiety symptoms are likely a function of the fact that her core emotional self is feeling overwhelmed by deep existential conflicts, it seems highly likely that she will be defensive about exploring such issues, especially when she is feeling the pressure to make a life decision quickly (i.e., to transfer or not). Because of all of these factors, she likely will not have much tolerance for a slowly developing therapy (i.e., a therapy that does not help her feel grounded and better quickly). And yet there is the very real concern, which many therapeutic perspectives would emphasize, that a therapy that moves too quickly and a therapist who is too directive might short-circuit a key developmental task, that Tina needs to sort these issues out for herself, and that the job of therapy is to provide her with a context for doing so but not necessarily to be an advice-giving guide. The point here is that the decisions that will go into establishing a working relationship with Tina will have a number of potentially competing considerations that require thoughtful reflection. This point raises the question regarding the final elements of TEST RePP, which involve a description of the key processes and principles that ought to guide practitioners in their work.

Processes and Principles

The last two elements of TEST RePP remind practitioners of how to be guided by their knowledge systems. Historically, the emphasis on empiricism has been so strong in certain domains (i.e., academia) that the message seemed to be that rigid adherence to specific procedures enacted by a practitioner following a step-by-step treatment manual were the key to scientific treatments. Thankfully, it now appears that the majority in the field are moving away from the attempt to reduce the therapeutic process to a series of prespecified steps, like what one would do when baking a cake, and more toward a view that recognizes therapy as an organic process that should not be overly structured like some algorithmic recipe. The latter has long been the model of humanistic and psychodynamic practitioners and is now becoming the general way many cognitive–behavioral practitioners operate. For example, acceptance and commitment therapy, a new wave cognitive–behavioral treatment, emphasizes a set of guideposts for clinicians as they form a relationship and foster commitments toward valued goal states (Hayes & Spencer, 2005).

"Processes and principles" is an attempt to remind wise practitioners of the guideposts that are shaping their work and orient them toward the rest of the TEST RePP formulation. With regard to processes, I emphasize three broad domains of process that I encourage students to keep in mind as they make decisions about what to do in their psychological interventions: (a) awareness, (b) acceptance, and (c) active change. Central to all therapeutic encounters is assessment—problem formulation and fostering systematic awareness in relative parties regarding the nature of the problem and the variables that are contributing to it. Human behavior is enormously complex, and humans notoriously are unaware of how much they do not know or understand. Much of the work of a psychologist is the process of developing a shared formulation that fosters clarity about the current situation. As such, a key treatment process variable for the psychologist to keep in mind when making decisions is awareness, in terms of understanding what level of awareness the client has, how greater clarity might be achieved, and self-reflective awareness of the psychologist.

Although traditionally psychoanalytic practitioners deemed awareness (or insight) as fundamental to a successful intervention, it is now generally understood that treatment must be geared to more than fostering awareness. The other two process variables, acceptance and active change, are both quite complicated, but they can serve as guideposts to the process of therapy. For example, learning to accept the aspects of the world that cannot be controlled is now broadly recognized as a key ingredient to mental health. The rise of mindfulness as a key ingredient to many therapeutic perspectives is a testament to the centrality of enhancing capacities for acceptance. And for as long as people have being doing therapy, acceptance of past losses, unfinished business, failures, or traumas (usually via fostering a more compassionate attitude) and of warded-off feelings have been salient aspects of the therapeutic process.

Of course, sometimes people need to actively learn how to be different so that they are in a better place to flourish and avoid the vicious, maladaptive cycles associated with their distress and impairment. When this is the case, the focus of therapy is on fostering active change. Individuals often need to learn to do things differently, whether this involves altering a maladaptive habit, training themselves to think differently, or developing a new relational skill. Here, understanding the process of human change is crucial, including recognizing the client's stage of change, how gradual and dramatic change can happen, and how changes can be maintained. The twin processes of acceptance on the one hand and active change on the other can seem almost contradictory. However, it is worth noting that both psychodynamic (Wachtel, 2011) and cognitive–behaviorally oriented (Linehan, 1987) practitioners have helpfully pointed out that acceptance and change can be thought of as existing in dialectical relationship to one another. This dialectical emphasis offers a more useful holistic view of the two processes than when they are viewed separately or in conceptual contrast to one another.

With regard to Tina, issues of awareness, acceptance, and change are all very salient. Sooner rather than later she needs to develop a better way of understanding her character and her situation and the origins and nature of her anxious symptoms. It seems likely that she lacks awareness about many of the features that are contributing to her distress, and if so, this needs to be addressed. At the same time, she needs ways of coping with her immediate problems that will help improve her functioning. My approach would be to take an active stance, helping Tina in a fairly direct way to come as quickly as possible to the understanding of her situation that is spelled out in the formulation described earlier. That is, I would likely use the approach of a "therapeutic assessment" (Finn & Tonsager, 2002) to attempt to generate such an understanding. From there, a shared plan could be developed that teaches her evidence-based strategies to (a) reduce her test anxiety; (b) enable her to increase her social support; and (c) adopt a longer term, hopeful perspective about what she might learn about herself in the context of this difficulty with adjustment. If this stage was initially successful and her symptoms were stabilized, then a focus on her core identity, purpose in life, and relational style and needs could be employed to build a deeper, more aware and resilient character structure that would enable her to make more adaptive interpretations and decisions, both in the short and long term.

The final "P" in TEST RePP stands for principles. It serves two related functions. First, the goal is to remind budding practitioners that they are guided by principles—values, goals, and knowledge bases—and that effective clinical decision making involves a frame that keeps these ideas salient and keeps the practitioner reflective and aware of his or her actions. The second function of "principles" is to help elucidate the more specific guiding frames that inform practitioners regarding their practice. It encourages them to consult both the literature and existing practice guidelines in their work. A sample of key treatment principles is offered in Appendix 11.1.

SUMMARY

If we are to produce ethical, self-reflective, and effective professional psychologists, we must be able to teach them the capacity to deeply answer the questions "If this is the case, what should you do and why?" and "In that situation, why did you do what you did?" These basic questions provide the frame for thinking about clinical decision making, and it is crucial that practitioners of psychotherapy have solid justification systems that guide them.

The field of professional psychology has historically not attended systematically to the process of clinical decision making as much as other health care professions, such as nursing and medicine. In addition, the field has often been characterized as being split between empirical and romantic visions of practice, with the former emphasizing decisions grounded in data derived from the scientific method and the latter emphasizing the deep, intuitive skills of the seasoned practitioner. It is time that we transcend this old dichotomy and move toward a different conception of science and a more rationalist approach to intervention. It has always been the case that the only effective bridges between the worlds of research and practical knowledge are found in concepts and theories. Thankfully, for the first time, there are comprehensive, scientifically grounded visions for human psychology that effectively bridge to the world of practice. Thus, we are set for a new era of unification and synergistic growth between the fields of professional practice and human psychology.

This chapter has outlined some of those emerging perspectives and articulated how a unified view of practice and human psychology can give rise to a scientific humanistic perspective on decision making that speaks both to methodological issues of precision, reliability, and validity and to broader philosophical questions. There is also now a model for conceptualizing the human condition that transcends the traditional midlevel paradigms and affords practitioners a systematic approach to conceptualizing that is grounded in scientific rationality.

APA attempted to bridge the disputes between clinical researchers and practitioners with its guidelines for EBP, which emphasizes the three domains of best available research, clinical experience, and patient values in the particular cultural and policy context as being the primary sources that practitioners ought to be relying on when developing their interventions. However, more specificity is needed in helping students approach their clinical decision making about psychotherapy interventions. The reason for this is that the vast field of psychotherapy is conceptually fragmented at a multitude of levels. To address the conceptual fragmentation, a heuristic frame going by the acronym TEST RePP, which stands for "Theoretically and Empirically Supported Treatment and Relationship Processes and Principles," was developed that attempts to delineate the key conceptual elements that ought to guide decision making in developing and enacting such psychotherapeutic interventions. This perspective allows future practitioners to address the competing paradigms in the field, provides them with an integrative meta-perspective, and allows them to appreciate and consider major debates in the field of psychotherapy research (e.g., medical model vs. psychosocial process). We hope practitioners informed by this model will make more effective clinical decisions.

APPENDIX 11.1

The following list offers some of the key principles that guide effective psychotherapy. This attempts to breakdown the elements of TEST RePP in a way that is congruent with the empirical literatures in psychology and psychotherapy.

1. *Set an appropriate, ethical frame.* Psychotherapy is a relationship that is grounded in professional obligations and constraints, and it is crucial that all stakeholders involved understand the purpose and function of the relationship; issues of confidentiality; financial reimbursement; general focus of the work; and, where appropriate, expected time frame.
2. *Begin to foster a strong therapeutic relationship.* It is crucial that the psychologist exhibit a level of competence and respect toward the client such that the client feels valued and heard and believes the therapist can help where appropriate.
3. *Identify cultural context variables.* Consideration of the social construction of identities is crucial for both the therapist and the client. When the client and psychologist do not share the same broader cultural background, particular attention should be paid to how the influence of cultural context might lead to differences in communication patterns, expectations of roles, core values, and so forth.
4. *Identify client values and hopes.* The central goal of psychotherapy is to enhance adaptive ways of living, a central element of which is the client's value states of being.
5. *Identify risk of harm.* A fundamental tenet of practice is to minimize the risk of harm. A practitioner must be reflective about the possible ways an intervention might have unintended side effects. If there is anticipated possible harm, all parties should be informed, and that must be carefully weighed against probable benefits.
6. *Begin to formulate an ongoing case conceptualization.* A comprehensive assessment includes a general categorization of the major symptoms, character, key developmental factors, relevant biological and sociocultural variables, current relational context, and major stressors and affordances in the environment. In addition, a systematic approach to assessing relational style, identity, and presenting problem (i.e., diagnosis) should be included.
7. *Begin to identify realistic, adaptive treatment outcomes.* The therapist should work with the client to identify therapy goals in

the context of the client's values and stage of change within a holistic, biopsychosocial, developmental conceptualization. In cases of excessive maladaptive symptoms, these goals are often straightforward (e.g., reducing levels of depressive symptoms). Sometimes, however, goals need to be more focused on awareness (i.e., increasing values or clarifying identity issues) or acceptance of past losses or current injury.

8. *Tailor treatment to level of client functioning.* More than anything else, treatment outcomes are determined by the client's history, level of impairment, and attitude about therapy. It is crucial that the goals of therapy consider this fact. It is also recommended that therapists increase their levels of direction and guidance when impairment is high.
9. *Consider therapy as a nonlinear process of fostering awareness, acceptance, and compassion and of engaging in active efforts to change.* Although therapists should have a clear road map of their work, it is also the case that therapy is rarely a simple, linear, stepwise process. Instead, many times individuals have symptoms that are the consequence of tangled and confused psychological processes that require an unfolding of awareness, acceptance, and active change, in varied sequences.
10. *Reducing maladaptive levels of negative affect.* When the major treatment goals include reducing the levels of negative affect, the treatment plan should consider the following: (a) altering maladaptive antecedent cognitive appraisals, (b) identifying layers of emotional–experiential processing and preventing problematic avoidance (i.e., foster exposure and acceptance), and (c) facilitating action tendencies antithetical to the dysregulated emotion (teaching clients to relax when they are anxious or becoming active and to focus on mastery or pleasure when they are depressed).
11. *Altering problematic aspects of relationships and identity.* When the major treatment goals include altering aspects of identity and maladaptive relationship patterns, the practitioner should consider (a) patterns between old relationships and current relationships, looking especially for vicious relationship cycles; (b) role functions and conflicts relative to core relational needs; (c) developing awareness of purpose in life, existential narratives, and problematic core beliefs and considering ways to renarrate self or life in a healthier way; (d) fostering compassion for both self and other and flexibility in human relating; (e) making conscious defense mechanisms

and working toward restructuring maladaptive defenses; and (f) ways to increase agency, coherence in identity, or coping self-efficacy.
12. *Monitor changes in desired goals.* Once problem areas and treatment goals are identified, therapists should monitor changes in symptoms and problem areas (e.g., with appropriate test instruments).
13. *Monitor client satisfaction and attitudes about the therapist.* In addition to monitoring symptom outcomes, it is crucial that regular feedback is solicited about the satisfaction the client has with the therapist and the treatment. Ideally, there should be intermittent opportunities designed to solicit authentic opinions about the treatment.
14. *When there are ruptures or failure to make adequate progress, process this and be open to making changes.*
15. *Plan for termination, monitor changes, and taper therapy if necessary.* Therapy, especially when financed by an outside source, should be conducted in a time-sensitive way. It is the obligation of the health care professional to foster treatment advances as efficiently as possible and not to extend treatment beyond what is necessary.

REFERENCES

APA Presidential Task Force on Evidence-Based Practice. (2006). Evidence-based practice in psychology. *American Psychologist, 61,* 271–285. http://dx.doi.org/10.1037/0003-066X.61.4.271

Baker, T. B., McFall, R. M., & Shoham, V. (2009). Current status and future prospects of clinical psychology: Toward a scientifically principled approach to mental and behavioral health care. *Psychological Science in the Public Interest, 9,* 67–103.

Barlow, D., Allen, L. B., & Choate, M. L. (2004). Toward a unified treatment for emotional disorders. *Behavior Therapy, 35,* 205–230. http://dx.doi.org/10.1016/S0005-7894(04)80036-4

Bordin, E. S. (1979). The generalizability of the psychoanalytic concept of the working alliance. *Psychotherapy: Theory, Research & Practice, 16,* 252–260. http://dx.doi.org/10.1037/h0085885

Caldwell, A. B. (2004). My love affair with an instrument. *Journal of Personality Assessment, 82,* 4–10. http://dx.doi.org/10.1207/s15327752jpa8201_2

Duncan, B. (2013). What makes a master therapist? *Psychotherapy in Australia, 20,* 58–66.

Eysenck, H. J. (1952). The effects of psychotherapy: An evaluation. *Journal of Consulting Psychology, 16,* 319–324. http://dx.doi.org/10.1037/h0063633

Feinstein, D. (2008). Energy psychology: A review of the preliminary evidence. *Psychotherapy: Theory, Research, Practice, Training, 45,* 199–213. http://dx.doi.org/10.1037/0033-3204.45.2.199

Finn, S. E., & Tonsager, M. E. (2002). How therapeutic assessment became humanistic. *The Humanistic Psychologist, 30,* 10–22. http://dx.doi.org/10.1080/08873267.2002.9977019

Gambrill, E., & Dawes, R. M. (2003). Ethics, science, and the helping professions: A conversation with Robyn Dawes. *Journal of Social Work Education, 39,* 27–40.

Garb, H. N. (2005). Clinical judgment and decision making. *Annual Review of Clinical Psychology, 1,* 67–89. http://dx.doi.org/10.1146/annurev.clinpsy.1.102803.143810

Gladwell, M. (2005). *Blink: The power of thinking without thinking.* New York, NY: Little, Brown.

Hayes, S. C., & Spencer, S. (2005). *Get out of your mind and into your life: The new acceptance and commitment therapy.* Oakland, CA: New Harbinger.

Henriques, G. R. (2003). The tree of knowledge system and the theoretical unification of psychology. *Review of General Psychology, 7,* 150–182. http://dx.doi.org/10.1037/1089-2680.7.2.150

Henriques, G. R. (2004). Psychology defined. *Journal of Clinical Psychology, 60,* 1207–1221. http://dx.doi.org/10.1002/jclp.20061

Henriques, G. R. (2008). The problem of psychology and the integration of human knowledge: Contrasting Wilson's consilience with the tree of knowledge system. *Theory & Psychology, 18,* 731–755. http://dx.doi.org/10.1177/0959354308097255

Henriques, G. R. (2011). *A new unified theory of psychology.* New York, NY: Springer. http://dx.doi.org/10.1007/978-1-4614-0058-5

Henriques, G. R. (2013a). Evolving from methodological to conceptual unification. *Review of General Psychology, 17,* 168–173. http://dx.doi.org/10.1037/a0032929

Henriques, G. R. (2013b). Vertical and horizontal integration in psychotherapy. *The Neuropsychotherapist, 2,* 120–121. http://dx.doi.org/10.12744/tnpt(2)120-121

Henriques, G. R., & Sternberg, R. J. (2004). Unified professional psychology: Implications for the combined–integrated model of doctoral training. *Journal of Clinical Psychology, 60,* 1051–1063. http://dx.doi.org/10.1002/jclp.20034

Henriques, G. R., & Stout, J. (2012). A unified approach to conceptualizing people in psychotherapy. *Journal of Unified Psychotherapy and Clinical Science, 1,* 37–60.

Insel, T. (2013, April 29). *Director's blog: Transforming diagnosis.* Retrieved from http://www.nimh.nih.gov/about/director/2013/transforming-diagnosis.shtml

Kahneman, D. (2011). *Thinking, fast and slow.* New York, NY: Farrar, Straus & Giroux.

Kimble, G. A. (1984). Psychology's two cultures. *American Psychologist, 39,* 833–839. http://dx.doi.org/10.1037/0003-066X.39.8.833

Lambert, M. J., & Bergin, A. E. (1994). The effectiveness of psychotherapy. In A. E. Bergin & S. L. Garfield (Eds.), *Bergin and Garfield's handbook of psychotherapy and behavior change* (4th ed., pp. 143–189). Oxford, England: Wiley.

Lilienfeld, S. O., & O'Donohue, W. T. (2012). *Great readings in clinical science: Essential selections for mental health professionals*. Upper Saddle River, NJ: Pearson.

Linehan, M. M. (1987). Dialectical behavior therapy for borderline personality disorder. Theory and method. *Bulletin of the Menninger Clinic, 51*, 261–276.

Magnavita, J. J., & Anchin, J. C. (2014). *Unifying psychotherapy: Principles, methods, and evidence from clinical science*. New York, NY: Springer.

Marquis, A., & Douthit, K. Z. (2006). The hegemony of "empirically supported treatment": Validating or violating? *Constructivism in the Human Sciences, 11*, 108–141.

Martell, C. R., Dimidjian, S., & Herman-Dunn, R. (2010). *Behavioral activation for depression: A clinician's guide*. New York, NY: Guilford Press.

Melchert, T. P. (2014). *Biopsychosocial practice: A science-based approach to behavioral healthcare*. Washington, DC: American Psychological Association.

O'Donohue, W. (1989). The (even) bolder model. The clinical psychologist as metaphysician-scientist-practitioner. *American Psychologist, 44*, 1460–1468. http://dx.doi.org/10.1037/0003-066X.44.12.1460

O'Donohue, W. T., & Henderson, D. (1999). Epistemic and ethical duties in clinical decision-making. *Behaviour Change, 16*, 10–19. http://dx.doi.org/10.1375/bech.16.1.10

PDM Task Force. (2006). *Psychodynamic diagnostic manual (PDM)*. Silver Spring, MD: Alliance of Psychoanalytic Organizations.

Radin, D. I. (2011, November). Predicting the unpredictable: 75 years of experimental evidence. *AIP Conference Proceedings 1408*(1), 204–217. doi:10.1063/1.3663725

Shealy, C. N. (2004). A model and method for "making" a combined–integrated psychologist: Equilintegration (EI) theory and the beliefs, events, and values inventory (BEVI). *Journal of Clinical Psychology, 60*, 1065–1090. http://dx.doi.org/10.1002/jclp.20035

Stam, H. J. (2004). Unifying psychology: Epistemological act or disciplinary maneuver? *Journal of Clinical Psychology, 60*, 1259–1262. http://dx.doi.org/10.1002/jclp.20069

Wachtel, P. L. (2010). Beyond "ESTs": Problematic assumptions in the pursuit of evidence-based practice. *Psychoanalytic Psychology, 27*, 251–272. http://dx.doi.org/10.1037/a0020532

Wachtel, P. L. (2011). *Therapeutic communication: Knowing what to say when* (2nd ed.). New York, NY: Guilford Press.

Wampold, B. E. (2001). *The great psychotherapy debate: Models, methods, and findings*. Mahwah, NJ: Erlbaum.

Whitaker, R. (2010). *The anatomy of an epidemic: Magic bullets, psychiatric drugs, and the astonishing rise of mental illness in America*. New York, NY: Crown.

INDEX

Abbass, A., 163
actuarial prediction, 36–38
adaptive treatment, 148
addictive disorders, 177
ADHD (attention-deficit/hyperactivity disorder), 277, 283
adversial collaborations, 129
affect, negative, 304
affective disorders, 177
Agency for Healthcare Research and Quality (AHRQ), 108, 115
Allison, Tom Spencer, 267
Ambady, N., 35
ambulatory monitoring, 154
American Psychiatric Association, 128, 130
American Psychological Association (APA)
    and clinical practice guidelines, 11, 105, 108–110, 116, 125–126
    Ethics Code of, 256, 258, 276
    Task Force on Evidence-Based Practice, 25, 65, 126, 196, 224, 289
analytic processing. *See* Slow thinking mode (System 2)
analytics, 28–29
Anchin, J. C., 41, 80
anchoring bias, 5, 39–40
Andersson, G., 151
Anker, M. G., 228
antidepressants, 128, 152
antisocial personality disorder, 197
anxiety disorders, 194
APA. *See* American Psychological Association
Apgar, Virginia, 52
Ariely, Daniel, 25, 39
Association for Counselor Education and Supervision, 163
associative processing. *See* Fast thinking mode (System 1)
Athay, M., 153, 225
attention-deficit/hyperactivity disorder (ADHD), 277, 283
attributional bias, 7, 11, 40

automatic processing, 69–74, 76–78
automatic thoughts (cognitive therapy), 83
availability heuristic, 40, 47, 135, 224
avoidant personality disorder, 210
awareness (process variable), 299

Baker, T. B., 279
Bardenstein, K. K., 224
Bargh, J. A., 30, 78
Barlow, D. H., 149, 155, 165
Barnum effect, 45
base rate neglect, 48
Bayesian approaches to clinical decision making, 50–51
Bazian Limited, 116
Beck, A. T., 286
behaviorism, 283. *See also* Cognitive and behavioral therapies
Bell, H. H., 66
Benjamin, L. S., 198
Berger, T., 162
Best Practices in Clinical Supervision (Association for Counselor Education and Supervision), 163
Betan, E., 189
Beutler, L. E., 155, 164, 195
bias
    analysis of, 252
    anchoring, 5, 39–40
    attributional, 7, 11, 40
    biological, 11
    and clinical practice guidelines, 109, 116–118
    confirmation, 5, 40–41, 43, 50, 128
    in deliberative decision making, 76
    function of, 71
    gender, xiii
    hindsight, 45, 259
    inevitability of, xiii
    minimization of, 27
    overconfidence, 6, 46–47
    publication, 49, 116, 132
    recall, 47
    and risk management, 253
    safeguards against, 189

bias, *continued*
    selection, 5, 48–49
    survivorship, 49
    in System 1 thinking, 34
Bickman, L., 153, 225–229, 232
Big Data (Viktor Mayer-Schonberger &
    Kenneth Cukier), 16
"Big data," 16, 32
biofeedback, 152
biology, 8–9, 11
blended treatment, 157
Blink (Malcolm Gladwell), 30, 35
Bloom, Benjamin, 261
*Board of Psychology v. Tom Spencer
    Allison*, 267
Bodenhausen, G. V., 78
borderline personality disorder, 5, 40,
    44, 47, 48, 189, 196, 197, 210
Bordin, E. S., 291
Borkovec, T. D., 196
Breda, C., 228–229
Buchanan, T., 152

care, standard of, 255–257
case conceptualization, 160–162,
    205–216, 303
case management models, 187–188
Caspar, F., 147–148, 162, 167
Castonguay, L. G., 195, 196
Caudill, C. O., 256
CBTs. *See* Cognitive and behavioral
    therapies
CFS (contextualized feedback
    system), 228
chaos theory, 176
character adaptation system theory
    (CAST), 281–285, 289, 291–292
children, treatment of, 265
chronic fatigue syndrome, 177
Claxton, K., 15
clinical decision making, 3–16, 23–55.
    See also High-stakes clinical
    decision making; *specific headings*
    and actuarial prediction, 36–38
    analytics for, 15
    approaches for enhancing, 50–54
    basics of, 38–39
    and big data, 16
    and decision theory, 5–6
    elements of, 31–33

errors commonly influencing, 39–50.
    See also Bias
and evolutionary basis of decision
    making, 8–9
and expertise. *See* Clinical expertise
fast vs. slow thinking in, 33–36
heuristics for, 3–4
knowledge of, 12
pillars of effective, 9–12
pragmatics of, 27–28
rationality and emotionality in,
    29–31
risk management in. *See* Risk
    management
schemata and prototypes in, 14
shared, 15
sunk costs in, 4–5
uncertainty of analytics in, 28–29
clinical expertise, 23–27
    definitions of, 25–26
    development of, 4, 10–11
    in three-circle model of evidence-
        based practice, 106–107
    training and experience required for,
        24–25, 34
clinical judgment, 257–259
clinical practice guidelines (CPGs),
    105–121, 125–142
    advantages of decision making with,
        118–119
    and American Psychological Asso-
        ciation, 11, 105, 108–110,
        116, 125–126
    and bias, 109, 116–118
    criteria for, 108–109
    and hierarchy of evidence, 136–138
    history of, 109–111
    implementation of, 119–120
    Institute of Medicine standards for,
        105, 111–115, 126–134
    limitations of, 108
    as link between research and
        practice, 106–107
    overview, 106
    selection of appropriate, 134–136
    systematic reviews of, 108–109, 113,
        115–116
    and treatment efficacy, 138–142
Clinical Practice Guidelines We Can Trust
    (Institute of Medicine), 111

clinical prediction
   actuarial prediction vs., 36–38
   effectiveness of, 35
clinical support tools (CSTs), 156
clinical training, 158–164. *See also*
      Teaching clinical decision making
Clinical Versus Statistical Prediction (Paul Meehl), 35
Clinician's Guide to Evidence-Based Practices (J. C. Norcross, T. P. Hogan, & G. P. Koocher), 25
cognitive and behavioral therapies (CBTs)
   for anxiety disorders, 194
   patterns in, 216
   processes in, 299, 300
   psychoanalytic treatment vs., 180
   research support for, 138, 141
   semantic meaning in, 283
   theory in, 64
cognitive bias. *See* Bias
cognitive capabilities, 254
cognitive continuum theory, 77
cognitive dissonance theory, 227
cognitive restructuring, 194
cognitive theory, 82–83
Cohen, J. T., 15
coherence, 160
COIs (conflicts of interest), 112, 128–129
collaborative problem solving, 158, 164
collaborative shared decision-making model, 178–180, 183–187
combined–integrated approach to training, 274–275
Comer, J. S., 149, 155, 165
common factors in psychotherapy, 291
comorbidities, patient, 177–178, 196
complexity theory, 176
complex trauma, 177
computer-assisted testing, 151–152
computer-based training, 159–162
confirmation bias, 5, 40–41, 43, 50, 128
conflicts of interest (COIs), 112, 128–129
Conklin, C., 189
consultation, 154–155, 264, 284
contact and communication technologies, 156–157

contextualized feedback system (CFS), 228
Conway, M. A., 78
cost–benefit analysis, 7
countertransference–transference reactions, 188–189
CPGs. *See* Clinical practice guidelines
Creighton, L. A., 69
Critchfield, K. L., 196
"Criteria for Evaluating Treatment Guidelines" (APA document), 110
critical thinking, 249–253
Croskerry, P., 68, 72, 90, 91
Cross, G., 10, 52
Crossing the Quality Chasm (Institute of Medicine report), 52
Csikszentmihalyi, Mihaly, 30
CSTs (clinical support tools), 156
Cuijpers, P., 139
Cukier, Kenneth, 16

Dahlin, M., 151
data
   "big," 16, 32
   in clinical decision making, 226–229
   defined, 32
   and knowledge databases, 150
   patient, 151–155
Dawes, Robyn, 278
de Andrade, A. R., 228–229
decision analysis, 26
decision-making research, 253–255. *See also* Clinical decision making
decision theory
   history of, 13–14
   influence of, 9
   overview, 5–6
   study of, 12
default-interventionism model, 77
deliberative processing, 69, 73–78
depression, 44, 46, 65, 128, 140, 288
DeRubeis, R. J., 135, 152
Diagnostic and Statistical Manual of Mental Disorders (DSM), 71, 287
diagnosticity, 51
diagnostic labels, 5
dialectical behavior therapy, 159, 196, 197, 216
divorce, 35, 52, 260, 265

dodo bird effect, 291
dopamine, 30
Doverspike, W., 256
DSM (*Diagnostic and Statistical Manual of Mental Disorders*), 71, 287
dual process model, 79–94
   applications of, 79
   automatic processing and decision making in, 69–74, 76–78
   clinical recommendations, 89–94
   clinical vignette, 79–89
   deliberative processing and decision making in, 73–78
   development of, 68
   overview, 68–78
dual process model of explicit and implicit theory, 79–94. *See also* Theory
   applications of, 79
   clinical vignette, 79–89
   recommendations with, 89–94
Dumont, F., 92
Duncan, B. L., 228

eating disorders, 177
EBM (evidence-based medicine), 107
EBP. *See* Evidence-based medicine
ecological momentary assessment (EMA), 154
efficacy, treatment, 138–142
egocentrism, 43
Ellis, E., 254
EMA (ecological momentary assessment), 154
EMDR (eye movement desensitization and reprocessing), 194
eMedicine Clinical Knowledge Database, 150
emotional reasoning, 252
emotions
   awareness of, 254
   in clinical decision making, 29–31
empathy, intellectual, 250
empirical evidence, 9–10
empirically grounded relational principles, 193–217
   across treatment approaches, 195–196
   for case conceptualization and interventions, 205–216

   case examples, 205–216
   in moment-by-moment therapy process, 201–205
   norms in, 201
   principles of, 196–198
   and structural analysis of social behavior, 198–201
empirically supported treatments (ESTs). *See also* Evidence-based practice
   and clinical practice guidelines, 106
   treatment efficacy of, 138
empiricism (philosophy), 286
endowment effect, 42
Ensworth, Heather, 266
Ensworth v. Mullvain, 266–267
Epstein, S., 78
e-SOFT (System for Observing Family Therapy Alliances), 158–159
ESTs. *See* Empirically supported treatments
e-texts, 149–150
ethical frameworks, 12
ethical violations, 258
EU (expected utility) theory, 180
EUV (expected utility value), 74–75
Evans, J. St. B. T., 69, 76, 77
Evans, W. J., 162–163
evidence
   empirical, 9–10
   hierarchy of, 136–138
evidence-based medicine (EBM), 107
evidence-based practice (EBP). *See also* Empirical evidence
   defined, 13
   history of, 285–290
   for posttraumatic stress disorder, 10
   and teaching clinical decision making, 285–290
evolutionary psychology, 8–9, 280
expected utility (EU) theory, 180
expected utility value (EUV), 74–75
experiential practitioners, 64, 283
experiential processing. *See* Fast thinking mode (System 1)
expertise. *See* Clinical expertise
explicit theory, 64–65
external review, 114
external validity, 137
eye contact, 4

eye movement desensitization and reprocessing (EMDR), 194
Eysenck, H. J., 295

fair-mindedness, 251
"Faith in reason" (trait), 251
family systems therapists, 64
fast thinking mode (System 1), 33–36
　biases with, 53
　overview, 14
feedback systems, 153. *See also* Measurement feedback systems
FFT (functional family therapy), 232–236
FFT-CFS (Functional Family Therapy Clinical Feedback System), 232–236
FFT-CMI (Functional Family Therapy Clinical Measurement Inventory), 232
fibromyalgia, 177
fight–flight response, 34
financial conflicts of interest, 128–129
Finding What Works in Health Care: Standards of Systematic Reviews (Institute of Medicine), 111
Fischer, U., 72
Fiske, S. T., 27
Fitzgerald, F. Scott, 44
fixed frames, 43–44
flow, 30
Foundation for Critical Thinking, 249–250
Four Horseman of the Apocalypse (algorithm), 52
Frank, Jerome, 291
Frederickson, J., 163
Friedberg, R. D., 224
functional family therapy (FFT), 232–236
Functional Family Therapy Clinical Feedback System (FFT-CFS), 232–236
Functional Family Therapy Clinical Measurement Inventory (FFT-CMI), 232
Furr, J. M., 28

Galinsky, A. D., 258
Gallinger, L., 154
gambler's fallacy, 41–42

game theory, 13
Gawronski, B., 69
GDP (guideline development panels), 111–113, 126–131
gender bias, *xiii*
Gervind, E., 151
Gladwell, Malcolm, 30, 35, 50
Goethe, Johann Wolfgang von, *xi*
Goodman and Gilman's Pharmacological Basis of Therapeutics (L. Brunton, B. Chabner, & B. Knollman), 149–150
Gosch, E., 28
Gottman, J. M., 40
Gottman, John, 52
GRADE (Grading of Recommendations Assessment, Development, and Evaluation), 116
Graves' disease, 44
Grawe, K., 153
The Great Psychotherapy Debate (Bruce Wampold), 288
Greenberg, R. P., 154
Gregory, R., 154
Groopman, J., 27, 28, 38, 53
guideline development panels (GDP), 111–113, 126–131

Hammond, K. R., 77
Harmon, C., 228
Harwood, T. M., 155, 164
Hassin, R. R., 30
Hautle, I., 162
Hawkins, E. J., 228
Health Insurance Portability and Accountability Act (HIPAA), 164, 256
Heim, A. K., 189
Henderson, D., 283, 284
Henriques, G. R., 283
Henry, W. P., 196
heuristic(s), 3–6
　availability, 40, 47, 135, 224
　defined, 26–27
　errors with, 39
　function of, 71–72
　representative, 5, 48
　and teaching clinical decision making, 274–275
Higgs, J., 254

high-stakes clinical decision making, 175–190
  aids for, 183
  case management models for, 187–188
  collaborative shared decision-making model for, 178–180, 183–187
  and expected utility theory, 180
  managing countertransference–transference reactions in, 188–189
  overview, 176–177
  with patient comorbidities, 177–178
  pattern recognition in, 188
  quadratic decision-making model for, 181–183
  risk management in, 187
  and safeguards against cognitive biases, 189
  simplified decision-making model for, 180–181
hindsight bias, 45, 259
HIPAA (Health Insurance Portability and Accountability Act), 164, 256
Hogan, T. P., 25
Hollon, S. D., 152
Holmes-Rovner, M., 180
hormone replacement therapy (HRT), 137
How Doctors Think (J. Groopman), 27
humanistic psychologists, 64, 283, 294, 299
humility, intellectual, 250
hyperthyroidism, 44

illusory correlations, 46
ILT (instructor-led training workshops), 159
implicit theory, 65–68
information, 32
insight, 299
Institute of Medicine (IOM), 12, 52, 105–107, 111–115, 126–134
instructor-led training workshops (ILT), 159
integrative psychotherapy, 64
intellectual courage, 250
intellectual empathy, 250
intellectual humility, 250

intellectual integrity, 250–251
intellectual perseverance, 251
internal validity, 137
Internet, 149–151
Internet-based testing, 151–152
Internet-based training system (ITS), 158
interpersonal psychotherapy, 65, 79, 138, 194, 216
interpersonal reconstructive therapy (IRT), 210–214
interventions, 205–216
intuition, 30–31, 34–35, 51, 80. *See also* Clinical prediction; Fast thinking mode
intuitive processing. *See* Fast thinking mode (System 1)
IOM. *See* Institute of Medicine
IRT (interpersonal reconstructive therapy), 210–214
ITS (Internet-based training system), 158

joint collaborative care meetings, 186
Jones-Smith, E., 64

Kagan, Jerome, 11
Kahneman, Daniel, 6
  on clinical expertise, 26, 179
  on clinical prediction, 37–38
  on clinicians and algorithmic thinking, 52
  development of decision theory by, 13–14
  on evidence, 50, 53
  and heuristics, 26
  and priming, 11
  System 1 and System 2 thinking developed by, 33–36
Karlin, B. E., 10, 52
Keillor, Garrison, 47
Kelley, S. D., 153, 225, 228–229
Kendall, P. C., 28
Kiesler, D. J., 80
Kimble, G. A., 276
Klein, G., 26, 66, 70, 179
Knight, Frank, 13
knowledge, 32, 294
knowledge databases, 150
Koocher, G. P., 25

Lake Woebegone effect, 47
Lambert, M. J., 33, 47, 228
Lammers, J., 258
latent semantic analysis (LSA), 161
Lehrer, J., 29
licensing boards, 245–246, 256, 258
Lilienfeld, S. O., 274–275
Linardatos, E., 128
Linehan, M., 196
Lohr, S., 32
LSA (latent semantic analysis), 161
Luhrmann, T. M., 43

Maggio, L. A., 149, 150
Magnavita, J. J., 41, 188, 225, 274–275
malpractice, 258–259
Manring, J., 154
Månsson, K. N. T., 151
manuals. *See* Treatment manuals
Maslow, A., 31
Matthews, A. M., 128
Mayer-Schonberger, Viktor, 16
McFall, R. M., 279
measurement feedback systems (MFS), 153, 223–241
  benefits of, 225
  in clinical decision making process, 236–239
  in functional family therapy, 232–236
  future directions of, 239–240
  OQ-Analyst, 229–230
  overview, 226–229
  Partners for Change Outcome Management System, 231
  Systemic Therapy Inventory of Change, 230–231
medical model of treatment, 287, 296
Meehl, Paul, 35, 37, 132
memory, 47–48
mentalization, 31
metacognition, 254
metacommunication, 80–82, 84
methodological view of science, 278–281
MFS. *See* Measurement feedback systems
Miller, K. L., 162–163
Miller, S. M., 162–163
Miller, Scott, 33
mindfulness, 92

Minnesota Multiphasic Personality Inventory—2 (MMPI-2), 46, 280, 285
moment-by-moment therapy process, 201–205
Morgenstern, Oskar, 13
Mosier, K. L., 72
Mullvain, Cynthia, 266
multiple personality disorder, 40
multiple relationship violations, 267–268

Najavits, L. M., 66, 93
Naked Statistics: Stripping the Dread From the Data (C. Wheelan), 47
narcissism, 5, 40, 43, 196
narrative fallacy, 46
narrative therapists, 283
National Guidelines Clearinghouse, 108
National Institute for Health and Clinical Excellence (NICE), 127, 129–130
National Institute of Mental Health (NIMH), 12
naturalistic decision making (NDM), 70
negative affect, 304
Neumann, P. J., 15
neurofeedback, 153
Neuropsychotherapy (K. Grawe), 153
neuroscience, 11, 30–31
Newnham, E. A., 239
The New Unconscious (R. R. Hassin, J. S. Uleman, J. A. Bargh), 30
NICE (National Institute for Health and Clinical Excellence), 127, 129–130
NIMH (National Institute of Mental Health), 12
nonmaleficence, 258
Norcross, J. C., 25
Norman, G., 90, 91
Norsworthy, L. A., 228

O'Donohue, W. T., 24, 283, 284
Of Two Minds: An Anthropologist Looks at American Psychiatry (T. M. Luhrmann), 43
online supervision, 162–164
online testing, 151–152
online textbooks, 149–150

optimal decision making, 9, 13, 31–33, 54, 73, 225
OQ-Analyst (computer feedback program), 229–230
outcome research, 109
overconfidence bias, 6, 46–47

Page, A. C., 239
paranoid personality disorder, 29, 197
Parkinson's disease, 44
Partners for Change Outcome Management System (PCOMS), 231
passive-aggressive personalities, 197
patients
　data of, 151–155
　values and preferences of, 106–107, 181
pattern recognition
　in high-risk cases, 188
　overview, 38–39
Patterson, R. E., 66
PCOMS (Partners for Change Outcome Management System), 231
peer consulting, 154–155
personality disorders (PDs), 177, 196–198. *See also specific disorders, e.g.:* Borderline personality disorder
personality systematics, 188
PICOTS (populations, interventions, comparisons, outcomes, time, and settings), 133–134, 137–138, 141
Pierce, B. J., 66
Pincus, A. L., 80
posttraumatic stress disorder (PTSD), 10
practice parameters. *See* Clinical practice guidelines
prescriptive indices, 134
priming, 11
probability, 42, 50–51, 155–156
prognostic indices, 134
prototypes, 14, 38, 39. *See also* Bias; Heuristics
psychiatry, 43–44, 49
psychoanalytic treatment, 64, 180
Psychodynamic Diagnostic Manual, 287
psychodynamic psychologists, 64, 194, 283, 287, 300
psychoeducative information, 151

Psychology's Ghosts: The Crisis in the Profession and the Way Back (Jerome Kagan), 11
psychopathy, 5
psychosocial learning, 297
psychotherapy
　common factors in, 291
　definitions of, *xi–xii*
　integrative, 64
　interpersonal, 65, 79, 138, 194, 216
　supportive, 139
　and theory, 63–64
　unified theories of, 280–281, 290–292
Psychotherapy Training e-Resources, 159–160
PTSD (posttraumatic stress disorder), 10
publication bias, 49, 116, 132

quadratic decision-making model, 181–183

randomized controlled trials (RCTs), 137, 194–195
rationalism (philosophy), 286
rationality, 29–31
Rationality and the Reflective Mind (Keith Stanovich), 33
rational processing. *See* Slow thinking mode (System 2)
RCTs (randomized controlled trials), 137, 194–195
recall bias, 47
recency effect, 7, 47–48
recognition-primed decision making (RPD), 70–72
record keeping, 264
Reese, R. J., 228
referrals, 44
reflective processing. *See* Slow thinking mode (System 2)
reflexive processing. *See* Fast thinking mode (System 1)
reframing, 44
Reid, W. H., 256, 257
reimbursement policies, 108
relational processes in therapy. *See* Empirically grounded relational principles
relational psychoanalysis, 79n3

representative heuristics, 5, 48
research. *See also* Evidence-based practice
   components of best available, 106–107
   decision-making, 253–255
   outcome, 109
Riemer, M., 226, 228–229
risk-averse psychologists, 260–261
risk-managed psychologists, 261–264
risk management, 245–269
   case examples, 246–248, 265–268
   and clinical judgment, 257–259
   and critical thinking, 249–253
   and decision-making research, 253–255
   in high-stakes clinical decision making, 187
   overview, 14, 259–260
   by risk-averse psychologists, 260–261
   by risk-managed psychologists, 261–264
   and standard of care, 255–257
Roberto, M. A., 26
Rosen, C. S., 10
Rosenthal, R., 35, 128
Rothert, M. L., 180
Rousmaniere, T., 163
RPD (recognition-primed decision making), 70–72
Rummel, N., 164
Russell, E. J., 152

Sackett, D. L., 107
Sapyta, J., 226
SASB (structural analysis of social behavior), 198–201, 216
schemas, 82, 216
schemata, 14
scientific humanistic philosophy, 276–278
selection bias, 5, 48–49
selective treatment, 148
SEUT (structural analysis of social behavior), 73–75
severe mental illness, 177
Sexton, T. L., 224
Shanteau, J., 25
Shapiro, J. P., 224
shared clinical decision making, 15

Shoben, E. J., Jr., 63, 65, 67
Shoham, V., 279
Siegle, G. J., 152
simplified decision-making model, 180–181
Singer, J. A., 78
Skagius Ruiz, E., 151
Slade, K., 228
sleep disorders, 177
Slone, N. C., 228
Slovic, P., 73, 78
slow thinking mode (System 2), 33–36
   biases with, 53
   overview, 14
Smith, M., 254
social capabilities, 254
Society for Psychotherapy Research, 157
Socrates, 249
Sood, E., 28
Spada, H., 164
Sparks, J. A., 228
splitting, 184
standard of care, 255–257
Stanovich, Keith
   on Bayesian instincts, 51
   classification of System 1 and 2 thinking by, 33, 36
   on clinical prediction, 35, 37
   and decision making errors, 42, 45, 46
   default-interventionism model, 77
   and dual process models, 69
   and heuristics, 26, 27
   on optimal decision making, 31
Stanton, M., 176
Stapel, D. A., 258
stepped care, 156
STIC (Systemic Therapy Inventory of Change), 230–231
Stout, J., 283
Strangers to Ourselves: Discovering the Adaptive Unconscious (Timothy Wilson), 30
Stricker, G., 240
structural analysis of social behavior (SASB), 198–201, 216
subjective expected utility theory (SEUT), 73–75
Sullenberger, Chessy, 8
Sumner, W. G., 249

sunk-cost effect, 4, 48
sunk-cost fallacy, 5
supervision, 154–155, 162–164
supportive psychotherapy, 139
survivorship bias, 49
System 1. *See* Fast thinking mode
System 2. *See* Slow thinking mode
systematic reviews (SRs), 108–109, 113, 115–116
System for Observing Family Therapy Alliances (e-SOFT), 158–159
Systemic Therapy Inventory of Change (STIC), 230–231

Tavris, C., 252
Taylor, S. E., 27
teaching clinical decision making, 273–302
   and evidence-based practice, 285–290
   and heuristics, 274–275
   integrative model for, 281–285
   and methodological view of science, 278–281
   and paradigms in psychotherapy, 290–292
   scientific humanistic approach to, 276–278
   TEST RePP model for, 292–301
technology in clinical decision making, 147–167
   acceptance of, 165
   advantages of, 149
   ambulatory monitoring, 154
   and clinical training, 158–164
   contact and communication technologies, 156–157
   future developments, 166–167
   and health care, 15–16
   information available on Internet, 149–151
   patient data, 151–155
   probability calculations in, 155–156
   psychoeducative and therapeutic information, 151
   risks with, 165–166
   skillful use of, 165
   video recordings, 154–155, 158–159
Tell, R. A., 128
termination, therapy, 266, 305

TEST RePP (Theoretically and Empirically Supported Treatment and Relationship Processes and Principles), 292–301
"The autonomous set of systems" (TASS), 90
Theoretically and Empirically Supported Treatment and Relationship Processes and Principles (TEST RePP), 303–305
theory, 61–68. *See also specific theories and models, e.g.*: Dual process model of explicit and implicit theory
   of automatic processing, 69–74, 76–78
   definitions of, 294
   of deliberative processing, 73–78
   explicit, 64–65
   implicit, 65–68
   role of, 11
   role of, in psychotherapy, 63–64
therapeutic alliance, 196–198, 291, 297–298, 303
therapeutic ruptures, 305
Thinking, Fast and Slow (Daniel Kahneman), 14, 33
"Thin slicing" (information processing), 35
Todd, A. R., 78
Toland, M. D., 228
Tracey, T. J. G., 25, 50
training, clinical, 158–164. *See also* Teaching clinical decision making
trauma symptoms, 194
treatment efficacy, 138–142
treatment guidelines. *See* Clinical practice guidelines
treatment manuals, 28
Trierweiler, S. J., 240
The Trust (malpractice carrier), 259
Turner, E. H., 128
Tversky, Amos, 13, 26
Type 1. *See* Fast thinking mode
Type 2. *See* Slow thinking mode

Uleman, J. S., 30
uncertainty tolerance, 52–54, 187, 253
unified theories of psychotherapy, 280–281, 290–292

U.S. Agency for Health Care Policy and Research, 109
U.S. Department of Veterans Affairs (VA), 109, 118

VA (U.S. Department of Veterans Affairs), 109, 118
videoconferencing, 157
video recordings, 154–155, 158–159
virtual reality, 164
von Neumann, John, 13

Wade, C., 252
Walfish, S., 47
Wampold, Bruce, 288–289, 291
web assessment, 151–152
web-based training, 159–160
webinars, 157

Weigold, A., 152
Weigold, I. K., 152
Welsh, R., 176
West, Richard, 33
Westen, D., 189
Wheelan, C., 47, 49
Whipple, J. L., 228
Williams, M. H., 256
Wills, C. E., 180
Wilson, Timothy, 30
wisdom, 33, 34, 78

Youth Outcome Questionnaire (Y-OQ), 230

Zittel, 189
Zur, O., 256

ABOUT THE EDITOR

Jeffrey J. Magnavita, PhD, ABPP, is a nationally recognized psychologist, psychotherapist, and clinical theorist who has been in clinical practice for 3 decades. He is the author and editor of eight professional books on psychotherapy, personality theory, and the treatment of personality disorders, as well as numerous chapters and articles. Dr. Magnavita has been recognized for his work, including the American Psychological Association's (APA's) Award for Distinguished Professional Contribution to Independent or Institutional Practice in the Private Sector. He is featured in two APA videos demonstrating his unifying approach to psychotherapy. He also served as the president of the APA Division of Psychotherapy in 2010 and is the producer of the video series Psychotherapists Face-to-Face (http://www.divisionofpsychotherapy.org/face-to-face/).

Dr. Magnavita's work focuses on the unification of clinical science and he is the founder of the Unified Psychotherapy Project (http://www.unifiedpsychotherapyproject.org/) and the coeditor of the *Journal of Unified Psychotherapy and Clinical Science*. He is trained in a number of modalities and approaches to clinical treatment, and his work seeks to combine the best of all approaches to maximize treatment outcomes. His most recent research interest is decision making and the use of technology in mental health practice. Dr. Magnavita served as a member and then vice chair of the APA Steering Committee tasked with the development of Clinical Practice Guidelines and is a lecturer in the Department of Psychiatry at Yale University. His most recent volume, with Jack C. Anchin, is *Unifying Psychotherapy: Principles, Methods, and Evidence From Clinical Science*.